BORN IN THE USA

HOW A BROKEN MATERNITY SYSTEM MUST BE FIXED TO PUT MOTHERS AND INFANTS FIRST

MARSDEN WAGNER, MD, MS

UNIVERSITY OF CALIFORNIA PRESS
BERKELEY LOS ANGELES LONDON

University of California Press, one of the most
distinguished university presses in the United States,
enriches lives around the world by advancing scholarship
in the humanities, social sciences, and natural sciences.
Its activities are supported by the UC Press Foundation
and by philanthropic contributions from individuals and
institutions. For more information, visit www.ucpress.edu.

University of California Press
Berkeley and Los Angeles, California
University of California Press, Ltd.
London, England

First paperback printing 2008

Library of Congress Cataloging-in-Publication Data
Wagner, Marsden, 1930–.
    Born in the USA : how a broken maternity system
must be fixed to put mothers and infants first / Marsden
Wagner.
        p.   cm.
    Includes bibliographical references and index.
    ISBN-13: 978-0-520-25633-0 (pbk. : alk. paper)
    1. Obstetrics—United States.   2. Childbirth—United
States.   3. Maternal health services—United States.
4. Midwifery—United States.   I. Title.
RG518.U5W34   2007
362.198'200973—dc22   2006018090

Manufactured in the United States of America
17   16   15   14   13   12   11
10   9   8   7   6   5   4   3   2

CONTENTS

BORN IN THE USA

PREFACE

To remain silent and indifferent is the greatest sin of all.
ELIE WIESEL, NOBEL PRIZE WINNER

You can't change the status quo by being appropriate.
SUSAN SARANDON, ACTOR

Much of what is in this book will come as a shock to women and families in America. There are two reasons for this. The first is that accepting that our present maternity care system is as abusive as documented here is a hard pill to swallow. No society wants to believe itself capable of putting its most vulnerable members—pregnant women and babies—at such risk. The second reason is that the American obstetric profession has managed to keep a big secret from the public for fifty years.

When I was a medical student, decades ago, I was shocked when I first became aware that obstetricians don't attend women during their labor but instead rush in at the last moment to catch the baby (and the money). I talked about the situation with other students, and we all thought it was a terrible scandal, particularly since the laboring women had never been told that their doctors were not going to be there. But at the same time we were learning to be doctors ourselves, and that meant we were learning that great power is available to doctors who are willing to play by the rules—and rule number one is never talk about medical mistakes or bad practices.

Think about it: How often have you heard of a medical whistle-blower? It is a rare occurrence in medicine, and it is a rare occurrence in maternity care, where medical students, obstetricians, midwives, nurses, and everyone else in the field is under pressure to keep their mouths shut or risk losing their ability to practice. For me, however, there came a time when it was no longer possible to stay silent. The final straw was my horror at the widespread use of a drug called Cytotec for inducing labor—a drug that is not approved by the Food and Drug Administration (FDA) for this purpose and has resulted in unnecessary complications and even death for women and their newborns. As it became clear in the 1990s that the use of Cytotec to induce labor was not going to stop and was for the most part being kept secret from the American public, I knew it was time to pick up the whistle (or pen) and start blowing.

In blowing the whistle on American maternity care, I have an important advantage in that I have a range of experiences in the field. After some years of clinical practice as a perinatologist (obstetrics and neonatology), I became interested in science and engaged in two years of full-time study as a National Institutes of Health Scholar to become a scientist specializing in perinatal epidemiology (the scientific evaluation of events surrounding childbirth). The fact that I have both clinical and scientific experience has been especially helpful in my role as whistle-blower, as there is often tension between practitioners and scientists.

In part, the tension is caused by the misconception among those outside the medical field (and among some inside the field) that the two areas are closely related—that medical doctors are also trained in science. This is not true. There is a fundamental difference between the practice of medicine and the practice of science. To generate hypotheses, scientists must believe that they don't know, whereas to have the confidence to make life-and-death decisions, practicing doctors must believe that they *do* know. Medical doctors receive little or no training in scientific methodology, either in medical school or as residents in specialty training. For this reason, it can be difficult for practicing obstetricians to understand the basis on which scientists give advice. In my experience, the tension between practitioners and scientists can be constructive, as long as mutual respect remains, and I have come to believe that no group of practitioners can do without close collaboration with scientists. However, we are not there yet in American maternity care, and many of the serious problems described in this book are directly and indirectly the result of practitioners going seriously astray because they do not have adequate direction from scientists.

Like many medical scientists who started as practitioners, I have continued some clinical practice to keep my clinical thinking realistic and up to date. I travel frequently to hospitals and clinics where I speak, work with groups of staff, and consult on individual cases.

When evaluating maternity services, I have also drawn on my years of experience as a public health specialist—in the Department of Public Health for the state of California and on an international level with the World Health Organization. Working in health policy has shaped my perspective by forcing me to consider issues such as cost, training, manpower, and distribution of services—issues that, whether or not we like it, profoundly affect what happens to a woman receiving maternity care and her family.

More recently, I have also worked as an expert witness or consultant on a number of maternity care legal cases. This too has broadened my perspective on our maternity care system and has given me the opportunity to get to know firsthand some of the families who have been damaged by it. Some of their real-life stories have been used as examples in this book. I have also drawn on cases I have encountered in hospital consultations and on cases I have learned of through doctors, midwives, and families who have contacted me over the years. Though I feel concrete examples are critical to getting the message across, I have changed names and other details to protect the privacy of these families.

I believe that an important part of the struggle for control of maternity care described in this book is gender-specific—that there has been a paternalistic takeover of territory that rightly belongs to women and that did belong to women until relatively recently. For this reason (as well as for convenience), I've chosen to use the pronoun "he" when referring to obstetricians, though approximately 38 percent of American obstetricians are women.

Finally, though I am writing a book about childbirth, I acknowledge that I, like every other man involved in maternity care, will always be essentially an outsider on this subject, since I will never give birth. I once asked a well-known feminist and scientist, a friend of mine, if I could be a feminist. She replied, "I have bad news and good news. The bad news is, no, as a man you can never be a feminist. The good news is if there could be male feminists, you would certainly be one."

ONE MATERNITY CARE IN CRISIS: WHERE ARE THE DOCTORS?

We do not see childbirth in many obstetric units now. What we see resembles childbirth as much as artificial insemination resembles sexual intercourse.
RONALD LAING, PSYCHIATRIST

Scene: A large hospital in Oregon. (This is a real-life story, as are the other stories in this book.)

Grabbing the telephone from the maternity ward secretary, the nurse blurts out, "Doctor, I have tried and tried to find the baby's heart beat and then I got my charge nurse who tried and tried. We can't get a fetal heart tone at all. We need you. Please come quick!"

The obstetrician replies, "Right. I'm leaving home now. I'll be there in fifteen minutes, depending on traffic." Click.

"But doctor, what should we do in the meantime?! Oh damn, he's gone."

The nurse rushes back to the labor room, where a woman lies moaning in pain, her face pale and sweaty, classic signs of shock. The nurse throws yet another blanket on and turns up the flow of oxygen in the mask over the woman's face. Sadly, the nurse never consults another doctor, even though there is another obstetrician in the doctor's lounge just down the hall, perhaps because, in general, nurses are discouraged from consulting another doctor if it is a private patient.

The woman's obstetrician arrives twelve minutes later and quickly determines that there are indeed no fetal heart tones, and the woman is in shock. He realizes this is almost certainly a case of uterine rupture, a situation where the woman's uterus, after an especially hard contraction, blows out like a tire. Uterine rupture is a known risk of Cytotec, the drug he has

1

used to induce the woman's labor. Now it is his face that turns pale as he finds himself confronted with the most feared of all birth catastrophes—one that could kill the woman and the baby. "Set up for emergency C-section," he shouts.

It takes twenty minutes to prepare the operating room for an emergency cesarean section, enlist the obstetrician in the lounge to assist, find the anesthesiologist, and get scrubbed. By the time the laboring woman's belly is finally cut open, the baby is floating free in the abdominal cavity, having escaped from the uterus through a large rip in the uterine wall.

Handing the deep blue, flaccid baby to the waiting neonatologist, the obstetrician orders, "Now let's cut out the damaged uterus."

The assisting obstetrician objects: "But we can repair it."

"No, it's quicker and easier to just remove it."

"But the husband is just outside the operating room door," replies the assisting obstetrician. "We should at least discuss it with him. Removing the uterus means they can't have another baby."

Perhaps because he doesn't want to face the husband, the obstetrician stops all discussion by turning back to the operating table and starting the removal of the damaged uterus.

Meanwhile, the neonatologist has determined that the baby is brain-dead, after nearly one hour without sufficient oxygen, due to the damaged uterus. The baby is rushed to the nearest neonatal intensive care unit, but dies twenty-four hours later. The mother is hemorrhaging from the ruptured uterus and receives a blood transfusion.

The outcomes of this story were tragic. A women nearly died and a family was left with a dead baby and no possibility of having another baby in the future. Most tragic of all, it need never have happened.

We doctors have a fancy word for the appalling outcomes in a case like this: they are *iatrogenic,* or caused by the doctor. Cytotec is a popular drug among obstetricians who use it to induce labor, even though it has not been approved by the drug manufacturer, or by the FDA, for that purpose, and to date there is no scientific evidence showing that it is safe for that purpose.[1] On the contrary, in 1999, two years after this incident took place, studies proved conclusively that, while the risk of uterine rupture is higher than normal when Cytotec is given to "ripen the cervix" and induce labor, the risk of rupture is significantly greater still when it is given to a pregnant woman (like the woman in Oregon) who has had a cesarean section in the past and already has a weakness in the wall of her uterus at the scar.[2]

Here is another story. This one is about a recent "normal" birth in Northern California.

Ms. C chose Dr. E, an obstetrician, to care for her during her pregnancy and birth. She wanted to have a natural birth and his printed flyers advertised that he "believes pregnancy is not an illness," "works toward making pregnancy a happy experience," and "provides natural delivery methods."

A week before Ms. C's due date, Dr. E proposed that he induce labor with the powerful intravenous drug Pitocin. "Come to the hospital Friday at 7 A.M., and you'll have a baby by dinnertime," he said. What Dr. E did not add was "and I'll be home for dinner."

Inducing labor is medically indicated in rare cases, such as when the patient shows signs of preeclampsia (persistent, severe high blood pressure, edema or swelling due to an accumulation of fluid in the ankles, and protein in the urine)—or when the pregnancy is more than two weeks overdue and there are definite signs of fetal distress. In Ms. C's case, there were no medical indications for inducing labor. Ms. C and her husband refused Dr. E's offer and repeated their desire to let nature take its course.

A week later, Ms. C went into spontaneous labor and was admitted to the hospital at 11 P.M. Dr. E was informed by phone, but perhaps because it was 11 P.M., he did not come in to examine her. Over the phone he ordered the nurse to start Pitocin in the morning to "augment" or speed up the labor, though there was no medical reason to do so, as Ms. C's labor had not slowed or stopped.

The next day, at 8:30 A.M., Dr. E visited Ms. C in the hospital for the first time, nine and a half hours after her admission and two hours after a nurse had started her on a Pitocin intravenous drip. During that time, no other doctor had seen Ms. C, and she was not told she was being given Pitocin.

At 8:40 A.M., and again at 8:43 A.M., there were signs of distress on the electronic fetal heart monitor. Ms. C's chart indicates that her nurses were aware of these signs, but there is no indication that a doctor was called.

When drugs such as Pitocin are used to induce or augment labor, the pain of labor typically becomes much worse than normal.[3] At 8:50 A.M., an anesthesiologist gave Ms. C an epidural block to relieve her pain. Administering an epidural block is a delicate procedure that involves putting a needle into the spinal cord just far enough for the tip to be in the spinal fluid and injecting an anesthetic. An epidural blocks all sensations below the injection site, leaving the lower half of the body without feeling.

Nurses notes indicate that at 8:55 A.M., Ms. C was completely dilated— a sign that it was time for her to push the baby out. However, Ms. C was not told that birth was imminent. A nurse called Dr. E, and on the phone he gave the order, "tell her don't push." But the urge to push is spontaneous and out of the woman's control—like trying not to vomit when the urge to vomit comes. For the next hour and forty-four minutes, the nurses tried to keep the baby from being born before the doctor arrived by urging Ms. C not to push and by pushing on the baby's head to hold it back. Nurses' notes indicate that Dr. E was called several times during this period and urged to come quickly. Nurses also gave Ms. C oxygen while she waited and told her it was for the baby, so we can assume that they were aware that holding the baby back was putting the baby at risk.

Ms. C had made it clear to Dr. E before she went into labor that she and her husband wanted a natural birth without surgical interventions, such as an episiotomy (the practice of cutting the vagina open supposedly to create more room for the baby). During her labor, Ms. C reinforced this point. She repeatedly told a nurse, "I do not want an episiotomy." Dr. E rushed in at 10:39 A.M., more than two hours since his last visit, and gave her an episiotomy, for no apparent reason and without telling her what he was doing. Since she was numb from the waist down, she did not know he was cutting her. When she reminded him that she did not want an episiotomy, he said, "too late." Dr. E then used a vacuum extractor to pull the baby out—again, for no apparent reason. (Dr. E claimed the reason was "fetal distress," but there were no signs of fetal distress on the electronic monitor just before the birth.)

These two birth stories—one with a disastrous outcome, one not at all unusual—illustrate many of the egregious errors that go on in maternity care in the United States. The fundamental flaw: in America, we have highly trained surgeons called obstetricians regularly "attending" normal, or low-risk, births.

The United States and Canada are the only highly industrialized Western countries in the world where this is true.[4] And Canada is rapidly converting to the system used in all other industrialized Western countries, including Australia, the Netherlands, Great Britain, all Scandinavian countries, Germany, and Ireland, and in many other countries, where more than 75 percent of all births are assisted by trained midwives. It is a midwife who provides prenatal care, a midwife who admits a woman to the hospital when labor begins (or goes to her home), a midwife who attends the labor, a midwife who assists at the birth, and a midwife who discharges the woman from the hospital. In these countries, obstetricians serve as specialists. They are essential members of the maternity care team, but they play a role only in the 10 to 15 percent of cases where there are serious complications. Most women have babies without ever setting eyes on a doctor.

In the United States, the numbers are reversed. Obstetricians "attend" 90 percent of births and have a great deal of control, essentially a monopoly, over the maternity care system.[5] Obstetricians are taught to view birth in a medical framework rather than to understand it as a natural process. In a medical model, pregnancy and birth are an illness that requires diagnosis and treatment. It is an obstetrician's job to figure out what's wrong (diagnosis) and do something about it (treatment)—even though, with childbirth, the right thing in most cases is to do nothing. To put it another way, having an obstetrical surgeon manage a normal birth is like having a pediatric surgeon babysit a normal two-year-old. Both will find medical solutions to normal situations—drugs to stimulate normal labor and narcotics for a fussy toddler. It's a paradigm that doesn't work.

This book will show that by embracing a medical model of birth and allowing obstetricians control of our maternity care, we Americans have accepted health care for women and babies that is not only below standard for wealthy countries but often amounts to neglect and abuse.

Let's take a look at the stories above.

The birth certificate says that the obstetrician in Oregon "attended" the birth, but this is obviously a misstatement. It is a well-known fact among health care providers that in U.S. hospitals, "attending" obstetricians are almost never in attendance during a women's labor, except for occasional drop-in visits, and are often not even in the hospital building.[6] An episode of the award-winning TV series *ER* showed a woman in labor having convulsions. The emergency room doctor asks the nurse where the woman's obstetrician is. The answer: "Across town in his office seeing patients." If a pregnant woman in America signs on with an obstetrician thinking she will have him around during her labor, she is almost certainly in for a rude awakening.

Doctors are not inclined to discuss the consequences of their absence, but a recent study shows a 12 percent increase in neonatal mortality in babies born between 7 P.M. and midnight and a 16 percent increase in neonatal mortality for babies born between 1 A.M. and 6 A.M.. Researchers believe the increased deaths may be attributed to "the availability and quality of physicians, nurses and support personnel, as well as the accessibility of diagnostic tests and procedures."[7]

A review of litigation cases in obstetrics and gynecology, commissioned by the prestigious Institute of Medicine in Washington, D.C., reported that nearly two-thirds of labor and delivery injuries were caused by problems in medical management—that is, failure to adequately supervise or properly monitor.[8] In the Oregon story, the obstetrician's "failure to adequately supervise and monitor" meant that treatment was delayed during a crisis—a crisis that was brought on by the use of Cytotec, a drug that has not been sufficiently studied to have been proven safe. Does that amount to neglect? I think it *is* neglect on at least two levels. To begin with, the physician ignored the most basic principle of medical practice: *First, do no harm.* Second, the woman was given a powerful drug, then left to go through the second stage of labor (when the risk of developing complications increases) without a doctor's continuous attendance but in the care of a nurse who was responsible for several women in labor and could check in only from time to time, as is usual in hospital maternity care,

It is no surprise that patients are neglected in a system where an obstetrician tries to be all things to all women. An American ob/gyn must be a primary care provider assisting normal, healthy pregnancies and births, a specialist in complications of pregnancy and birth, a counselor and family planning provider, a specialist in gynecological diseases, and a highly skilled surgeon. No other specialist anywhere in health care tries to maintain competence in so many areas. It is not humanly possible. Can an obstetrician do a major gynecological surgical procedure—such as a six-hour "pelvic clean-out" on a woman with extensive cancer—and then rush to his office and do a good job of quietly and patiently counseling a healthy pregnant woman about her sex life? Not likely.

In America, obstetricians' plates are full to overflowing. There is no way they can do it all. And of all the things they try to do, the most difficult thing to fit into their busy schedules is normal childbirth, which lasts twelve hours (on average) and, as we all know, can happen night or day, seven days a week. As in these stories, the actual attendant for the majority of births in the United States is a labor and delivery (L&D) nurse with a telephone.

On average, L&D nurses receive only six weeks of on-the-job training in L&D nursing after completing their basic nursing training. They have no autonomy, and so if problems develop they can do nothing without a doctor's orders. At the same time, L&D nurses are held responsible for accurately judging the moment of birth. If a nurse calls the doctor too soon, she may be accused of wasting the doctor's time. If she calls the doctor too late and the doctor misses the birth, the doctor is equally unhappy. It is no wonder that the thirty thousand L&D nurses working in American hospitals are frustrated and exhausted.[9]

In most hospitals, L&D nurses are asked to closely monitor several women in labor simultaneously. Some level of neglect is inevitable in this situation. When you consider the fact that nurses work eight-hour shifts, the chance that a women in labor will receive continuous, one-on-one care in the hospital is reduced to zero. This is distressing, since many studies have shown that one-on-one, continuous care by the same person throughout labor means a shorter labor, less pain, fewer complications, and better safety for mother and baby.[10] Hospitals and health maintenance organizations (HMOs) say they don't have the money to provide continuous care to women giving birth. Yet somehow they *do* have the money to purchase and maintain expensive electronic fetal monitors and use them on all women—even those having low-risk births, without drugs to induce labor—despite the fact that there is no scientific evidence that routine electronic fetal monitoring improves birth outcomes.[11] Most hospitals believe in machines, not bodies and not human contact, and that is where the money goes.

Now let's look at Dr. E's management of Ms. C's birth in the second story. There are many reasons it is justified to call it abusive. First, Ms. C was given Pitocin for no apparent reason other than the doctor's convenience. Speeding up labor with Pitocin induction has been shown to carry the risk of overly rapid uterine contractions, which can mean insufficient oxygen for the baby and brain damage, as well as another serious risk, uterine rupture, which can be fatal for the woman and the baby.[12] Because the risks are severe, women receiving Pitocin must be closely monitored by the doctor. Dr. E ordered the drug without even examining Ms. C and didn't see her until after she'd been on it for two hours. Furthermore, it is likely that it was the Pitocin that caused Ms. C's labor pains to increase to a level where she needed an epidural, which carries its own risks—such as a sudden fall in blood pressure (depriving the baby of oxygen) as well as the risk to the woman of paralysis or death resulting from the anesthesia.[13] The epidural also meant that Ms. C was robbed of the opportunity to feel the birth of her baby.

A second reason Dr. E's treatment of Ms. C must be considered abusive is that she was given an unnecessary episiotomy. Though it is a common procedure in the United States, episiotomy is actually called for only in rare cases, such as when the baby's head has come out but the shoulders are stuck. There are numerous scientific studies on the risks of episiotomy. One of the proven risks is long-term painful sexual intercourse, a condition which Ms. C has suffered from since this birth.[14]

Pulling the baby out with a vacuum extractor meant even more unnecessary risks, such as an increased risk of permanent urinary and fecal incontinence for Ms. C and an increased risk of brain hemorrhage for her baby. It is ironic that Dr. E said he used an extractor out of concern for the baby, when any difficulties the baby was having almost surely resulted from Dr. E's delaying the birth; if Dr. E had honored Ms. C's body, the birth would have happened an hour and a half earlier.[15] With no other explanation available, it is fair to assume that the birth was delayed on Dr. E's orders, so he could rush in, catch the baby, and take the credit. Delaying birth for convenience is abusive. I first saw this happen as a medical student, and it is still common today, decades later. Based on his behavior, we can speculate that Dr. E was having a busy day (which explains why it took him so long to come when Ms. C was ready to give birth) and, though Ms. C and her baby waited for him, when he finally arrived he was in a hurry to get the birth over with.

Dr. E's management of the case is also abusive on a deeper level. When Dr. E gave Ms. C a drug without her knowledge, he violated her fundamental human right to be fully informed and to consent to any medical intervention prior to it being used on her body.[16] Beyond not giving consent, Ms. C and her husband had made it clear to Dr. E that they did not want Pitocin when he offered it a week earlier. Beyond not giving consent to an episiotomy, Ms. C explicitly said she did not want one. Ms. C was not informed of the risks of using a vacuum extractor nor was she asked for her consent. However, given that she had made her desire for a natural birth very clear, it is safe to assume that if she had been asked she would have refused.

Dr. E blatantly rejected his patient's wish for a natural childbirth, and instead applied a surgical routine that by every standard was unnecessarily aggressive and interventionist. He turned what could have been a happy family event into a miserable surgical event. After the birth, Ms. C tried repeatedly—and unsuccessfully—to get information from Dr. E about why so many interventions were used. After her attempts to get information failed, Ms. C felt so betrayed and abused by Dr. E that she and her husband looked for a lawyer who could help them get some degree of closure. However, because the baby was apparently okay, and Ms. C suffered "only" from sexual problems and mental anguish, no lawyer was willing to take the case. Dr. E's damaging style of practice in this case must be called dishonest and unethical—and, sadly, as this book will show, it is quite common in the American maternity care system.

In a country where consumer rights are taken seriously and legally pro-

tected, it's hard to accept that a doctor like Dr. E ca
"false advertising" and expect to get away with it. Bu
next chapter, obstetricians in the United States have g
and they have fought hard to prevent regulations and
them accountable for their actions. In forty-eight of th
and hospitals are under no obligation to disclose mat
(rates for cesarean section, labor induction, episiotom
public, which makes it very difficult for a women to find out in advance
how she is likely to be treated.[17] When something goes wrong with her
treatment, it is all but impossible to find out what happened or who is to
blame—without filing a lawsuit. A severe lack of information is one of several reasons that in the United States obstetricians are sued more than any
other medical specialist.[18]

The maternity care problems discussed in this book have profound costs
for our society. Organized obstetrics groups such as the American College
of Obstetricians and Gynecologists tell us that we have the "Cadillac" of
maternity care. This is certainly true in one respect, since we pay much
more per capita for maternity services than any other country in the world
does. There are also good data showing that when obstetricians attend
normal births, maternity services are far more expensive than when midwives attend normal births.[19]

But are we getting more bang for all those bucks? Are we number one in
providing high-quality care? Hardly. Twenty-eight countries have lower
maternal mortality rates (women dying around the time of birth) than we
do,[20] and for more than twenty-five years, the number of women dying
around the time of birth in the United States has been increasing.[21] Every
year, at least one thousand women—that is, three jumbo jets full of our sisters, daughters, and mothers—die around the time of childbirth, and at
least half of those deaths could have been prevented. Forty-one countries
have lower infant mortality rates (babies dying before their first birthday).[22]

As you'll see in the coming chapters, our lousy track record is not caused
by poor training. Obstetricians in the United States receive high-caliber education and training, and most also have good intentions. The problem lies not
with individual doctors but with a system in which stretched-thin doctors
have an unjustified monopoly and women and babies are left to pay the price.

It is important to note that in every country that has a lower maternal
mortality rate than the United States—or a lower infant mortality rate—
it is midwives, not obstetricians, who manage normal pregnancies and
births.[23] In some of these countries a significant percentage of births take

homes and out-of-hospital birthing centers.[24] Studies that allow us to compare low-risk births attended by obstetricians and low-risk births attended by midwives show midwives to be safer, less expensive, and more likely to facilitate a satisfying experience for the mother and family.[25] In the United States, however, most obstetricians are vehemently opposed to midwives and have gone to great lengths to drive them out of business. Far beyond a mere territorial battle between two groups of health care professionals, the persecution of midwives in this country has taken on the fervor of an old-fashioned witch hunt. The result is fewer options for women. In many regions of the United States, a pregnant woman who wants the care of a midwife can't get it unless she's willing to go outside mainstream health care channels, and, in some areas, even risk being persecuted and/or prosecuted herself. See chapter 5.[26]

Obstetricians have been telling women for decades that doctors are the only people who can provide them with a safe birth. Fortunately, as Abraham Lincoln said, you can't fool all of the people all of the time. More and more women are finding the courage not to believe everything obstetricians say. The percentage of births attended by midwives in the United States is increasing. Today, the number is 9 percent, up from 5 percent just ten years ago.[27]

There are other encouraging developments as well. Health care in the United States is driven by the bottom line, and more and more HMOs are coming to realize that having midwives attend low-risk births saves money. Not only are midwives paid less than half what obstetricians are paid, but the number of risky, expensive, *unnecessary* interventions is cut in half as well.[28]

Another hopeful sign: in 1999, a new edition of *Danforth's Obstetrics,* a popular textbook, devoted the entire first chapter to the value of practicing "evidence-based obstetrics and gynecology," that is, practicing medicine that comes as close as possible to what scientific studies show to be most beneficial and least risky for patients. The next year, a new edition of *Williams Obstetrics,* perhaps the most widely read obstetric textbook in the United States, followed suit. This emphasis on science was continued in the 2005 edition of *Williams,* leaving no doubt that obstetrics standard-bearers see it as the right direction for the field. As we will see in later chapters, today's actual obstetrics practices have a long way to go to meet the new standard, but a commitment in theory from the obstetrics establishment is certainly an important move in a positive direction.

Perhaps most promising of all, more women in the United States are coming to see the crisis in maternity care as a women's issue. It's about a woman's rights to control what happens to her body and to have access to the best health care options available. For some time women have lobbied for the right to prevent—or end—an unwanted pregnancy, but a woman's right to control a wanted pregnancy and birth has received less attention. Now women's groups are taking on a wide range of issues related to maternity care, such as the need for transparency and accountability.

One example: after considerable struggle, women's groups in New York State got legislation passed requiring hospitals to report to the public on their maternity care practices, including the percentage of births by cesarean section. Several years after the law was passed, it became clear that few hospitals (if any) were complying with the law. An advocacy group called Choices in Childbirth brought the situation to light, which resulted in a public investigation. In their findings, New York City investigators expressed outrage at the high birth intervention rates in city hospitals and recommended that the law be amended to make failure to disclose required information a finable offense.[29]

Of course, it is also important to remember that maternity care is not just a women's issue—the level of interest and commitment of fathers to the birth of their children, generally, could not be higher. I am frequently reminded of the importance of childbirth to the father when I hear once again that one of those most macho of men, a professional sports star, missed an important game because he rushed home to be with his wife during the birth of their child. It's just about the only excuse coaches and teams accept for an athlete's absence, and I have never once heard of a complaint.

In every country in the world where I have seen real progress in maternity care, it has been women's groups working together with midwives, nurses, doctors, doulas, scientists, journalists, lawyers, and politicians that made the difference. In the United States, the movement for demedicalizing and humanizing birth is gaining momentum. The Coalition for Improving Maternity Services (CIMS) has taken the lead and now has more than fifty member organizations and more than ninety thousand individual members. Their mission: "to promote a wellness model of maternity care that will improve birth outcomes and substantially reduce costs."[30] These are the principles underlying this model:

· Normalcy: treat birth as a natural, healthy process.

· Empowerment: provide the birthing woman and her family with supportive, sensitive, and respectful care.

- Autonomy: enable women to make decisions based on accurate information and provide access to the full range of options for care.

- First, do no harm: avoid the routine use of tests, procedures, drugs, and restrictions.

- Responsibility: give evidence-based care solely for the needs and in the interests of mothers and infants.[31]

It's hard to find fault with these simple but profound concepts, yet they stand in sharp contrast with the reality millions of American women experience each year. If these principles were in place, neither of the real-life stories recounted in this chapter would have happened; women would not be faced with rates of cesarean section and drug induction of labor that are twice as high as science tells us are appropriate, using evidence-based care; and women and families would be free to have the childbirth of their choice.

This book is designed to further an understanding of problems in the maternity care system in the United States. In order to make changes, however, we need to begin envisioning solutions as well. I believe we can learn a lot by studying successful strategies developed in other countries and by looking at regions of the United States, such as New Mexico and Oregon, where important advances have been made. I will share my thoughts on best practices in obstetrics in chapter 8. The final chapter of the book will look at the movement for humanizing birth in the United States and suggest ways that all interested parties—from policy makers to pregnant women—can play an active role.

TWO TRIBAL OBSTETRICS

Keep medicine a profession instead of a service.
EDITORIAL, ACOG JOURNAL "OBSTETRICS AND GYNECOLOGY" (AUGUST 2002)

Nature is a bad obstetrician.
CANADIAN OBSTETRICIAN

While lecturing to a roomful of doctors, I will sometimes say, "I remember the first time I killed a patient." The hostility in the room is immediate and palpable. I have committed treason. Although no doctor can practice for many years without at some point making a mistake that results in the death of a patient, when it happens, most doctors either go into intense denial or quickly come up with ten reasons why they are not at fault. My statement that I made a serious error goes against an unspoken rule among physicians—we must never admit to mistakes because it undermines our belief in ourselves and puts us in jeopardy of litigation. It also has the undesirable effect of reminding the doctors in the room that they too make mistakes. There is a saying: "It is better to beg forgiveness than to ask permission." But physicians seem to believe the opposite. Some are finally learning to ask permission (fully informed consent is the law) but they have not gotten around to asking forgiveness for their mistakes. Being a doctor is never having to say you're sorry.

As a result of my error, I went through a long soul-searching. I came to terms with my humanity and attempted to learn from the tragedy. The next time I encountered the same clinical situation, I immediately remembered the mistake—I had not done a tracheotomy quickly enough when a patient had a swelling obstructing the throat—and chose a different course, so that the second time around the patient didn't die.

There are serious problems with allowing doctors to deny that they sometimes make mistakes. Not only do they set themselves up to suffer from hubris, they create a situation where the concept of "clinical experience" can become nothing more than making the same mistakes over and over again with increasing confidence. Physicians do not learn from mistakes because they never make them. Another drawback: if doctors don't make mistakes, there's no need for them to accept responsibility for their practices. Under the current medical ethos, most doctors feel no guilt when their choices have a negative impact on patients.

I have had many discussions with obstetricians about the iatrogenic deaths of women and babies from rupture of the uterus after Cytotec induction in cases where the woman had previously had a cesarean section. It was a common practice in the 1990s and even the American College of Obstetricians and Gynecologists (ACOG) now strongly recommends against it. Yet I have heard no discussion among obstetricians (or from ACOG) of this mistake. When obstetricians discuss induction of labor with Cytotec, listen carefully. It is sad to say, but I have detected almost no remorse for this decade of scientifically unjustified practice, nor compassion for the women who suffered uterine rupture or lost their babies—no apologies, no sense whatsoever of obstetric responsibility, no mea culpa, only you-a culpa. Instead, it is common to hear attempts to justify the practice. Put simply, the response has been widespread denial.

That Cytotec induction was used for years on women with a previous cesarean section, long before adequate scientific studies determined that it was killing women and babies, could be an opportunity to learn from a terrible mistake. The situation serves as a prime example of why we need the FDA, why we need scientists, and why we must have evidence of safety before rushing to try a "hot" new drug or technology. But unless obstetricians can admit they made a mistake, there will be no lesson.[1]

If we accept Santayana's maxim that those who fail to remember the past are condemned to repeat it, we should not be surprised that this use of Cytotec represents one of many widespread iatrogenic tragedies in the history of obstetrics. I will discuss some of the more recent cases involving X-rays and drugs in chapter 4, but an earlier example is instructive as well. It dates back to the end of the eighteenth century, when women first began having babies in hospitals. There was an epidemic of women dying in hospitals during childbirth from an infection known as "childbed fever." In 1795, the Scottish scientist Alexander Gordon, through systematic observations in hospital wards, proved the deaths were the result of doctors touching the bodies of one laboring woman after another, without washing their hands, thus transferring deadly bacteria. Gordon was ignored. Fifty years later, in 1843, Oliver Wendell Holmes, a famous American medical doctor and professor at Harvard, published an essay agreeing with Gordon. Holmes's essay was also ignored. In 1847, the director of a maternity hospital in Vienna, Ignaz Semmelweiss, brought about a 6 percent drop in maternal mortality simply by requiring hand washing by all staff, doctors included. His reward? He lost his job and was driven out of town by hostile obstetricians who refused to believe the deaths of so many women could be their fault.

It was not until the 1880s, ninety years and many thousands of deaths after Gordon determined the cause of the epidemic, that hospitals and governments in the United States and Europe instituted regulations forcing doctors to wash their hands, leading to the abrupt end of "childbed fever."[2]

When I mention epidemics resulting from faulty obstetric practices, many obstetricians are not contrite but angry with me for suggesting that members of their profession are not infallible. Obstetricians are not used to being challenged in this way by their peers. Among other doctors, obstetricians are treated as the supposed experts on pregnancy and birth, and that includes the family physicians who do maternity care. But, as we will see later in this chapter, the American Academy of Family Physicians recently parted company with ACOG when the latter organization made scientifically unfounded recommendations regarding vaginal birth after cesarean that have a negative impact on family physicians and families.

When doubt is expressed by a patient, it is all but intolerable. You can't imagine how upset many doctors become when a patient seeks a second opinion. They put a good face on it, but I've met countless physicians who feel that the doctor-patient relationship has been destroyed if a patient expresses less than 100 percent faith in their judgment. It's hard not to tease a group that takes itself so seriously. I like to wear a button that says, "Trust me, I'm a doctor."

To understand how obstetricians come to believe that they are infallible, it is worthwhile to take a look at their training. The education students receive in medical school is not only medical, but social. We are taught how to behave as doctors and think as doctors. And we internalize the medical hierarchy.

I remember coming to class late one day in medical school. The professor was already demonstrating on a patient in the front of the lecture hall. He looked up when I came in, and said "Dr. Wagner, since you are late, come down and examine this patient." (I was not yet a doctor, but part of the indoctrination process is calling students "doctor" so they get used to thinking of themselves in that elevated position.) I replied, "I'm sorry, but I have forgotten my tools." The professor slammed his fist on the lectern and shouted, "You are not a carpenter or plumber, you are a doctor! They are not tools, they are instruments." Without thinking, I blurted out, "But I always thought doctors were one kind of plumber."

I received the lowest possible passing grade in that course. When I complained that I had earned a better grade, the professor replied, "What do you care what your grade is? You're only going to become a general practitioner and for that you don't need top grades." In truth, I had not decided to become a general practitioner, and the professor knew it. Saying that I had was a way of putting me down, as many medical school faculty members consider general practice to be at the bottom of the medical practice hierarchy, with lower status than any specialty.

Another classic demonstration of the medical hierarchy, which is well known by doctors and nurses but practically hidden from patients, is the dress code. In any given hospital or medical school, there are telltale signs that indicate exactly who's who. Believe it or not, all white coats are not alike. When I was in training at the UCLA hospital, medical students wore long unbuttoned white coats, for example, while interns wore short white coats with mandarin collars that buttoned down the side. "Residents"—graduated physicians in specialty training—wore short unbuttoned white coats, and faculty wore long white coats buttoned closed. Attending physicians wore no white coats at all. Medical school and specialty training are full of subtle lessons like these on status and hierarchy, on lording it over those under you and being subservient to those above, on "kissing up and kicking down."

This hierarchy is reinforced within each specialty—including obstetrics. Over the years, I have also come to see that, in many respects, organized obstetrics has the characteristics of a primitive tribe.[3] There is a long period of preparation for "manhood"—beginning with four fiercely competitive years in an undergraduate college, after which students start yet another four years of intense study in medical school. At UCLA, the medical school I attended, this phase of a doctor's life begins with an initiation ceremony—a rite of passage. Each student receives a symbol of his new status as a pledge in the tribe: the great white coat.

After eight years of undergraduate and medical school, initiates embark on a year of internship, and then go on to three or more years of specialty training in obstetrics and gynecology. It is no accident that those in specialty training are called "residents," as their duties demand that, for all practical purposes, they reside at the hospital due to long workdays and frequent on-call duty nights and weekends. In this phase of education, a doctor-in-training's world shrinks even further. He becomes more and more removed from normal life. Every day he is surrounded by elders whose job it is to teach him to think like an obstetrician. When his indoctrination is sufficient, he will go through his final initiation rite—examination by a "board" of elders and "board certification" as a member of the tribe. By the end of this educational purgatory, tribe members have developed strong feelings of loyalty to the tribe as a whole and to the tribal chieftains. From this point on, the greatest offense a tribe member can commit is not incompetence but disloyalty.

Armed with arrogance and a sense of entitlement, the young doctor enters the insular, protected world of obstetrics. He goes to local meetings of obstetricians or regional meetings of ACOG, and perhaps even occasionally attends national meetings of this organization. As he builds his practice, the young doctor will also be invited to obstetric "meetings" sponsored by pharmaceutical companies—meetings held on a cruise ship or at a ski resort, with a few hours each day devoted to lectures and the rest of the time for play.

In each of these various meetings, the obstetrician hears only the current obstetric dogma. As in everything else, there are fads in obstetrics and every dogma has its day. Participants may gain a bit of new knowledge at these meetings, but the key message is always, "We obstetricians know what we're doing, and we're doing it right." This is the important function known as "preaching to the choir." I have given many lectures at all kinds of obstetric meetings, and the fact that some of the ideas I present are outside the present obstetric orthodoxy always comes as a shock to the audience. As a clinician/scientist/epidemiologist, I give presentations that suggest a need to change certain practices. The response is always revealing. Typically, most doctors are so mired in and blinded by the obstetric establishment point of view that they react as if I have done a no-no in church by not reassuring them that all is well in our closed little world. But there are always some whose faces show confusion and concern as it begins to dawn on them that all might not be as right as they've been led to believe.

Obstetricians also spend much of their time in, and are heavily influenced by, hospitals. They go to a weekly "obstetric grand rounds," a meeting to discuss cases with the other obstetricians on the staff of that hospital. A hospital is itself a closed society, and in my view, it is one of the last bastions of feudalism in our culture—complete with rigid regulations, hierarchies, and fiefdoms. Whether you're a doctor or a patient, when you go to a hospital in the United States, you leave a one-person, one-vote world (messy, noisy, infuriating, but democratic) and enter a world where fear is the primary management tool and censorship and misinformation are standard practice. The maternity wards of America's fabled democratic society are anything but democratic.

In U.S. hospitals the hierarchies are absolute. Carrying on from medical school, obstetrics medical ethos dictates a clear ranking of all maternity care players—with obstetricians at the top, then hospital administrators, then midwives and nurses, and, at the bottom, patients. Naturally, those at the top tend to feel that any admiration or adulation directed to them is well deserved and they develop a certain scorn for those below. But in a hospital, this hierarchy is not just about status; it is about authority and control. I was once part of a group that, while preparing for an international conference on maternity care, drafted a document on humanizing birth that included the statement "Doctors and midwives must work together as equals." The obstetric organizations that participated in the conference approved the entire document with the exception of those last two words. *As equals* was unacceptable within their hierarchy.

Still, the relative ranking of players in a hospital has never been so clear to me as it was when I experienced it as a layperson. Several years ago, while at a party, my partner twisted her leg while we were dancing, and her kneecap popped out, causing her extreme pain. I rushed her to the ER, where she was placed on a rolling table in a small room, and we were told to wait for the doctor. (I did not tell anyone that I am a physician.) She was completely miserable, so I climbed up on the table to hold her and comfort her. A nurse came by and told me to get off the table, even though we were alone in the room. Two hours later, a doctor applied a cast to my partner's leg, with the assistance of another nurse, and the two whispered to each other, giggled, touched, and carried on an open sexual flirtation while they worked. Their flirting didn't bother me, but it occurred to me that according to some unwritten hospital rule it was okay for doctors and nurses to display intimacy but not for patients to do so. I've come to believe that every doctor needs to experience being a patient in a hospital when the staff doesn't know the patient is a doctor so that he can see what it feels like to be at the bottom of the pecking order, instead of at the top.

Part of the reason for this belief in the hierarchy is that, in my experience, many practicing medical doctors live an insular life. They are not only limited in their contact at work, they tend to lead relatively insular personal lives as well. They, like other people providing individual services of a personal nature (police officers, mental health or family counselors, and so on),

TABLE 1. THE RECIPROCAL NATURAL CHILDBIRTH INDEX

Add points as indicated if the woman:

Goes into labor Friday afternoon	5
Checked (or husband checked) cervix at home	5
Arrives in a late-model Volvo station wagon	5
Has a hyphenated last name	5
Husband has one too	10
Is insured by a managed health care plan	5
Has more than 4 years of college	5
Either parent is a physician	each, add 5
Either parent is an attorney	each, add 10
Insists on calling all staff members by first names	5
Brings own naturopath to assist	5
Has a written birth plan, per page add	5
Spends more than half of labor in shower	5
Brings own Walkman	5
Brings New Age tapes, each tape add	5

Discussion: We have found that a Reciprocal Natural Childbirth Index score of 30 or greater should earn the woman in labor immediate consideration for cesarean section. In fact, since you can get a score of 30 without even being in labor, someone with a high enough score could be offered a C-section at her convenience during regular working hours.

SOURCE: A. Berg, "The Reciprocal Natural Childbirth Index," *Journal of Irreproducible Results* 36, no. 2 (March/April 1991): 27. (Yes, such a journal does exist.)

seem to hang around with their own kind. They rarely have close friendships with people outside their own vocation. I believe this is at least in part because they have to keep "secrets" in their work. They can't share the truth of their experience with their clients/patients, so they learn not to share their experience with other outsiders as well. In daily practice, obstetricians usually talk only with other obstetricians or, when they must, with those they control—nurses, office staff, patients. Being an authority figure in such a cloistered world has inevitable results, the most common being a feeling that it's "us versus them." And too often "us" rapidly becomes superior to "them."

A professor of obstetrics at an Ivy League university medical school posted a copy of a "Reciprocal Natural Childbirth Index" (supposedly as a joke) on his office wall (see table 1). This table heaps contempt on women whose ideas and preferences for giving birth inconvenience the doctor. Many obstetricians find the table hilariously funny. Isn't it frightening that the ultimate weapon obstetricians use to punish overly "independent" women is to cut into their bodies, using a surgical procedure (cesarean section) only obstetricians can perform, which completely deprives the women of control over their own bodies?

Another story of contempt: Early in my career, I heard several women in a local hospital where I was working complaining that a certain obstetrician treated them in an aggressive and mean way. I dismissed their complaints, until one day, by accident, I saw the doctor with a patient when he didn't know I was there, and I was shocked to see him shouting at her and calling her deprecating names. Over time, through informal chats with him, I learned that he had a very low opinion of women, seeing them as inferior and irrational, and I came to understand that he truly hated women. This confused me. Why would he choose to go into obstetrics and gynecology? Then I got it. He had found the perfect way to punish women. Sound ridiculous? Ask the women who have suffered through unnecessarily rough pelvic exams. Over the years, I have run across other obstetricians who hate women and this horrible hypothesis has been confirmed, although my impression is that most obstetricians have a gentle manner with the women under their care.

At the other end of the continuum are obstetricians who cherish women. These are the obstetricians who practice obstetrics for many years. They don't mind long waits with women in labor or being on call 24/7, and still experience wonder with every birth. However, given the strain of the job, it is not unusual for obstetricians in the United States to take the first opportunity to drop obstetrics and limit their practice to gynecology—perhaps handing obstetrics cases off to a younger partner.

With few exceptions, obstetricians are not evil people. They are hardworking and want the best for their patients. But years of isolation in the obstetric world leaves them believing the obstetric establishment point of view—that they should control maternity services. Obstetricians internalize this as the official truth. They don't sit down and decide, "I'm going to speak for the obstetric establishment." They unconsciously internalize a set of assumptions, and one of the most potent assumptions is that pregnancy and birth are medical events and so maternity care should be seen in obstetricians' terms, not women's terms. Individual obstetricians are human beings, no more, no less. They have all the imperfections and neuroses everyone else has. But when individuals get together in groups, strange things can happen. There is a process of natural selection that allows a certain type of obstetrician to rise to a position of authority in organized obstetrics. Whether driven by a need for power, admiration of peers, or feelings of self-importance, the people at the top in organized obstetrics in the United States have gotten there by convincing others that they are best able to protect and promote the obstetric monopoly.

Given the constricted, adversarial nature of a doctor's world, it's not surprising that, despite good intentions, it's difficult for physicians to maintain real compassion for patients. Some obstetricians achieve it but, in my experience, they are in the minority, and it is difficult for women to identify these obstetricians through the smokescreen of hype and falsehoods that envelops the field. The world of doctors and hospitals functions satisfactorily, in general, for cases of serious illness and major injury. In these cases, a medical approach focused on diagnosis and treatment is appropriate, as is spending time in a hospital with other sick and injured people where care routines focus less on emotional and social needs than on heroic treatment of physical ailments. But the way things are done in the medical realm is totally inappropriate for normal life events such as birth and death.

Generally speaking, most of us would prefer not to have a surgeon taking charge during a normal life event. And obstetricians are surgeons, a fact you forget at your peril. To slice a woman's body open, the surgeon must maintain a dispassionate distance from the woman, which, when achieved, makes it difficult to feel compassion. It makes no sense for a gynecological surgeon to assist during normal pregnancy and birth—unless doctors' tasks are to be divvied up by dividing the human body into territories. Some countries, such as the Netherlands, are considering a new system that would make gynecology and obstetrics two separate specialties. Gynecologists would provide reproductive health care to women who are not pregnant. Obstetricians would provide care to pregnant and birthing women with medical complications. And birthing women with no complications would be cared for by midwives (as they are currently in these countries), whether they are giving birth at home or in a hospital.

It's interesting to note that the word *obstetrician* comes from the Latin for standing in front of (the female genitals), and that is what a gynecological surgeon does: stands in front of a woman, between her legs. This requires that the woman be on her back. It is no coincidence that in the United States, where gynecological surgeons are also obstetricians and bring their surgical mindset and methods when they attend normal births, women are put in the worst of all positions for giving birth—"lithotomy" or "on the back." The doctor is close to the woman's genitals and far away from her head and heart—symbolic of the focus of obstetrics.

Another point to understand about surgeons is that they believe in surgery—"if in doubt, cut it out." There are many examples of surgeons choosing to "cut it out" when the scientific evidence says that's not a good idea. One recent example is surgery for the pain and stiffness caused by arthritis in the knee resulting from old age, in which the smooth surfaces of the knee joint become roughened. Incisions are made in the knee, an instrument is inserted into the knee joint and the rough areas are shaved off and flushed out. Sounds like a good idea. But a study proved otherwise. Half the patients in the study had the surgery and the other half had a sham procedure (patients were sedated and surgeons pretended to operate). Subsequent tests revealed that the operation did not help knee function and most of those who got the sham surgery reported feeling just as good as those who had the real operation. This surgery is done on at least 225,000 middle-aged and elderly Americans each year at a cost of more than a billion dollars to Medicare, the Department of Veterans Affairs, and private insurance companies.[4]

That obstetricians are surgeons who believe in surgery is further illustrated by a study that asked women health practitioners and laywomen if they would choose to have a surgical birth (cesarean section) rather than a vaginal birth if there was no medical indication of a need for cesarean. Four percent of midwives said they would; 5 percent of laywomen said they would; and 46 percent of women doctors said they would.[5] That women doctors would choose cesarean section for themselves, without any medical indication, shows the extent to which they believe in surgery and in the obstetric hype about how safe elective cesarean section is, even though scientific evidence shows clearly that vaginal birth is safer for the woman and the baby except in certain emergency situations.

Interestingly, while the rate of cesarean section performed in the United States has nearly doubled since 1980,[6] the trend among other medical specialists is toward doing less surgery. It is becoming common to hear other types of surgeons quote a very different saying—"A good surgeon knows when to operate and a better surgeon knows when not to operate"—and express concern, if not contempt, for the surgical excesses of obstetricians.

While obstetricians tend to lose compassion for their patients over the course of their education and practice, their desire to protect their tribe (and with it their own self-interest) tends to grow stronger. One of the most convincing demonstrations of the power of tribal loyalty in obstetrics is Mafia-like "omertà": tribal members are taught never to speak about the tribe or any of its members in public in a negative way. Never. We may talk to one another about the terrible way a certain tribal member practices obstetrics, but only in private.

In every tribe—from the U.S. Marine Corps to a local fraternal lodge—the tribe and its leaders take care of their own people first; everything else is secondary. In return, each member of the tribe has an absolute duty to support the tribe and follow its rules. Loyalty, of course, can be a good thing, but like many good things, it can also be misused or misplaced. When loyalty is misplaced, as often happens in obstetrics, we have cronyism, which can lead to behaviors that are detrimental and even dangerous to patients and the community. For many obstetricians, cronyism is a way of life and they call it loyalty.

In Oakland, California, in 2001, a woman and her baby died after Cytotec was used to induce her labor. Preparing to report on the case for the local affiliate of a national television network, a journalist contacted a number of local obstetricians. Some of them told the journalist "off the record" that they do not use Cytotec for induction themselves because of the known risks, but not a single obstetrician was willing to go on camera. Omertà. This response from local doctors was typical, as any journalist will tell you.

The same is true in a court of law. When an obstetrician is charged with malpractice, it is extremely unlikely that another local doctor will be willing to testify against him. Lawyers must go outside the community to find a doctor willing to testify. Why? Because an obstetrician knows that if he testifies in court against another obstetrician, he will be shunned (and worse) by the tribe. And when someone has spent so many years becoming a doctor, that price is simply too high. As we will see in chapter 7, the organized medical establishment has found a number of ways to prevent doctors from assisting lawyers in malpractice cases.

Hospitals have their own brand of omertà. Hospitals have perinatal "peer review" committees that investigate obstetric cases in which something has gone wrong, but these committees are made up of other tribal members in that hospital and always meet behind closed doors. Even if a case goes to court, it is virtually impossible to find out what was said, because hospital peer review findings are inadmissible as evidence. As further protection, most hospitals have people on staff whose job it is to convince patients who might have cause to sue that a doctor has not made a mistake. I have also noticed that these "patient liaison" people, like some nurses and other non-physician hospital staff, are often so eager to be liked by tribal members that their loyalty can go to extremes. They seem to seek an "affiliate" membership of sorts, perhaps hoping that a bit of the glory will rub off on them, or hoping to convince themselves and others that they are made of the same stuff as tribal members.

I saw the hospital omertà in action at a regional level when I was invited to speak at a large obstetric meeting attended by doctors from a number of private hospitals in the area. In my presentation, I showed a slide of the cesarean section rates for each hospital, and some rates were shockingly high—up to 60 percent of all births. The next day there was an uproar in the local obstetric community, not about the shameful number of unnecessary surgeries or the disparity between their cesarean rates and what scientific evidence shows is acceptable, but about the fact that someone had given me, an outsider, those hospital data. The critical question: Who broke the hospital omertà? In that area, hospitals are required to report cesarean section rates to the local health department. However, in typical allegiance to the tribe (rather than to the public they are paid to serve), the public health officials had promised the hospitals that they would not leak the rates to the public. The hospitals believed that the health department had betrayed them. They were outraged. But, as it happened, the public health department was not the source of my data.

There are many fascinating examples of ways that organized obstetrics puts the interests of tribal members before the interests of patients. One that is particularly blatant is ACOG's Committee Opinion number 207, "Liability Implications of Recording Procedures or Treatments," published in September 1998. The opinion addresses the issue of hospital births videotaped by the family. It includes the statement, "Recording solely for the purpose of patient memorabilia or marketing is not without liability—the Committee strongly discourages any recording of medical and surgical procedures for patient memorabilia." In essence, ACOG is recommending that doctors and hospitals refuse to allow women and families to videotape their babies' birth for fear of litigation. In ACOG's world, protecting its members is a higher priority than women's rights or family values. Its fear is so strong, it cannot accommodate the need of families to record one of the most important events in their lives. For this reason, recommendations from this organization cannot be considered the gospel. We must always consider them carefully in the light of their primary purpose—protecting the welfare of the tribe.

Here is another example of how tribal interests are protected in obstetrics. On a *Dateline NBC* program that focused on the widespread use of Cytotec for induction of labor—a use not approved by the FDA—an ACOG representative was asked whether an obstetrician should always tell his patient if a drug is not approved by the FDA before administering it. The representative responded that to do so or not is at the discretion of the individual obstetrician. The answer was a cop-out. The organization did not want to go on record as opposing Cytotec for induction, because many members of the tribe use it all the time for this purpose. At the same time, it did not want to look foolish by saying that women do not have the right to informed choice and it's fine for obstetricians to ignore FDA recommendations.[7]

Naturally, tribal protection goes on at a national level as well. In the spring of 2002, ACOG hosted a meeting of the U.S. Safe Motherhood Coalition at its headquarters in downtown Washington, D.C. Safe Motherhood's mission is to lower maternal mortality rates, a particularly important effort in the United States, where for twenty-five years maternal mortality rates have been going up, not down. Furthermore, public health officials know that our rates are underreported. In one state in one year, one-third of the maternal deaths had not been reported, and one official suggests, "The actual pregnancy-related death rate could be more than twice as high as that reported."[8]

Sitting around the table with the obstetricians from ACOG at the Safe Motherhood Coalition were representatives of several midwifery organizations that are members of the Coalition. Most of the midwives had come to the meeting on shoestring budgets and were staying with friends because they could not afford to stay at a hotel. At the meeting, ACOG had the gall to announce that it was dropping out of the Coalition due to "lack of funds." Certainly, this national obstetric organization in its large, well-appointed headquarters does care about women dying around the time of birth. So why did it drop out? Is it possible that it cares more about tribal issues, such as liability risks to obstetricians if maternal deaths are monitored too closely?

Obstetricians are terribly frightened of having the deaths of their patients investigated. Not long ago, I talked with an obstetrician who at one time was a professor of obstetrics at a highly respected university hospital. He is known for writing and speaking on the importance of evidence-based obstetric practice, so he must be seen as among the more progressive American obstetricians. Yet, when I asked him if he would like to see a maternal death audit system developed in the United States (this idea is covered further in chapter 7), he responded by telling me about a lawyer in Texas who somehow got information from a maternal death audit and used it to get big bucks for the family of the dead mother. We must never underestimate the power fear of litigation holds over obstetricians. In my experience, as a motivational force it overshadows their desire to lower the maternal mortality rate.

Occasionally, a group of obstetricians does try to get a handle on maternal deaths in their locale. A study reported in the year 2000 looked at ten hospitals in greater Chicago where the maternal mortality rate was twice as high as the national rate reported by the Centers for Disease Control and Prevention. The doctors looked at each case individually and found that 37 percent of the deaths were preventable, and, of those preventable cases, 80 percent of the time the cause of death was one or more mistakes by doctors and nurses. (Unfortunately, as is nearly always the case, the study made no attempt to determine how many of the deaths were related to obstetric interventions such as induction of labor, epidural block, and cesarean section.) The paper laments the fact that in the United States, maternal mortality committees that carefully review all maternal deaths are now largely defunct, and urges that these committees be revived.[9] There are conscientious, concerned obstetricians out there trying to do something about the maternity care system, but it is an uphill battle, to say the least, as many of their colleagues would prefer to believe there is nothing wrong and will go to great lengths to perpetuate the myth.

While the obstetrics establishment is masterful at protecting tribal members, it is equally effective at controlling them. It has devised a number of ways to make sure members comply with the obstetric omertà and other unwritten tribal rules, the most common being the threat of punishment. And the punishment can be severe. An offending doctor can be completely ostracized. Other doctors in the community may stop referring patients to him. He may be brought before a hospital peer review committee, where, behind closed doors in a tribal kangaroo court, he will face everything from humiliation to loss of staff privileges, making it impossible to practice. Put simply, an offending doctor can be thrown out of the tribe.

I know an obstetrician who witnessed blatant malpractice while assisting at surgery, and the case resulted in a dead baby. In private, she told me that she was shocked by what she saw. But when I asked what she was going to do about it, she said, "Nothing." Now I was shocked, as I knew her to be a caring, compassionate, competent obstetrician. "Why do nothing?" I asked. She explained that hers was a small city, and all the obstetricians knew one another. If she stepped out of line, she would put her practice in serious jeopardy and the women she served could lose her services. On the other hand, by doing nothing, she allowed the obstetrician guilty of serious malpractice to get off without so much as a reprimand and to remain in practice in that community. Don't underestimate the power of the tribe.

I have personally experienced the wrath of the tribe when I have disobeyed the obstetric omertà. While I was with the World Health Organization, I spoke in Scotland at a public meeting on maternity care. During my talk, I mentioned that data show that in Scotland (as in the United States) birth occurs much less frequently on weekends than during the week, and suggested that perhaps Scottish doctors were influencing time of birth for reasons of convenience.[10] The following Sunday, a leading newspaper in Edinburgh ran an article quoting me on this topic of birth by day of the week and convenience.

The next day, the director of health for Scotland called my boss at the World Health Organization to insist that I be reprimanded, if not fired, and to demand that I publicly retract what I had said. My boss called me in and asked if I could produce data to substantiate my statements. I showed him the data, and he called the director in Scotland, quoted the data, and said that there would be neither reprimand nor retraction. (The data on time of birth in Scotland indicating convenience had existed for some time, but no one had spoken about it in public.) Because the obstetric tribe in Scotland couldn't employ the usual methods of tribal punishment (that is, bring me before a hospital committee), they tried another age-old tactic. They tried to get me in trouble with my boss.

ACOG also uses fear of litigation to control doctors and hospitals. If doctors and hospitals go against one of their recommendations, they are more vulnerable to litigation. At a policy level, ACOG uses another brand of fear to control women, politicians, and the media. They justify many of their statements (for which there is little or no scientific support) by calling their position a matter of "safety." One example: in its 2002 publication *Guidelines for Perinatal Care,* ACOG states that home birth is "not safe." The publication doesn't even try to reference data, because the statement flies in the face of overwhelming scientific evidence showing that planned births at home and in out-of-hospital birth centers are perfectly good options for the vast majority of women.[11] This irresponsible talk of safety is misleading, most importantly, to women and their families. If the obstetric tribe says that out-of-hospital birth is not "safe," the implication, of course, is that a hospital birth is safe, which is not true. Newborn babies die in hospitals every day, sometimes because someone made a mistake. When the obstetrics establishment implies that this doesn't happen, the family naturally feels deceived when it does happen.

Another way that organized obstetrics uses tribal loyalty is to protect its territory, that is, to maintain its monopoly in American maternity care. I saw this in action at a local level when I visited Des Moines, Iowa, to speak at an evening meeting of the local medical association. Every person in the room was a doctor. In my talk, I said that I found it tragic that the only out-of-hospital birth center in the area that offered midwifery care—an important and safe option for women—was in danger of closing. The general practitioner who provided backup consultation (required by law in Iowa) was retiring and not one other doctor was willing to replace him.

During the general plenary discussion following my talk, a doctor stood up and said, "Regarding that birth center, doctor, you just don't get it. We don't want the competition. We want that place closed, and we have seen to it that it will close. You can be sure no doctor in this area will give backup." (This is how doctors talk behind closed doors.) The birth center did close soon thereafter. For me, the saddest thing about that meeting in Des Moines was that during the break after my talk, several doctors told me that they personally believe there should be an out-of-hospital birth center, but they didn't dare break rank and provide backup.

One of the most interesting recent examples of tribal protectionism and the ability of the obstetrics establishment to maintain its monopoly is ACOG's practice bulletin number 5, "Vaginal Birth after Previous Cesarean Section (VBAC)," issued in July 1999. Prior to the publication of this ACOG bulletin, there had been general consensus, even among obstetricians, that women should be encouraged to try VBAC. The federal Department of Health and Human Services even had a stated goal to increase the rate of VBAC births. The discussions leading up to this practice bulletin began in the 1990s, when cases of uterine rupture during labor among women who had previously had cesarean sections increased at an alarming rate. (As we saw in chapter 1, uterine rupture is an obstetric catastrophe, with a high risk of death for the baby and a significant risk of death for the woman.)

The phenomenon was almost certainly related to the fact that the percentage of births in which powerful drugs, such as Cytotec, were used to induce labor had doubled, given that studies show there is an increased risk of uterine rupture with pharmacological induction. But instead of acknowledging and addressing this connection by recommending that obstetricians not use Cytotec for induction, the organization recommended that a woman not be permitted to attempt a vaginal birth after previous cesarean section unless she was in a hospital where an obstetrician and anesthesiologist were always present. In other words, instead of preventing uterine rupture, ACOG said that we should surround the woman with experts to deal with the rupture when it happens. This is like trying to solve the problem of children drowning at summer camp not by teaching the children to swim, but rather by putting a couple of life preservers in the lake.

The language of the bulletin makes it clear that fear of litigation is at the root of ACOG's policy on VBAC. Near the beginning, the document mentions that "physicians in the United States are facing increased medical-legal pressures" in general, and then focuses on VBAC litigation, saying, "Increasingly, these adverse events during trial of labor have led to malpractice suits." The fear is further revealed in figure 1, which points out the need to "counsel the patient regarding the benefits and risks of VBAC," but does not point out a similar need to counsel the patient regarding the benefits and risks of the other choice, cesarean section.

ACOG's recommendation on VBAC has a huge impact on maternity care in the United States. Where VBAC in compliance with ACOG's recommendation is not a possibility, such as in areas that have only a small local hospital, it means that every time a women has a cesarean section, all subsequent babies must again be born by cesarean section, resulting in a geometrical increase in the rate of cesareans. This is borne out by the rapid increase in the rate of cesarean section births in the United States, which is now approaching one-third of all births. The ACOG policy denies this rapidly increasing group of women who have previously had cesarean sections a choice of where they will give birth. If they want a VBAC, they will not be able to give birth at home, in an out-of-hospital birth center, or in a small local hospital.

Now, in many areas of the United States, no hospital or doctor will allow women to attempt a VBAC, despite evidence that it is no more risky than a repeat cesarean section birth. A study of eighteen thousand women shows that 75 percent of VBACs are successful (no surgical intervention needed).[12] In addition, a National Institutes of Health study on VBACs found that uterine ruptures occurred in fewer than 1 percent of those who attempted VBAC.[13] Because of all these data, the National Institutes of Health recommends that women be given the choice of having a VBAC. But many obstetricians are unwilling to take the legal risk of going against ACOG. In some states, the choice is effectively made for them, because malpractice insurance companies in the state will no longer cover claims resulting from VBAC. According to one insurance company CEO, physicians are for the most part pleased with their decision to drop the coverage "because it simplifies things for them."[14]

It is disturbing to find that a policy with such a serious impact on women is not backed up by scientific evidence. There are no studies showing that fewer women and babies die in certain types of hospitals. One study, which, ironically, ACOG included in its reference list, looked at VBACs and repeat cesarean section births in three types of hospitals—community, regional, and tertiary care (large regional referral hospitals)—and found no difference in mortality rates between the two procedures by type of hospital.[15]

Another problem with the ACOG recommendation on VBAC is that it is based on the unproven assumption that a cesarean section can be accomplished faster if a women undergoes labor at a large specialty-care hospital. It sounds logical, but in truth it takes considerable time to prepare for the operation and transport the woman to the surgical ward when she is already on a labor ward in the hospital. A study conducted at a large specialty hospital found that in 52 percent of emergency cesarean sections done because of fetal distress on women already in that hospital, the time between the decision to do a cesarean section and the incision exceeded thirty minutes.[16] One reason for the delay, of course, is that the doctor is not on the premises but is instead monitoring the labor by telephone. ACOG's recommendation "to have a physician immediately available" must be taken as inadvertent criticism of a system in which a laboring woman's doctor is not usually available and must be called and asked to come in when there is an emergency.

The elegant solution to the issue of VBAC is not to take away valid choices for woman and families, as ACOG recommends by insisting that a woman having a VBAC be transported at the beginning of labor to a big hospital away from her home, family, friends, and primary care physician. Instead, it is to create an effective communication and transport system, as highly industrialized countries where mortality rates are lower than ours have done. When there is good communication between a woman's local care providers (at home, in a birth center, or in a small hospital) and a larger regional hospital, if the woman needs to be transported for surgery, in most cases the "decision to incision" time need be no greater than if she were laboring in the specialty hospital and needed to be transported from the delivery ward to the surgical ward.

The ACOG recommendation on VBAC illustrates a double standard often found in the organization's recommendations. Policies that have no evidence to support them but are "doctor-friendly" (of benefit to obstetricians)—such as VBAC only in hospitals with surgeons standing by—are recommended by the organization. Other solutions to the problem that are not obstetrician-friendly—such as facilitation of communication, collaboration, and transportation between local hospitals and big regional hospitals—are not recommended even though they would benefit many women.

Very rarely, ACOG is forced to make a recommendation that is not doctor-friendly, such as when it finally recommended against using Cytotec induction in VBAC cases. But that was only after overwhelming scientific evidence of serious risks and years of damage to women and babies.

ACOG's practice bulletin on VBAC includes a number of recommendations for managing VBACs. When we take a closer look at who made the recommendation that limits where VBAC births can occur—the recommendation we've been discussing—we find that it was placed in a category "Level C." The summary says that Level C recommendations are not based on scientific evidence but rather are based "primarily on consensus and expert opinion." So who are the experts and who was involved in the consensus? I contacted ACOG, but the organization was unwilling to say. Evidently, this particular tribe does not accept that in a democratic society transparency in these matters is a necessity.

When a policy affects the care of a large group of women, we might hope that a "consensus" would include not only obstetricians but also midwives, nurses, family physicians, perinatal epidemiologists, and consumers. This is particularly important when a recommendation, such as this one, is of the "you need more of us" variety. Since ACOG's policy gives an advantage to obstetricians and a disadvantage to family physicians, midwives, and many women, the recommendation could easily be seen as self-aggrandizing for obstetricians—or, worse, an attempt to drum up more business.

The following editorial was published in the *Lancet:*

Advocacy guidelines developed by a single-specialty group in isolation may be counterproductive, because those disciplines and professions that were not involved in the development of the guidelines but may be required to implement the recommendations mount their attacks and lodge their disclaimers. Some of the guidelines may be of the Good Old Boys Sat at Table (GOBSAT) variety, based on received wisdom rather than current scientific evidence, and may be biased by undeclared conflicts of interests. . . . Studies have shown that the balance of disciplines within a guideline-development group has considerable influence on the guideline recommendations. Widespread multidisciplinary participation is essential not only to ensure that the guideline is valid, but also that it is valued by all the members of the multidisciplinary team, in order to be incorporated successfully into practice.[17]

Since ACOG's VBAC guideline was made public, other interested parties—midwifery organizations, family practice organizations, women's groups—have come out against it.[18] While visiting hospitals in Maine, I was told by a leading family practitioner that small hospitals and family practitioners in that state are violently opposed to the recommendation but are too afraid to go against it because of fear of litigation. More recently, the American Academy of Family Physicians released its own report on VBAC. Based on a more careful and thorough review of the literature than the ACOG recommendation, the Academy's report explicitly states that there is no scientific evidence to support the ACOG restriction on VBAC location. It goes on to recommend, just as the National Institutes of Health does, that women be given the right to choose VBAC, regardless of place of birth.[19] But while progress is being made to overcome the scientifically unjustified ACOG restriction on VBAC, the attitude of the hospitals in Maine is a good example of how ACOG—not women, not insurance companies, not HMOs, not government agencies—controls American maternity care.

Why does ACOG have so much power? Because it is very effective at protecting and promoting an obstetric monopoly—and simply because it assumes power. In a citizen petition delivered to the FDA in November 2000, ACOG argued its case for Cytotec induction (which will be covered in detail in chapter 4). In a transparent attempt to establish power over the FDA, the petition states: "The American College of Obstetricians and Gynecologists is an organization representing more than 41,000 physicians dedicated to improving women's health care. ACOG is also the body which establishes standards of care for the ob-gyn profession." First the petition says how big ACOG is and then says that the organization sets standards. Who says? No one, not any government agency or any other official, has assigned ACOG standard-setting responsibility. Practicing obstetricians in this country are under no official obligation to be members of ACOG (many are not). They are not obligated even to read this organization's recommendations, much less required by any law or regulation to abide by them. ACOG has simply pronounced, "We set the standard." ACOG no longer has the moral authority to set standards in maternity care, however. It has made too many self-aggrandizing and self-protective recommendations (e.g., against home birth, videotaping birth, and VBAC) that limit the freedom of American women and families.

Another important reason organized obstetrics dominates in the United States is the sins of omission of many of its members. The chairman of obstetrics at a large university hospital on the Eastern seaboard confided to me one day that he hates ACOG and all it stands for. He agreed with me that its recommendations are sometimes unscientific. But he has never said these things in public—one of the reasons he has made it up the ladder. Many obstetricians tell me in private that they disagree with the current obstetric dogma but they do not speak out. The silence of all these lambs allows their organization to proceed merrily on with its reactionary, sometimes destructive agenda.

To understand the absolute monopoly ACOG has established in American maternity care, it is helpful to look more closely at this organization. The American College of Obstetricians and Gynecologists is not a "college" in the usual sense: it is not an institution of higher learning. Nor is it a scientific body. With few exceptions, its members and leaders are not scientists but medical practitioners, and there is nothing in ACOG's mission statement about science. The ultimate proof that ACOG is not a scientific body? Too many of its policies and recommendations are not based on real science. For example, in May 2002, ACOG issued a news release with the title "Cytotec Given Orally Found Safe and Effective to Induce Labor." The release reports on a study of 107 women randomly assigned to two groups.[20] It is impossible to measure safety with such a tiny sampling. It would take at least thirty times that number to have enough statistical power to draw conclusions about the serious risks of induction with this drug. Putting the word *safe* in the title of the news release is a gaffe that demonstrates ACOG's lack of understanding of scientific methodology.

In truth, ACOG is a "professional organization," which amounts to a trade union. Like every trade union, ACOG has two goals—to promote the interests of its members and to promote a better product, in this case, the well-being of women. But if there is conflict between these two goals, the interest of its members comes first.

ACOG, and all the other national obstetric organizations in other countries, belong to an umbrella international organization called the International Federation of Gynecologists and Obstetricians (FIGO). FIGO has no authority over ACOG; it can only make recommendations. Interestingly, I have rarely heard a practicing American obstetrician who is not involved in international activities even mention FIGO. ACOG collaborates with FIGO on key activities in other countries, but I have not seen any evidence that FIGO recommendations have any effect on maternity care policy in the United States One example: the FIGO Committee for the Ethical

Aspects of Human Reproduction and Women's Health stated in a 1999 report, "Performing cesarean section for non-medical reasons is ethically not justified" (see chapter 3).[21] But the following year, the president of ACOG published a paper urging that women have the right to choose cesarean section for no medical reason.[22] So organized obstetrics at the international level is not able to apply any brakes on organized American obstetrics.

Sheltered by the all-powerful ACOG, with no authority to answer to and surrounded by people they control (midwives, nurses, clerks, patients), living in an obstetrician's world is like living as an animal with no natural predators. No one challenges obstetricians. I've seen the effects of this in all aspects of the profession, but it is especially frightening in a court of law. The tried and true defense for obstetricians who are sued is "only we can judge what we do." I will never forget two obstetricians practicing in partnership in a small rural town in Idaho—the only obstetricians in town. When testifying in a deposition in preparation for a court case, they were questioned about giving a patient a dose of Cytotec for induction that was two to three times the maximum dose generally used. They replied that the dose was the standard of practice in their community. When asked where this standard of practice came from, the two obstetricians replied simply, "We are the standard of practice." This insistence that only members of the tribe can understand what tribal members do and why they do it results in standards of practice that tribal members want—doctor-friendly practices. What it comes down to is that what is euphemistically called a "standard of practice" in a given community simply means whatever the local doctors do, regardless of whether or not it is good practice as defined by scientific evidence—a frightening level of power and control.

When obstetricians in the United States come together to strategize and decide how best to keep the wolves at bay, they tend to focus on two perceived threats: HMOs and lawyers. (I recently saw a printed flyer in a doctor's office waiting room that defended rising medical costs by blaming "greedy lawyers.") However, most obstetricians are in essence practitioners, and their vision is limited. They do not see that, in the long run, the real threat is that women in the United States will find out that much of what obstetricians do—from putting a women flat on her back during labor and birth to cutting her vagina open—is done for the doctor's benefit, not the patient's.

A couple of years ago, I was interviewed by an obviously intelligent journalist for *NBC Dateline* television. At the end of the program, when we were off camera, she looked at me with alarm and said, "But doctor, if what you are saying is true, we women can't really trust obstetricians. We must find out for ourselves what our situation is, what the science says about our situation, and whether or not what this obstetrician says is right for this situation."

I answered: "That's exactly right. You must take responsibility not only for your own body for also for the care given to it."

"My God," she said, "I've never realized that before."

"And that's why we need journalists like you to tell the truth to women."

"Yes, I understand."

Another real-life threat to obstetric territory is that health insurance companies and the government will discover just how many billions of dollars are wasted as a result of the obstetric monopoly. Though VBAC rates have dropped to single digits since ACOG's recommendation on VBAC, in a Healthy People 2010 report, the U.S. Department of Health and Human Services set a goal to triple the VBAC rate—acknowledging the cost to pregnant women and heath care resources of a policy that promotes unnecessary cesarean sections.

I recently testified before a state legislative committee in California on pending midwifery legislation. Among other things, I said in my statement that midwives are perfectly capable and that planned home birth is a healthy option for many women. I then presented scientific evidence to support both statements. I finished by suggesting that if anyone said otherwise to the committee, they should ask, "Where are your data?"

Thirty minutes later, a representative from the California Medical Association stood before the same committee and said that midwives are less safe than doctors for low-risk pregnant women and that home birth is not safe. Lo and behold! One of the legislators on the committee immediately asked, "And does the California Medical Association have any data to support your statements?" Not surprisingly, it did not (there are none). Instead, the spokesperson retreated to the familiar position: Trust us, we're the California Medical Association. That legislator took note, and the midwifery legislation was eventually passed. Slowly but surely, times are changing.

American maternity care, then, is under the control of tribal obstetrics. A small group, most of them men, are controlling birth in such a way as to preserve their own power and wealth while robbing women and families of control over one of the most important events in their lives. We cannot expect ACOG to significantly change the way it operates; an organization built on special privileges is too invested in maintaining its privileged position to engage in soul-searching or self-examination.

Power without wisdom is tyranny. There are plenty of intelligent obstetricians who have lots of knowledge, but intelligence and knowledge do not guarantee wisdom. I have known wise individual American obstetricians, but I see no evidence of wisdom in organized obstetrics in the United States. The maternity care we have in what we like to believe is our free country is obstetric tyranny.

THREE CHOOSE AND LOSE: PROMOTING CESAREAN SECTION AND OTHER INVASIVE INTERVENTIONS

Today, many if not most obstetricians do not attend births: they perform fetal extractions through the vagina or through an abdominal cut.
FAITH GIBSON, MIDWIFE AND AUTHOR

And let the angel whom thou still hast served
Tell thee,
Macduff was from his mother's womb
Untimely ripp'd
SHAKESPEARE, "MACBETH," V, VII, 43

After more than a decade of trying to bring down the number of cesarean sections (C-sections), some obstetricians are now reversing themselves and promoting more of them. In fact, a growing number of American obstetricians now urge women to "choose" a cesarean even when there is no medical indication that they need one.

The following statement is from a popular book titled *The Girlfriends' Guide to Pregnancy:*

> With a scheduled cesarean section, you and your doctor have agreed to a time at which you will enter the hospital in a fairly calm and leisurely fashion, and he or she will extract your baby through a small slit at the top of your pubic hair. There are a lot of reasons to schedule a cesarean section. . . . Other women elect to have a cesarean because they want to maintain the vaginal tone of a teenager, and their doctors find a medical explanation that will suit the insurance company.[1]

This illustrates the degree to which our society at large condones the concept of women choosing C-section, as well as doctors committing insurance fraud. A recent president of the American College of Obstetricians and Gynecologists (ACOG) took it a step farther in a paper titled "Patient Choice Cesarean," in which he calls this major abdominal surgery "a life-enhancing operation."[2]

C-section is an essential surgical procedure that, when properly applied, can save the lives of women and babies. But giving pregnant women the option of choosing to have a birth by C-section when it's not medically necessary is another matter entirely. Put simply, C-section, even when it is "elective" (done by choice and not the result of a risky situation or an emergency), increases the chance that the woman and/or the baby will die. Contrast this last sentence, which is based on scientific evidence, with the glowing statement, quoted in the previous paragraph, on the advantages of choosing C-section.

Obstetricians have a number of reasons for encouraging women to have C-sections. First, though, we must recognize that when they say they are doing it because it is a woman's right to choose any kind of birth she wants, that is blatant spin-doctoring. It is ridiculous to suppose that obstetricians have suddenly discovered women's rights. For proof we need only remember the ACOG recommendation discussed in chapter 2 in which doctors and hospitals are strongly urged to refuse when a family requests permission to make a birth video.[3] This is clear evidence that we can count on organized obstetrics to put fear of litigation ahead of family values and women's rights.

Why would obstetricians use the rhetoric of women's rights to get what they themselves want, a surgical birth? There are three compelling reasons. First, scheduling C-sections allows obstetricians to maintain their present overextended style of practice and bring the most time-consuming piece of it under control. It means that they can split their time between seeing patients in the office, doing gynecological surgical procedures in the hospital, and attending births, on a timetable of their choosing, and reduces the chance that they will be required to attend births at inconvenient times. For some, it is perhaps their only chance to have a decent personal life. Vaginal birth takes twelve hours on average and happens whenever— twenty-four hours a day, seven days a week. C-section takes twenty minutes, and most of the time it can be conveniently scheduled. Doctors may deny that they promote elective C-section for convenience, but their position is not believable. I appeared recently on the television program *Good*

Morning America to debate the president of ACOG. When I suggested that obstetricians sometimes do things for their own convenience, the ACOG president indignantly replied that obstetricians never do things for their own convenience. But there is proof. Federal studies that analyze birth certificates tell us that the percentage of U.S. births that happen Monday to Friday, nine to five, is rapidly increasing. Even "emergency" C-sections are more common Monday to Friday, nine to five.[4]

The second reason obstetricians want more women to have C-sections is to avoid litigation. Obstetricians are desperate to stay out of courtrooms where, unlike in hospitals, they are vulnerable and are not "top gun."

The third reason for promoting more C-sections relates to the present crisis in American obstetrics. Politicians, HMOs, and the American public are rapidly realizing that it is wrong to have highly trained surgical specialists caring for healthy pregnant women and catching perfectly normal babies at low-risk births. Midwives cost much less and, unlike labor and delivery nurses, have had years of training. When obstetricians promote C-sections, they are protecting their territory by encouraging women to choose the one type of birth that only they can provide.

So when obstetricians succeed in talking women into choosing C-sections, in one fell swoop they gain enormous convenience, may reduce their risk of litigation, and win a point over the competition.

These are the big reasons obstetricians want to perform more C-sections. There are also several subtle but pervasive factors underlying this trend. For one, because obstetricians have been trained to manage the small percentage of cases of high-risk birth where things can and do go wrong, they end up afraid of birth. It's like an auto mechanic who sees only the Fords that have broken down and have been brought to his shop, so he ends up thinking that all Fords are in imminent danger of breaking down. He forgets that he never sees all the Fords on the road that are running just fine.

This fear of imminent trouble leads obstetricians to jump in and intervene too early with procedures that create complications, necessitating more procedures. One intervention leads to another in a cascade of interventions that all lead to Rome—C-section. In the past decade, the classic example of such a cascade is an induction of labor with powerful drugs, which leads to increased labor pain, which leads to an epidural block to relieve the pain, which leads to a slowing of labor, which becomes "failure to progress," the number one diagnosis used to justify pulling the baby out with forceps or a vacuum extractor or performing C-section.

Another factor in the wave of high-tech, high-interventionist births is that medicalized birth is all obstetricians know, and fish can't see the water they swim in.[5] Most obstetricians have experienced only hospital-based birth managed within a medical model. They have never seen natural birth. So they cannot see the profound effect their interventions are having on the entire process. This is put well in a World Health Organization (WHO) publication:

> By medicalizing birth, that is by separating the woman from her own environment and surrounding her with strange people using strange machines to do strange things to her, the woman's state of mind and body are so altered that her way of carrying through this intimate act must also be altered. It is not possible for obstetricians to know what births would have been like before these manipulations—they have no idea what non-medicalized birth is. The entire modern published literature in obstetrics is based on observations of medicalized birth.[6]

Another subtle factor driving some obstetricians to promote invasive interventions such as C-section is their fundamental belief in machines and technology and lack of belief in women and their bodies. Obstetricians tend to have blind faith in technology and the mantra technology = progress = modern. Here examples abound. Most obstetricians routinely use an electronic fetal heart monitor to observe the baby's heartbeat during labor in spite of clear scientific evidence that a good old-fashioned stethoscope is just as reliable.[7] When estimating the length of a pregnancy by measuring the fetus as seen in an ultrasound picture became popular in the 1980s, obstetricians dropped the tried-and-true method of asking the woman about her last menstrual cycle. But scientific evidence shows that when predicting the expected date of birth, ultrasound scanning is no more accurate than using the date of the woman's last period.[8]

Women's bodies work best for giving birth when they are standing, sitting, or squatting. But when the obstetrics establishment began to realize that putting a woman on her back inhibited the birth process, instead of encouraging women to simply take a more natural vertical position, it set about designing a variety of high-tech adjustable birthing beds or chairs. These furnishings are typically made of metal, are mechanically complex, and allow for a number of positions. Each one costs thousands of dollars. And a beanbag chair works better than any of them, because the woman can mold the chair to fit her own body. But, of course, with a beanbag chair, or with the woman in a vertical position, the obstetrician would have to be below the woman. I once visited a public maternity hospital where large numbers of women were in labor. When I suggested to the chief nurse who was showing me around the ward that they consider using vertical birth positions, she replied, "But that would require the doctors to get down on the floor. They would never consider doing that."

Here is one last example of the lengths to which the medical-industrial complex will go to mechanize normal human functions. As we've seen, there are serious risks in using powerful drugs to induce labor or stimulate uterine contractions. There is another method for stimulating contractions that involves no risk whatsoever, but that is rarely, if ever, used in hospital obstetrics, perhaps because it is "too natural." For centuries, midwives have relied on the woman's partner, the midwife, or the woman herself to stimulate the woman's nipples to promote uterine contractions. In 1990, an obstetrician working with a commercial firm sought FDA approval for a nipple stimulation device that includes an electric pump and a "suction hood" that fits over the nipple.[9] In machines we trust.

Throughout the twentieth century, this arrogant belief that obstetricians know better than nature has led to a series of failed attempts to improve on biological and social evolution, some of which we will examine more closely in later chapters. Doctors replaced midwives in the United States for low-risk births, and then later science proved that midwives were safer. Hospitals replaced home as the setting for low-risk births, and then later science proved that planned out-of-hospital births are as safe as hospital births and involve far less unnecessary intervention. Hospital staff replaced the family as the primary support providers for a woman in labor, and later science proved that a birth is safer when the family is present. The practice of taking newborns away from mothers in the first twenty minutes after birth replaced the practice of leaving babies with their mothers, and later science proved the importance of mother-baby bonding during this time. Putting normal newborns in a central nursery replaced rooming babies in with their mothers, and later science proved that rooming-in is superior. Man-made milk replaced woman-made breast milk, and later science proved that breast milk is far superior to any infant formula. If more obstetricians experienced an earthquake, a volcano, or a tsunami, perhaps they would realize that their ideas of controlling nature are ineffective, pathetic, and— most important—dangerous.

Beyond a general preference for technology over natural processes, there are social and economic factors that influence whether or not an obstetrician decides to do a C-section. These have been explored in at least seven different studies in the United States, and have shown that the women most likely to receive C-sections are white, married, have private health insurance, and give birth in private hospitals, despite the fact that poor women have more health problems and are more likely to have complications justifying medically indicated C-sections.[10] These studies suggest that women in this group are more likely to have C-sections in part because of their attitudes about pain and vaginal tone. They also suggest that these women are more likely to want the convenience of a scheduled surgery, and, finally, because their private insurance is likely to pay a doctor who is in private practice in a private hospital, they do not have to fear that the surgery won't be covered. Women in this group are also more likely to be highly educated and are more likely to sue, encouraging doctors to perform "defensive" C-sections.

It is important to add that not every obstetrician is trying to promote C-section. For example, Jan Christilaw, a woman obstetrician, commented on the rising C-section rate in an article titled "Too Posh to Push?" She says, "This is a way of remedicalizing birth. I think birth is such an important cultural process that to divorce ourselves from its natural course is horrific."[11]

Jan Christilaw's phrase *remedicalizing birth* is a reference to an interesting series of philosophical shifts in the way obstetrics has been viewed in the United States over the last few decades. In the 1980s, there was a shift toward a medical approach that resulted in the national C-section rate increasing from 16 percent to 23.5 percent of all births. The extent to which American obstetricians embraced a medical model of birth is illustrated by the fact that the prestigious *New England Journal of Medicine* saw fit to publish a paper in 1985 seriously recommending that all pregnant women be given a "prophylactic C-section." The paper went on to say that should a woman be so foolish as to insist on a normal birth, she must then "be required to sign a consent form for the attempt at vaginal delivery."[12]

In the 1990s, a group of obstetricians and public health scientists became concerned, and the federal government set a goal of reducing the C-section rate to 15 percent by the year 2000. The effort brought the rate down to 21 percent. But in 1999, an obstetric backlash began with four leading obstetricians in Boston proclaiming that the government's effort to reduce the C-section rate could endanger mothers and babies. They stated that "there is no evidence" to support the government target of 15 percent, completely ignoring the evidence-based recommendations made by the WHO.[13] The media picked up on this paper. In January 1999, the *New York Times* published an article titled "Warning on Drop in Cesarean Births." In late

2000, *Newsweek* published an article discussing the obstetric backlash.[14] After that, editorials began to appear in the *New England Journal of Medicine* warning of the risks of promoting C-section,[15] but the national C-section rate has nevertheless risen from 21 percent to more than 30.2 percent in the last five years. Thus, obstetricians are "remedicalizing" birth.

Cesarean section is also convenient for the woman, of course, but that alone would not make most women want one. To choose to have a C-section when it's not medically necessary, a woman must be convinced that it is safe for her and especially that it is safe for her baby. Obstetricians who promote C-section choice have gone to much effort to torture the scientific data on the risks of this surgery until it confesses to what they want it to say: that C-section is safer than normal (vaginal) birth. As we will see, it absolutely is not.

One example of the obstetric hype in popular and professional magazines regarding C-section is a claim that 60 percent of women who have a vaginal birth will later suffer from leaking urine (urinary incontinence) and leaking stools (fecal incontinence). Strangely, even obstetricians believe this hype. A survey found that 68 percent of British obstetricians believe than an elective C-section can reduce the risk of urinary incontinence and 78 percent believe an elective C-section can reduce the risk of fecal incontinence.[16]

This illustrates an important lesson: Doctors must learn to read articles in their professional literature much more carefully. First, in the paper quoted as showing an increased risk of urinary and fecal incontinence after vaginal birth, the urinary incontinence was often pre-existing—29 percent of women reported that their urinary incontinence started during pregnancy, before they had a vaginal birth. Furthermore, the hype lumps all women who had a vaginal birth together instead of dividing them into risk groups, as the researchers did. Urinary incontinence has been found to correlate with having a large number of births, having babies that weigh more than ten pounds, having the vagina cut open with an episiotomy, and having the baby pulled out with forceps or vacuum extraction. If the woman does not fall into any of these risk categories, she has no increased risk of urinary incontinence after a vaginal birth. Similarly, the risk of fecal incontinence increases twenty-two-fold with a midline episiotomy.[17] Furthermore, a gynecologist in Texas who specializes in repairing pelvic floor damage has found forceps delivery and episiotomy to be two of the biggest risk factors that lead to damage of the pelvic floor, which leads to urinary and fecal incontinence.[18] Another study, conducted in 2005, looked at 143 pairs of biological sisters. In each pair, one sister had had a vaginal birth and the other sister never had a baby. The women completed questionnaires about urinary incontinence and were also given examinations for incontinence. Of the women who had given birth, 49.7 percent suffered some urinary incontinence, but so did 47.6 percent of their sisters who had not given birth. The researchers concluded that family factors are more relevant in urinary incontinence than whether a woman has had a vaginal birth.[19] This study supports what scientists have been saying about this matter— that a comparison of the risks of normal birth versus C-section can be reliable only if both sets of risks are carefully evaluated.

Cesarean section presents many risks for a woman. Even an elective C-section, with no emergency, has a 2.84-fold (almost three times) greater chance than vaginal birth of resulting in the woman's death. This fact is based on data from more than 150,000 nonemergency, elective C-sections, giving more than enough statistical evidence of this danger.[20] It can be reliably estimated that at least twelve American women die every year because of *unnecessary* elective C-sections.

Women choosing C-section also face many other risks that come with major abdominal surgery—anesthesia reactions and/or accidents, damage to blood vessels with massive hemorrhage, frequent infections, accidental extension of the uterine incision, damage to the bladder and other abdominal organs, and internal scarring with adhesions, leading to painful bowel movements and painful sexual intercourse.[21] Surgery is risky—period. Recently, a woman in Iowa was referred to a university hospital during labor because of possible complications. At the university hospital, doctors decided to do a C-section. After the surgery, the woman was resting in her hospital room when she went into shock and died. The autopsy showed that the surgeon who did the C-section had accidentally nicked the woman's aorta, the biggest artery in the body, leading to internal hemorrhage.[22]

Beyond immediate risks to her health and the health of her baby, when a woman chooses C-section, she decreases the chance that she will be able to get pregnant again and increases the chance that if she does get pregnant, the pregnancy will occur outside the uterus, a situation that never results in a live baby and is life-threatening to the woman. Furthermore, the risk of having an unexplained stillbirth doubles when a woman has had a previous C-section. Having a C-section greatly increases the risk that in a future pregnancy the placenta will detach before the baby is born or the uterus will rupture—both conditions that carry a high risk of brain damage or death to the baby as well as posing a significant risk to the woman's life.[23]

There is another set of risks to the baby. Recently, on the *Good Morning America* television program, I debated the idea that women should be offered the option of choosing a C-section with the then president of ACOG. He said, "For the baby, the risks are higher for vaginal birth than for elective C-section." It is shocking that the head of a national organization of obstetricians is giving such blatantly scientifically false information to the American public. A C-section can save a baby's life in an emergency, but when there is no medical indication and the C-section is simply the woman's choice, there is no scientific evidence to suggest any benefit to the baby and plenty of data showing risks to the baby. There is no question that a woman who chooses C-section when there is no medical need for it puts her baby in unnecessary danger.

To begin with, in 2 to 6 percent of all C-sections, when the doctor cuts open the woman's uterus, he cuts into the baby. Depending on the severity of this accident, it may lead to further problems as well. Babies born from an elective C-section rather than vaginal birth are twice as likely to end up in neonatal intensive care and three times as likely to have serious pulmonary disorders in the newborn period.[24] Having an elective C-section also increases the risk that the baby will be premature. Respiratory distress syndrome and prematurity are both major causes of newborn mortality. If the woman and her doctor wait until the woman goes into spontaneous labor before performing an elective C-section, the risk of both these conditions is reduced.[25] But waiting until labor starts reduces the convenience factor. When an obstetrician doesn't wait for labor to start, it is clear that convenience has taken priority over the baby's safety.

Because there are now many challenges in our healthcare system to a woman having a vaginal birth after previous C-section (VBAC), once a woman has a C-section, there is an extremely high chance that any future babies she has will be born by C-section as well. So we must add to these serious risks to the baby the risks to any future babies the woman may have.

The fact that women are choosing C-section strongly suggests that women are not being told the truth about all the risks to themselves and to their babies.

Physicians and others in the obstetrics profession have debated the question: Is it ethical to give women the option to choose a C-section when it is not medically indicated? Although I agree that women should have absolute control over their own bodies, does it logically follow that they should be able to choose any medical procedure they want? I don't believe it does. When a woman comes to an obstetrician demanding female circumcision (clitorectomy) of her daughter, should the doctor do it? Most American women would say no, and most obstetricians, including those promoting a women's "right" to have an elective C-section, would most probably also say no. Although this analogy is not perfect, as the woman is asking for elective surgery on her daughter rather than on herself, it is important in illustrating that there are limits to what a doctor is willing to do just because a patient requests it. We must not allow doctors to use "patient request" as an excuse for elective C-section. A doctor's own feelings about a patient's request always play a role in the doctor's willingness to carry out the request. There are many obstetricians who refuse to perform "patient's choice" C-sections without medical indications.

In an article in an obstetric journal, the president of ACOG urged doctors to encourage women to choose C-section and cited Brazil as a wonderful example of a country that honors a woman's right to choose C-section.[26] Having consulted in Brazil many times, sometimes for periods of more than a month, I have seen with my own eyes that Brazil is a tragic example of what happens when doctors move away from medical indications for surgery—hospitals where 100 percent of births are by C-section, whole states where more than 50 percent of births are by C-section. And in areas where there are such extreme rates of C-section, the rate of women dying around the time of birth is, not surprisingly, going up.[27]

Obstetricians in Brazil have said for a long time that the women in Brazil want C-sections because, in their macho culture, they fear that they will lose their men if they don't have what the doctors call "honeymoon vaginas." Is this what we want in the United States? Ironically, excellent new research in Brazil now shows that most women do not want C-sections; they want to have normal births, but their doctors find excuses for doing C-sections anyway.[28]

"Choice" without full information is no choice. A deaf woman cannot make a choice between Mozart and Beethoven. The key ethical issue is not a woman's right to choose a major surgical procedure for which there is no medical indication, but her right to receive and discuss complete, unbiased information prior to any medical or surgical procedure. This requires mandatory full disclosure to the woman of all known risks of elective C-section before or on entry to the hospital (not when she is in the throes of labor or being prepared for surgery). This disclosure should be treated as seriously as the reading of *Miranda* rights to arrestees. This is a far cry from what happens today. Typically, when a woman enters the hospital, she is given a piece of paper to sign that is not written for her education or benefit but is designed to protect the doctor and the hospital from litigation by essentially giving them carte blanche to do whatever they want to her.

The information given to a woman who is deciding what kind of birth to have must come from a neutral, unbiased source such as the federal Centers for Disease Control and Prevention. Any information coming from professional organizations such as ACOG will unavoidably be biased. As we saw in chapter 2, the number one objective of every professional organization is to protect the interests of its members. Information generated by professional organizations that want to promote doctor-friendly data on procedures, like information generated by commercial firms that stand to profit, must be considered suspect. But these are the current sources for much of the information available to obstetricians. As a result, many obstetricians today are simply misinformed and are unqualified to provide full, unbiased information to women.

Ethically speaking, doctors also have rights with regard to medical care. It is well established in the United States that no doctor is obliged to provide services or perform procedures that are against his or her religious beliefs. So an obstetrician cannot use "she wanted it" as an excuse for doing a procedure he wanted to do anyway. A clinician's first obligation is to the well-being of his patient. If a woman asks for a C-section for which the doctor sees no medical indication and which, to the best of the doctor's knowledge, carries risks for the woman and her baby that outweigh any possible benefit, the doctor has the right, perhaps even the duty, to refuse to do the C-section. No one is holding a gun to the doctor's head.

This is why the International Federation of Gynecology and Obstetrics (FIGO), the umbrella organization of national obstetric organizations (including ACOG), issued a statement in 1999: "Because hard evidence of net benefit does not exist, performing cesarean section for non-medical reasons is ethically not justified."[29]

Currently more than one million C-sections are done in the United States every year, which amounts to more than 30.2 percent of all births.[30] Through an exhaustive scientific process, WHO has calculated that the optimal rate of C-section for saving the most women and babies is 10 to 15 percent.[31] There is no evidence that a rate of C-section over 10 percent saves lives.[32] All attempts to show fewer babies dying in highly developed countries when there are more obstetric interventions, such as C-sections, have failed. A U.S. National Center for Health Statistics study comments, "The comparisons of perinatal mortality ratios with cesarean section and with operative vaginal rates finds no consistent correlations across countries."[33]

A review of the scientific literature on this issue by the Oxford National Perinatal Epidemiology Unit found that a number of studies had failed to detect any relation between crude perinatal mortality rates and the level of operative deliveries.[34] In other words, scientific evidence shows that increased rates of C-sections are not saving more lives of either women or babies.

The WHO's optimal C-section rate was challenged and called "arbitrary" by American obstetricians in a 1999 article in the *New England Journal of Medicine*.[35] The authors of the article are not connected with the WHO and, to judge from their position, it appears that they did not take the time to learn how optimal C-section rates are determined.

The figure was ascertained during a WHO consensus conference attended by sixty-two participants from more than twenty countries, including representation from U.S. obstetrics.[36] Participants began with a thorough review of the scientific literature on the risks of C-section to women and babies and concluded that the optimal rate must be the minimal optimal rate. Then they studied variations in C-section rates across countries. As several countries that had low rates of maternal and infant mortality were found to have national C-section rates close to 10 percent of live births, this appeared to be a minimal optimal rate. Coupled with this, studies sponsored by the WHO that span many countries have found no evidence that C-section rates above this level decrease mortality rates. The overall recommendation was then modified from 10 percent to a rate of 10 to 15 percent because some hospitals have higher-risk populations, especially referral hospitals to which general hospitals send difficult or complicated cases. Participants concluded by consensus that a rate of 10 percent is optimal for hospitals serving the general population, and up to 15 percent is optimal for hospitals serving high-risk populations.

In 2004, twenty years after the WHO announced its recommendation regarding optimal C-section rates, the organization undertook a study to look at C-section rates in all countries and compare them with maternal mortality rates.[37] This study found that countries that have a C-section rate below 10 percent (as do most poor countries) have higher maternal mortality rates, and countries that have a C-section rate above 15 percent (as do some highly industrialized countries) also have higher maternal mortality rates. Thus the study confirmed the earlier WHO recommendation. Apparently, women's bodies and reproductive capacities do not change over twenty years. The study goes on to urge countries with C-section rates above 15 percent, such as the United States, to carefully evaluate their maternal mortality rates, including the contribution of C-section to maternal mortality. We can hope that this will raise awareness of the fact that the current C-section rate in the United States is double the optimal rate and the current U.S. maternal mortality rate is double that found in a number of other countries.

Interestingly, there is a small group in the United States that has a rate of C-section far below the national rate, with excellent results: the Zuni-Ramah Native American population. A study found a 7.3 percent C-section rate among this population in 1996.[38] And although many members of this group live in poverty and have a higher than average incidence of obstetric risk factors (such as many pregnancies and poor general health), no adverse outcomes were found from the low C-section rate. Researchers attribute the low C-section rate among the Zuni-Ramah to the "prominent involvement of family physicians and nurse-midwives, who have a significantly lower cesarean delivery rate and intervention rate," and to "almost universal acceptance of trial of labor after cesarean," and to "a cultural attitude toward childbirth and increased social support within the community." These are elements in maternity care that can be seen as more modern and advanced than the obstetric-based maternity care in the United States today. In chapters 8 and 9, we will look at how we can make all maternity care in the United States more like this group's.

Another important aspect of the debate surrounding C-section rates is cost. First, to say that vaginal birth is nearly as expensive as C-section, as some obstetricians have done, is absurd.[39] Although it is true that the practice style of many obstetricians in the United States results in vaginal births that are needlessly expensive owing to unnecessary interventions, a C-section has many associated costs that must be factored in. These include the cost of maintaining the operating room; fees for surgeons, assisting surgeons, and surgical nurses; and the costs of anesthesia, the anesthesiologist's services, surgical instruments, blood for transfusion, and a longer postbirth hospital stay.

The C-section rate in 2005 in the United States was 30.2 percent (a 46 percent increase in 9 years), which means there were approximately one million C-sections that year. If the rate had been 12 percent, the evidence-based rate found in those countries that have the lowest mortality rates for women and babies around the time of birth, there would have been only about a half-million C-sections that year, which leaves a half-million *unnecessary* C-sections. Since each C-section costs at least $5,000 more than a vaginal birth, we see that the United States spent approximately $2.5 *billion* more than necessary on births in 2004 because of uncalled-for C-sections.

Those are just direct costs. That $2.5 billion does not include the long-term costs of nonemergency C-section, which are huge. More C-sections mean more babies in intensive care with respiratory distress, more emergency surgeries for pregnancies outside the uterus, more emergency surgeries due to detached placentas and hemorrhaging, and more emergency surgery for ruptured uteruses. The true amount wasted on unnecessary C-sections is probably closer to twice the $2.5 billion figure.

The concept of women choosing C-section raises further questions. If surgery is done only because the woman requests it, who pays for it? If a woman decides to have cosmetic surgery, such as breast augmentation, most insurance companies and HMOs will not cover the cost. However, while it is next to impossible for a surgeon to find a medical reason to do breast augmentation, it's easy for an obstetrician to cover up an elective C-section with a medical justification. This is insurance fraud, and it happens frequently. When insurance companies unwittingly pay for elective C-sections, this inevitably causes insurance premiums to go up. So the cost of all those unnecessary C-sections is borne by the public, or by everyone who pays for health insurance. And even if a woman pays for an elective C-section performed by her private obstetrician in a private hospital, the public is still paying as well, because public funds helped pay for the education and training of her doctor and for the construction and running of the private hospital.

Some of these same issues regarding risks, information disclosure, ethics, and unnecessary costs apply to other invasive obstetrics interventions as well. When lecturing to a roomful of obstetricians, I often show a slide (see table 2) that lists common obstetric procedures and policies and shows how often they occur in the United States and how often they should occur based on scientific evidence.

Usually, quite a few obstetricians in the room become defensive when I present this table because it makes clear that their practice is a long way from the stated goal of obstetric textbooks: evidence-based practice. Every leading obstetric textbook today makes repeated strong statements about the importance of coming as close as possible to the scientific data. Obstetricians like to say they are scientific, but clearly many of them are anything but. Such a large gap between what obstetricians are doing and what science says they should be doing could not exist if many, if not most, obstetricians were not ignoring science and ignoring their own textbooks.

Now let's look at obstetric intervention rates in one metropolitan area—Seattle, Washington. Table 3 demonstrates the gap between obstetric prac-

TABLE 2. PRACTICE VS. SCIENTIFIC EVIDENCE IN THE UNITED STATES

Procedure	Practice	Evidence-based approach
One continuous attendant for all labor	< 10 percent	100 percent
Routine midwife care	5 percent	80 percent
Routine no food or drink	86 percent	no
Routine electronic fetal monitoring	93 percent	no
Routine intravenous drip	86 percent	no
Confined to bed during all or part of labor	69 percent	no
Lithotomy (on back with stirrups) near end of labor	nearly all	no
Episiotomy (cut vagina open)	35 percent	< 20 percent
Induce labor with drugs	44 percent	10 percent
Accelerate ongoing labor with drugs	53 percent	10 percent
Vacuum or forceps	13 percent	< 10 percent
Cesarean section	27 percent*	10−15 percent
Mother holds baby during routine exam of her newborn	seldom	yes

*This is the rate from 2002; the rate in 2005 was 30.2 percent.

SOURCES: Practice statistics are from "Listening to Mothers," a national survey of obstetric practices, published October 24, 2002, by the Maternity Center Association of New York City, and available at www.maternitywise.org. Evidence statistics are from I. Chalmers, M. Enkin, and M. Keirse, eds., *Effective Care in Pregnancy and Childbirth* (Oxford: Oxford University Press, 1989), and from the Cochrane Library (www.cochrane.org).

tices and scientific evidence at nineteen Seattle hospitals in the year 2000. In nearly every hospital in Seattle there is a big gap between what obstetricians do during labor and birth and what they should be doing, according to scientific evidence. Note specifically their practices with regard to the routine use of intravenous drip, drug induction of labor, routine electronic monitoring of the baby, and C-section. A woman in Seattle would be hard pressed to find a hospital where she could have a birth that is not high-tech and full of unnecessary invasive interventions.

One can see at a glance in both these charts that the big gap is the result of obstetricians doing too much, or intervening when it is not necessary and can even be dangerous. To understand why so much unnecessary technology is used during pregnancy and birth, it is instructive to understand how technology comes to be used in obstetrics in the first place. One might expect that the use of a new technology or drug would be preceded by careful scientific

TABLE 3. PRACTICE VS. SCIENTIFIC EVIDENCE IN NINETEEN SEATTLE
HOSPITALS

Procedure	Hospital practice	Evidence-based approach
Intravenous drip	Routine in 17 of 19 hospitals	not necessary
Drugs for induction and augmentation of labor	1 hospital: < 11 percent of cases 7 hospitals: 0–39 percent 5 hospitals: 40–59 percent 4 hospitals: > 60 percent	10 percent
Cytotec for ripening and induction	14 of 17 hospitals	never
Routine electronic fetal monitoring	17 of 19 hospitals: sometimes/often	never
Cesarean section	2 hospitals: 10–15 percent of cases 8 hospitals: 15–19 percent 9 hospitals: 20–28 percent	< 15 percent

SOURCES: Practice statistics are from the Childbirth Education Association of Seattle Hospital survey, 2000. For information on this survey, contact the Seattle Midwifery School, www.seattlemidwifery.org. Evidence statistics are from I. Chalmers, M. Enkin, and M. Keirse, eds., *Effective Care in Pregnancy and Childbirth* (Oxford: Oxford University Press, 1989), and from the Cochrane Library.

evaluation, followed by official approval and thoughtful requirements for educating doctors in its use. Sadly, the truth is something else entirely.

While I was attending a conference in Chicago in the mid-1990s, an anesthesiologist from Boston told the audience how she first heard the idea of using epidural block for normal labor pain. She said that a colleague called her one night and told her that he had tried it on ten women, it was fantastic, and she should try it too. So, as she proudly told the audience, the next day she tried it. During the discussion, I challenged her, saying that it appeared she was doing experiments on women without their permission. Confused and angry, she replied, "But that's how we make progress in medical care." She was clearly using the anti-precautionary approach to the introduction of new interventions—assumed safe until proven unsafe (see chapter 4). Still today, experimentation in the technique of epidural block is going on all across the United States on the bodies of women who are rarely told that they are experimental subjects.

So today another sign of the medicalization of birth is the epidemic of epidural block for normal labor pain, that is, the pain that accompanies "normal labor" in which there are no medical complications. Although hard data are scarce, the rate of epidural block is reported to be as high as 85 percent in some hospitals and is increasing throughout the country.[40] There are several reasons for this epidemic, but a primary reason is that the care an American woman receives when she comes to the hospital to give birth these days will substantially increase the pain of her labor. Scientific evidence shows that a women's labor pain is increased by undergoing labor in an unfamiliar place, being surrounded with unfamiliar people, having unfamiliar procedures done, and by being left unattended during labor. It is also increased when a women is put in a horizontal position and not allowed to walk about freely. In addition, having her "membranes" artificially ruptured has been shown to increase pain. (The membranes—the sac filled with amniotic fluid in which the fetus floats—breaks spontaneously during the course of labor and is sometimes artificially ruptured in the hope of speeding up labor, a procedure known as a amniotomy.) Finally, it is well known that inducing or augmenting labor with drugs significantly increases the woman's pain.[41] So a woman comes into the hospital in labor, has a number of things done to her that all increase her pain, and then she is offered an epidural. Women are naturally grateful to the staff for the relief of their pain, not realizing that the staff exacerbated the pain in the first place.

A women's perception of pain—how much is expected or tolerable—is strongly influenced by the culture in which she lives. Women in the Netherlands and in Japan do not view labor pain as negative or unacceptable, and there is no epidemic of epidurals for normal labor in either country.[42] In the United States, the way women perceive labor pain is strongly influenced by the way obstetricians perceive labor pain. The two great evils in a doctor's world are pain and death, and they see it as their job to fight them at all costs. The physiological fact that pain is an essential component of a normal labor, that it is necessary for the release of hormones that control the progress of labor, is either not understood by most American obstetricians or simply ignored. So, again, we have one intervention leading to another. When an epidural block removes all feeling in a women's lower body, the necessary hormones are not released and the labor does not progress normally, which leads to more interventions.

There are many less invasive, far safer methods of pain control that have been scientifically proven to be effective, but they are rarely encouraged as alternatives to epidural block in U.S. hospitals. These include water tubs and showers, acupuncture, hypnosis, transcutaneous electronic nerve stimulation (TENS), freedom of movement (including sitting up or walking around), and continuous one-on-one attendance by a midwife or doula.[43] Instead, epidural block has been given a "hard sell" by doctors, which includes promoting the procedure as safe.

Is epidural block safe? Epidural can hardly be called "safe" when close to one-quarter (23 percent) of women receiving it have complications.[44] The risks involved in epidural block are serious, starting with an increased possibility that the woman will die. Women who have epidural block for normal labor pain have risk of dying that is triple that of women who do not have epidural block for normal labor pain. In addition, for every five hundred epidurals performed, there will be one case in which the woman is temporarily paralyzed for hours or days, and for every half-million epidurals, there will be one case in which the paralysis is permanent.

A woman also has a 15 to 20 percent chance of developing a fever after receiving an epidural block. When a woman in labor develops a fever, it means that a diagnostic evaluation must be done to determine if there is an infection in her body or in the baby's body. These diagnostic procedures can sometimes be invasive, including doing a spinal tap on the baby, which is a painful and risky procedure in and of itself.

Another known complication of epidural block: between 15 and 35 percent of women who are given an epidural will suffer from urinary retention (inability to urinate) after the birth, a condition which, if it continues, necessitates putting a catheter in the bladder until bladder function returns.

Now let's look at the benefits of this widely used procedure. How effective is epidural block at relieving pain? Studies show that around 10 percent of epidural blocks don't work at all; there is no pain relief. Even when pain is blocked during labor, about one-third of the women given an epidural will trade a few hours of pain-free labor for days, weeks, or months of back pain after the birth. Studies show that 30 to 40 percent of women who receive an epidural during labor will have severe back pain after the birth, and 20 percent will still have severe back pain a year later.

The fact that when an epidural block is given labor does not progress normally has consequences as well. A great deal of scientific research has shown that women who receive epidural block for normal labor pain will have a significantly longer second stage of labor, and thus the epidural block means a four times greater chance that forceps or vacuum extraction will be used to extract the baby, and at least a two times greater chance that a C-section will be performed. One reason for the increased use of these interventions is that an epidural block interferes with the mechanisms that guide the rotation of the baby as it descends through the birth canal. As a result, an epidural block increases the chance that a fetus will end up in one of the more difficult positions for birth, such as the posterior position in which the baby is facing the wrong way as it descends and emerges.[45] These positions are generally more stressful for the baby, and, because they increase the chance that risky interventions will be performed, they can put the baby at greater risk.

Although many women might be willing to take risks with their own bodies for pain relief, very few women are willing to put their babies at risk. But that is what a women does when she agrees to an epidural. One common complication when a woman has an epidural is that there will be a sudden drop in her blood pressure, leading to a sharp drop in blood flow through the placenta to the fetus. This drop in blood flow can result in mild to severe lack of oxygen getting to the fetus, which if not quickly treated can result in brain damage in the baby.

Using a typical high-tech strategy, doctors will often use a second intervention to try to counter the bad effects of the first intervention, in this case the epidural block. They will give the woman a big dose of fluid through an intravenous drip (IV) to try to prevent a drop in blood pressure, but this technique does not always work. Studies have shown that in 8 to 12 percent of cases in which a woman is given an epidural block for normal labor pain, the electronic fetal heart monitor will show a severe lack of oxygen to the baby.[46] In a further study, after having an epidural, three-quarters of the babies of healthy women in normal labor had episodes of slowing of the fetal heart rate, a symptom of fetal distress. Because half of these episodes occurred shortly after an increase in the dose of the epidural or just after the epidural was "topped up," this suggests that the epidural was responsible for the fetal distress.[47]

There are also data that suggest an increased risk that the baby will show poor neurological function at one month of age when the mother is given an epidural block.[48] There have been some recent innovations in the way epidural blocks are given, such as changing the drugs injected or the drug doses, or performing a "walking epidural" (one in which the dosage and administration of the drug allows the woman partial use of her legs), but there is no evidence that these newer variations eliminate the risks to the woman and her baby.

As with C-section, one reason there is an epidemic of epidurals in the

United States is that women have not been told the facts about the risks to them and their babies before they are asked to give their consent. Indeed, at a meeting of obstetric anesthesiologists in Texas, a formal discussion was held on how to prevent information on the risks of epidural block from reaching the public. The rationale given was patronizing and not uncommon among physicians and others in obstetrics: "We don't want to scare the ladies."[49]

There are other examples of unnecessary invasive obstetric interventions. One is episiotomy, or cutting open the vagina during childbirth, which I believe can be considered female genital mutilation.[50] Many surgeons believe a surgical cut to be better than a natural tear, although scientific data has proven otherwise. The misperception stems from the fact that obstetricians are surgeons accustomed to sewing up openings that have been made with a scalpel—that is, cuts that are straight and clean—whereas tears are ragged and irregular. It is perhaps counterintuitive to surgeons that a tear is better than a cut. What they don't appreciate is that a tear follows the lines of the tissue, which can be brought back together like a jigsaw puzzle. An episiotomy cut, on the other hand, ignores any anatomical structures or borders and disrupts the integrity of muscles, blood vessels, nerves, and other tissues, resulting in more bleeding, more pain, more loss of muscle tone, and more deformity of the vagina with associated pain during sexual intercourse.

Episiotomy was first used in Europe in the 1740s when barber-surgeons began to attend births and was first popularized in the United States in the 1920s by Dr. Joseph DeLee, an obstetrician at the Chicago Lying-in Hospital who viewed childbirth as "a decidedly pathological process," comparing it to a "fall on a pitchfork." He proposed routine episiotomy to speed labor and reduce trauma, and because "virginal conditions are usually restored."[51] When childbirth in the United States was moved from the home to the hospital in the 1940s and 1950s, this surgical approach to birth accelerated and episiotomy became routine, with rates quickly rising to 60 percent of all births and 80 percent of first-time mothers.

Perhaps it is not surprising that episiotomy came into widespread practice, as it happened before the importance of using scientific evidence to justify interventions was appreciated. But the fact that it has remained in widespread practice, despite more than twenty years of increasing evidence of lack of efficacy and considerable risks, makes it a sad case study in inappropriate birth technology. In medicine, change comes slowly. In 1983, a landmark paper was published that reviews the English-language literature on episiotomy and calls into question the efficacy of the procedure.[52] In

1985, a WHO conference on appropriate birth technology evaluated this paper and other evidence, and concluded: "The systematic use of episiotomy is not justified. The protection of the perineum through alternative methods should be evaluated and adopted."[53]

But by then, routine use of episiotomy was firmly ingrained in obstetric practice. I remember visiting a large hospital in the 1990s, where I was told of an intern who performed an episiotomy *after* the baby was born. Why? Because he had been told that the procedure was to be done on all births, and there was no time to do it before the birth because the woman arrived at the hospital at the last minute.

In 1995, a review of the best episiotomy research by the Cochrane Library (a frequently updated, highly respected electronic library of reviews of the scientific evidence on different obstetric practices) found that when done routinely, the procedure increases the trauma and complications of birth.[54] Some hospitals began gradually to reduce routine episiotomy. At the University of California at San Francisco Hospital, the rate of episiotomy dropped from 80 percent to less than 10 percent during the 1990s. The number of third- and fourth-degree tears of the perineum in this hospital was cut in half, and the number of women with no episiotomy or tear tripled.[55] By the end of the 1990s, the rate of episiotomies at the Massachusetts General Hospital had fallen to between 10 and 15 percent.

But the practice of doing frequent episiotomies has continued in the face of the mounting scientific evidence against it and the example of leading teaching hospitals. In 2002, the episiotomy rate at the Mayo Clinic was still 60 percent for first babies.[56] A survey of obstetric practices, published in 2002, found a national episiotomy rate of 35 percent.[57]

Because episiotomy continues in widespread use, despite strong evidence questioning its usefulness, the Agency for Healthcare Research and Quality, a federal agency that conducts evaluations of contentious medical procedures, recruited a blue-ribbon panel of women's health researchers to conduct a new scientific review and analysis. The panel found that episiotomy is performed in about one-third of all vaginal births—which means that more than one million episiotomies are done every year in the United States. The rate varies around the country, but 70 to 80 percent of first-time mothers undergo episiotomies.[58]

This review by Hartmann and colleagues identified 986 studies on episiotomy conducted over the past fifty years, and culled from these twenty-six studies that provide the most reliable data on benefits and risks. They found that the three main supposed benefits of episiotomy claimed by proponents—prevention of bad (third-degree) tears, prevention of long-term damage to the floor of the woman's pelvis, and protection of the baby from the adverse consequences of an extended labor—are not supported by evidence. Their review and analysis showed that women who had episiotomies had a 26 percent greater chance of having a tear that required suturing (the surgical cut starts the break in the tissue, which is then more likely to extend by tearing, just as snipping a piece of fabric with scissors makes it easier to tear the fabric); had a 53 percent greater chance of having pain during sexual intercourse; and were twice as likely to suffer fecal incontinence. Dr. Hartmann told a journalist: "The evidence is clear: routine use of episiotomy is not supported by research and should stop. . . . Women need to know this information so they can talk with their care provider before they are in labor."

The general consensus now among perinatal scientists and obstetricians is that the ideal rate of episiotomy is 5 to 10 percent of all vaginal births. Episiotomies should be done only in urgent situations, such as cases of fetal distress due to a compressed umbilical cord, that require a hasty vacuum extraction.

Because obstetric interventions are introduced and disseminated in unsystematic, untested ways, it is no surprise that there is a big gap in the United States between what is being practiced in maternity care and what we know scientifically to be best. Perhaps even more frightening is the fact that there have been only a very few attempts to evaluate the long-term effects of interventions on the baby. As mentioned earlier, we know that there is a possible connection between a women having an epidural block during labor and reduced neurological functioning of the baby at one month of age. Two studies have shown that using drugs to manage pain during childbirth increases the chance that the baby will become addicted to drugs in adulthood.[59]

But there is much more that we do not know. For example, we have seen a rapid increase in the use of ultrasound to examine pregnant women in the last twenty years, but there has never been a large enough longitudinal, prospective, randomized trial to test the effects of ultrasound. So far research has suggested a connection between ultrasound of the fetus and later minimal neurological problems, but these findings have yet to be confirmed.[60] Other studies suggest that miscarriages and preterm labors increase with ultrasound, but again we must wait for further research to confirm these findings.[61] Finally, research now casts doubt on the efficacy of routine prenatal ultrasound. The author of a report on a large randomized trial involving 15,151 pregnant women concluded, "The findings of this study clearly indicate that ultrasound screening does not improve perinatal outcome in current U.S. practice."[62] Another large randomized trial found no benefit from routine scanning and concluded, "It would seem prudent to limit ultrasound examinations of the fetus to those cases in which the information is likely to be of clinical importance."[63] This situation was well summarized by a radiologist: "The casual observer might be forgiven for wondering why the medical profession is now involved in the wholesale routine examination of pregnant patients with machines emanating vastly different powers of energy which is not proven to be harmless to obtain information which is not proven to be of any clinical value by operators who are not certified as competent to perform the operations."[64] Two decades later, we don't know much more about routine ultrasound scanning during pregnancy and must continue to wait for a scientifically valid study that will reveal both safety (risk levels) and efficacy.

Procedures used today, such as ultrasound scanning, may seem harmless, but it is important to remember the history of obstetric practices and the fact that, in the 1930s, taking X-rays of pregnant women seemed harmless as well. In 1937, a standard obstetric textbook stated: "It has been frequently asked whether there is any danger to the life of the child by the passage of X-rays through it; it can be said at once that there is none if the examination is carried out by a competent radiologist."[65] A later edition of the same textbook stated, "It is now known that the unrestricted use of X-rays is harmful to mother and child."[66] The reason for this change was the report in 1956 on the connection between fetal X-rays and later cancer in the child.[67] Using the anti-precautionary approach and assuming the safety of any obstetric intervention is dangerous.

Today, there are essentially three approaches to "research" in obstetrics in the United States: non-science, false science, and valid science. The non-science approach, also known as "let's try it out," is what the anesthesiologist from Boston described, and it is by far the most common way obstetricians go about determining if a new procedure or drug is a good idea. (In chapter 4, we will see that doctors took this approach with the drug Cytotec, and that this approach, based on the anti-precautionary principle, is widespread in obstetrics.) When doctors take this approach, I often hear them call what they are doing "fine-tuning," as though they already know a lot about a new intervention and are just working out the last tiny details. But that is a euphemism, as there has been no primary research to fine-tune. "Trying it out" is not only unreliable, it's danger-

ous and demonstrates the wisdom of Benjamin Franklin's aphorism—
"Experience keeps a dear school, but fools will learn in no other." I rarely
hear doctors acknowledge that the women whose bodies are being used
without their informed consent to "fine-tune" a new intervention sometimes die from the fine-tuning.

The second approach to obstetric research is false science, which is usually conducted by an obstetrician or group of obstetricians who have found
an intervention they want to use, have been using it for a while on various
patients, and then afterward decide to try to "prove" that it's a good idea.
Medical schools do not usually train physicians in scientific methodology,
so most practicing doctors who undertake studies have little or no scientific
training and inevitably make mistakes, many of which stem from the fact
that the "researcher" is biased and believes that he already knows what the
study will find. This is the fundamental difference between a scientific approach and a clinical approach. To generate a hypothesis or a question, a
scientist must believe that he does not know the answer; otherwise, his bias
will contaminate the study. A practicing doctor, on the other hand, must
believe with certainty that he *does* know, because he must have the
confidence to make life-and-death decisions. Clinicians who do research
must have the ability to change their mindsets quickly and frequently from
clinician to scientist, and in my experience few have this ability.

Another common weakness in obstetric research is that once clinicians
take on a study, they are usually in a hurry. They want answers immediately,
and, as a result, studies are generally rushed and involve too few cases. In
some situations, a small number of cases can prove efficacy—that is, show
that a new drug or procedure works—but much larger numbers are needed
to determine the level of risk involved with a reasonable degree of statistical certainty. This is because the most serious obstetric risks (e.g., uterine
rupture, amniotic fluid embolism, brain damage, or death of the woman
and/or the baby) occur infrequently.

So, without knowing enough about scientific methods, doctors start collecting data on their patients. They may or may not get hospital approval
and they rarely get their patients' fully informed consent as participants in
the study. They keep the study "low-profile." Then, in spite of the fact that
the research methodology is faulty and the results are mostly or completely
invalid, the doctors may manage to get their study published in a "peer-
reviewed" journal, that is, a journal where submissions are reviewed by
other doctors who are also likely to lack adequate scientific training. Now
the study is big news. The "researchers" are famous in their little world and

may even get promoted—and other obstetricians will use their study as justification for their own practices.

Here is a real-life story that illustrates many of the issues involved in physicians conducting and relying on what amounts to false science. A chief of obstetrics at a large hospital in a medium-sized city—we'll call him Dr. S—decided to mount a study to look at using a prostaglandin drug (not Pitocin) to induce labor in women who had previously had C-sections, even though the drug's label specifically says that the drug should not be used in this way. Clearly, not enough was known about the safety of using this drug for labor induction after a previous C-section, which is why the label warned against this use. Dr. S later admitted that one of the primary reasons for doing the study was that doctors in that hospital wanted to use the drug and wanted something that would protect them from litigation. If they ran into trouble, the existence of a study would at least allow them to say, "We're researching it." As an afterthought, Dr. S decided that as long as they were going to do a study, they might as well have someone write a paper.

For the study to be official, Dr. S needed to have it approved by the hospital's institutional review board (IRB), and to be cleared by the IRB, certain research protocols must be followed. For example, the researchers must do a "review of the literature" to see what other studies have been published on the topic or related topics. Dr. S found a young obstetrician—we'll call her Dr. H—to join his study and do a lot of that scut work. Neither Dr. S nor Dr. H had any training in science, and they struggled to put together the IRB application.

Dr. H found only a few relevant previous studies. Naively, she put them together in a false "meta-analysis." When there are a number of small studies, and each one is too small to get a scientific handle on outcomes such as risks, one solution is to combine the results of the small studies into a meta-analysis. This can be a useful method of study, but there are many pitfalls to avoid. Too often, as in this case, a meta-analysis combines findings that were the result of very different methodologies, which is like mixing apples, oranges, and bananas, and has no scientific validity.

By combining study results in this way, Dr. H ended up with just over three hundred total cases. Since the most serious risk of using the drug for induction after previous C-section was uterine rupture (which has a high mortality rate), it can be calculated that a study would have to include at least 3,957 women to determine the safety of the drug with a reasonable level of certainty. Since this hospital handled only about twenty-five pregnant women per year who had previously had C-sections and were attempting VBAC, it would have taken the doctors 158 years to collect enough cases to prove that using the drug is safe. But this did not deter Dr. S. In fact, he later admitted that he knew from the start that he was not going to get a meaningful amount of data.

Working the system, Dr. S told various untrue stories about his study. He claimed that he told the women he recruited as subjects that they would be part of a study and further claimed that he told them they might be offered a drug that (to paraphrase) is not approved by the FDA, though he also told them that he and the other doctors at the hospital knew the drug to be safe and helpful. He told the hospital IRB something similar, though for their benefit, he did call the new drug "experimental" and indicated that the study would prove scientifically what doctors at the hospital already knew, that the drug is safe. Neither group was told the less palatable purposes of the study—that it was done to protect doctors using the drug from litigation, to advance the careers of Dr. S and Dr. H, and to promote the use of an obstetric intervention.

A hospital IRB is another example of the "peer-review" principle in medicine. The FDA mandates that an IRB of a hospital must include doctors from that hospital, as well as one administrator and one outsider from the community. The FDA also stipulates that it is the IRB's duty to guarantee that a study is scientifically valid and to protect the rights of the research subjects. A researcher must submit a research plan or protocol to the IRB for approval before starting. In this case, the doctors' research protocol was approved unanimously on the first try, despite the fact that it did not include an appropriate informed consent form and other essential elements. Any scientist reviewing this protocol would immediately have recognized the study as false science, but there were no scientists on the IRB.

Not long after the study began, a woman with a previous C-section came to Dr. S for maternity care. After a normal pregnancy, she was admitted to the hospital and, without her knowing it, she became part of Dr. S's study. (It appears that Dr. S's claim that all women were informed of the study was false.) Dr. S gave her the drug to induce labor, the drug led to overly strong contractions, a condition known as uterine hyperstimulation, and then to uterine rupture. As a result, the woman's baby was severely brain-damaged and died in infancy.

Several lessons can be learned from this example. First, "peer review" is not an effective method of quality control in approving obstetric research. When there are no trained scientists on an IRB, it is effectively a case of the blind reviewing the blind. Furthermore, today in American medical practice, *peer review* has become a catchword implying that this is a way of guaranteeing the validity of research papers and evidence. But the most respected leaders in medical scientific publishing warn us about peer review. An editorial in *The Lancet* comments: "'Peer review, a process that research has shown to be an ineffective lottery prone to bias and abuse.' Richard Smith, former editor of the *BMJ*. Smith is not alone in his utterances. *The Lancet's* editor and two former editors of *The New England Journal of Medicine* have publicly expressed similar views. In addition, what evidence is available from systematic reviews points to similar systematic manipulation of evidence by the pharmaceutical industry and sometimes also by governments. Moreover, there is a lack of convincing evidence that the editorial system works."[68]

We can also speculate that the IRB rubber-stamped the study application in this case because of hospital dynamics. Physicians generally dislike being regulated or controlled by their hospital administration, so the hospital administration must find ways to keep the physicians happy while also maintaining a reasonable system of quality assurance. One way to make physicians happy is to approve their study protocols. Published research also gives a hospital status and helps it attract doctors and patients. In addition, while the IRB is an agent of the administration in a hospital, most of the members are practicing physicians and are likely to want their own study protocols approved some day. So collusion among members is common— you approve my protocol and I'll approve yours. Finally, the physicians on the IRB were probably sympathetic when they heard the obstetricians in their hospital complaining that they needed to use this drug, but the FDA and the drug company said they shouldn't, because they had experienced similar frustrations.

This story is also an example of the way research can be abused and may be conducted for the wrong reasons, such as to advance physicians' careers or to protect physicians who are unwilling to adhere to regulations. It is extraordinary that in obstetrics, where most doctors have little or no training in scientific methodology, doing scientific research is nevertheless one of the important steps to climbing the career ladder.

The most important thing this story illustrates, however, is that the human rights of research subjects are being abused. The FDA has a list of eight kinds of information that must be given to a patient who is used as a research subject, so that the patient can make an informed choice about whether or not to participate in the study. Everyone who does research or approves research should know these eight FDA requirements by heart.

And yet the FDA has found it necessary to publish a list of the most common problems found when evaluating consent forms.[69] The forms (1) fail to include all eight required elements; (2) fail to state that the drug or procedure is experimental; (3) fail to state all the purposes of the research (i.e., they include only those purposes that the subject would consider most beneficial); (4) overstate facts or are overly optimistic in tone or wording; (5) fail to adequately describe the treatment alternatives available to the woman or the risks and benefits of the alternatives; or (6) fail to provide a contact for answers to questions about the research.

When the woman in Dr. S's study had a uterine rupture and lost her baby, the FDA sent someone to the hospital to investigate. They found a lot of inadequacies in the work performed by the hospital's IRB and found that the consent form used in Dr. S's study contained the first four of the six most common failures listed in the previous paragraph.

According to the federal government, the case presented here is not exceptional in obstetric research in the United States. So much of our medical research lacks adequate protection for "human subjects" that there is a special federal office set up to monitor research and deal with abuse cases. A document published by this special office says, "Despite their intentions to ensure compliance, it is not uncommon for federally funded research institutions to discover that their own policies for protecting human subjects are misunderstood, poorly implemented, or simply disregarded by their own clinicians and IRBs."[70]

Another related issue is "checkbook science," in which studies are conducted and papers are published that are intended not to expand knowledge or to benefit humanity, but rather to sell products.[71] Pharmaceutical companies and other health care industry interests hire public relations firms, which, in turn, hire medical writers to ghostwrite academic-style articles for medical school professors, who submit the articles to respected medical journals. When the paper is published, the headline refers to the new study as the "Harvard study," ensuring that the results will be taken seriously. For his part, the Harvard professor will receive a generous honorarium, such an all-expense-paid trip to another country, where the professor will play the role of the prestigious expert and speak on behalf of the new product at a major conference. In effect, the professor is a paid spokesperson, but he can honestly say that he is not paid by the company because the money comes from the public relations firm (which in turn is paid by the company).

In addition to these problems with how obstetric research is conducted in the United States, there are also many problems with the ways obstetricians interpret and use research. There are many examples in this book of obstetricians who have drawn false conclusions, used misleading language to manipulate research findings, acknowledged only the studies that support their position (and ignored the rest), and so on.

The third type of obstetric research—valid science—takes the form of randomized controlled experimental trials in which there is a sufficient number of cases to draw conclusions about serious risks, proper methodology is used, and researchers obtain proper informed consent from subjects. To examine this type of research, take a look at the Cochrane database (www.cochrane.org). The Cochrane database is assembled by a group of top-notch perinatal scientists from around the world who review the world's scientific literature and make recommendations on obstetric practices based on their reviews. This is valid science, and tragically there is far too little of it.

Several members of the Cochrane group published a textbook titled *A Guide to Effective Care in Pregnancy and Childbirth,* which focuses on valid science (findings from randomized controlled trials) and discusses their recommendations. At the back of the book are six tables that list obstetric practices. Table 1 includes practices for which effectiveness was demonstrated "by clear evidence from controlled trials," tables 2 through 5 show practices backed up by decreasing levels of valid science, and, finally, in table 6, we see practices for which "ineffectiveness or harm was demonstrated by clear evidence."[72] Of the 458 practices in the six tables, we can say that 260 practices (those in tables 4, 5, and 6) are not supported by adequate scientific evidence or scientific evidence indicates that they should not be done. It is extraordinary to note that among these 260 unsupported or harmful practices are a number of practices that are common in American obstetrics. Table 4 (on the next two pages) contains a partial list. As you read through the list, reflect on how many of these practices you have seen or experienced. (The statements, from *A Guide to Effective Care in Pregnancy and Childbirth,* of ineffective or harmful practices are in quotation marks. My comments are in italics following the statements.)

Compared to other medical specialties, the state of obstetric research is the worst by far. The Cochrane group has given the field of obstetrics an award called the "Wooden Spoon," which symbolizes its unique place as the medical specialty with the poorest quality of research and the least evidence-based practice.

Meanwhile, the rate of women dying around the time of birth in the United States is going up. It is difficult to draw conclusions from death

TABLE 4. OBSTETRIC PRACTICES THAT SHOULD NOT BE DONE

1. "Short periods of electronic fetal monitoring as a screening test on admission in labor." *Electronic monitoring doesn't improve the outcome of the birth and starts the cascade of unnecessary and risky interventions.*

2. "Early use of oxytocin (Pitocin) to augment a slow or prolonged labor." *Pitocin may or may not accelerate the labor but definitely accelerates the cascade of unnecessary and risky interventions.*

3. "Active management of labor." *A popular form of high-interventionist obstetrics, where* active *refers to the obstetrician, not the woman. Active management involves allowing only certain intervals of time to pass during certain stages of labor before prescribed interventions are applied. If you hear that an obstetrician likes active management, run.*

4. "Misoprostol (Cytotec) administered orally or vaginally for induction of labor." *The risks associated with this drug are covered in chapter 4.*

5. "Routinely involving obstetricians in the care of all women during pregnancy and childbirth." *The evidence shows that a woman is better off with a midwife than an obstetrician unless she has serious medical problems.*

6. "Fragmentation of care during pregnancy and childbirth." *Science shows that both the woman and the baby are safer with one caregiver throughout pregnancy, all of the labor, and birth.*

7. "Routine use of ultrasound for fetal measurement in late pregnancy." *If used selectively when problems appear, ultrasound testing can be valuable, but when such tests are routine, their value disappears and they serve only to give false diagnoses and provoke unnecessary risky interventions.*

8. "Screening for 'gestational diabetes.'" *The authors put gestational diabetes in quotation marks because there is no such thing as gestational diabetes. It is an invention of obstetricians that describes an elevated glucose level in the blood, a level that is normal in pregnancy and without serious consequences.*

9. "Withholding food and drink from women in labor." *This has become a routine practice because obstetricians are surgeons and manage birth as if it were a surgical procedure. It is far better for a laboring woman to eat and drink.*

10. "Routine intravenous infusion in labor." *This is another way obstetricians treat normal labor like surgery. An IV is not necessary, but it has great symbolic value to the doctors and nurses as it helps convert the birthing woman from a woman to a patient and makes her more compliant.*

11. "Wearing face masks during labor or for vaginal examinations." *This practice has been repeatedly proven to have no value in the prevention of disease or infection, except during vaginal exams and at the moment of birth when the attendant(not the others in the room) needs protection from possibly HIV contaminated blood. But it has great value in the medicalization of normal birth. In reality, it's pure Hollywood, doctors and nurses playing doctor and nurse. Putting masks on family members turns them into outsiders and makes them more afraid to intervene.*

12. "Routine directed pushing during the second stage of labor." *The second stage is the time just before birth when the cervix is fully dilated and the woman begins to feel the need to push. It's typical to hear nurses, under the direction of doc-*

tors, yelling at the woman, "Push!" or "Don't push!" Science shows that such directions are detrimental to the process, as natural pushing is completely involuntary. This is one of many examples of doctors thinking that they know more than nature does.

13. "Arbitrary limitation of the duration of the second stage of labor." *This is very important, because it's one of the most common and dangerous mistakes made in the management of childbirth in the United States. I have been in many hospitals with written regulations for the exact time limit allowed for the second stage, and when that time is up, doctors jump in with invasive, risky interventions. The diagnosis "failure to progress" is based on time limits and is one of the most common excuses offered for doing an unnecessary C-section. Valid science says that as long as the woman and baby are okay, a clock is not helpful.*

14. "Instrumental vaginal delivery to shorten the second stage of labor." *This refers to using a vacuum or forceps to pull the baby out because the doctor thinks things aren't going fast enough or wants the birth over for reasons of convenience. It is unnecessary in almost all cases and carries serious risks for both woman and baby.*

15. "Routine use of the lithotomy position (on back, feet in stirrups) for the second stage of labor." *This is the position used for gynecological exams and surgery, and obstetricians, who are also gynecologists, are comfortable with it. It is convenient for staff as well. But it is absolutely the worst position for facilitating normal progress of labor and birth and the position most likely to reduce the oxygen supply to the baby.*

16. "Routine or liberal episiotomy for birth." *The scientific evidence here is overwhelming—this practice is truly necessary in very, very few cases.*

17. "Routine restriction of mother-infant contact." *It is best never to take the baby away from the mother after birth, not even to do a pediatric exam, which can be done just as well while the mother holds the baby.*

18. "Routine nursery care for babies in hospital." *This is probably the biggest pediatric mistake of the twentieth century, causing more infectious epidemics and more cases of shattered mother-infant development with long-term consequences than anything else.*

19. "Wearing hospital gowns in newborn nurseries." *Again, this is a Hollywood act. There is plenty of scientific data proving that it's of no value.*

20. "Routine supplements of water or formula for breastfed babies." *These are done all the time, and they go against the Ten Steps to a Baby-Friendly Hospital. (Ten Steps to a Baby-Friendly Hospital is a WHO/UNICEF program to promote breast-feeding by changing practices applied to newborn infants in hospitals. For more information, including the ten steps, see www.babyfriendlyusa.org.) This practice is proven to reduce successful breast-feeding and breast-feeding has been shown scientifically to result in healthier babies with higher intelligence.*

21. "Restricting sibling visits to babies in hospital." *There is plenty of data that sibling visits are not a risk. Ironically, this practice is done to exclude dangerous germs from the hospital, but the dangerous germs are not brought in by children; instead, they are already in the hospital, carried by staff.*

SOURCE: Information in this list is from tables 4, 5, and 6 in M. Enkin et al., *A Guide to Effective Care in Pregnancy and Childbirth*, 3rd ed. (New York: Oxford University Press, 2000), pp. 487–507.

certificate data because only the immediate cause of death is listed, not the underlying causes. But if we look at the six leading causes of pregnancy-related death in the United States, three of them (hemorrhage, anesthesia, and infection) are likely to be the result of obstetric interventions. For example, the immediate cause of death is frequently given as hemorrhage, but we can speculate that in many cases the hemorrhage, as in the case in Iowa cited earlier, is associated with C-section. Research done in the United States and in Great Britain shows that the maternal mortality rate for C-section—combining emergency and elective—is four times higher than the maternal mortality rate for vaginal birth.[73] And the rate of women dying is still nearly three times higher when it is a routine or "elective" C-section without any emergency. Given that well over half of the C-sections performed in the United States these days are unnecessary, we must conclude that unnecessary C-sections are contributing to our increasing maternal mortality rates.[74] It is proven that using epidural block for normal labor pain carries an increased risk that a woman will die, and "anesthesia complications" is documented as one of the leading causes of maternal mortality in the United States.[75] So unnecessary epidural blocks are also contributing to the increase in deaths. There is good reason to believe that other obstetric technologies, such as drugs used to induce labor, contribute to the rising number of women dying during childbirth in the United States as well, and we will look closely at that in chapter 4.

For a time in the 1950s and 1960s, our maternal mortality rates were going down, but it has been shown that the decrease resulted from basic medical advances, such as the discovery of antibiotics and the ability to give safe blood transfusions. It was not due to high-tech obstetric interventions, though many obstetricians are inclined to give technology credit for the improvement.

More recently, there has been an increase in obstetric interventions and simultaneously an increase in maternal deaths and an increase in conditions such as autism, attention deficit disorders, and learning disabilities in children in the United States. A study commissioned by the California legislature and conducted by researchers in California reported in 2002 that the number of children with profound autism in that state has tripled in little more than a decade. Studies conducted by the federal Centers for Disease Control and Prevention show similar increases in autism in Georgia and New Jersey.[76] At this time we do not know the cause of autism nor do we know why an increasing number of children have the condition. However, we do know that this surge in autism coincides with a surge in ultrasound scanning, epidural block, pharmacological induction of labor, and C-section. Professional and community organizations that focus on these neurological disorders should be screaming for research to determine if there are correlations between obstetric interventions and these disorders.

I remember discussing labor induction using Cytotec with Dr. Luis Sanchos-Ramos, an obstetrician practicing in Florida, on a National Public Radio program in 2002. He said that he had used Cytotec on more than five thousand women to induce labor, and I asked him if he had done any follow-up on the children born from these five thousand Cytotec inductions. He admitted that he had not—and neither has anyone else. The gap between actual obstetric practices in the United States and what scientific evidence indicates obstetric practices should be continues and will be slow to change until there is sufficient pressure—from women, scientists, politicians, and the media—to force more evidence-based practices.

FOUR FORCED LABOR: INDUCTION OR SEDUCTION

Admission to the hospital places patients in a dependency relationship in which frightening questions of bodily integrity, of life versus death, are *not* negotiated, but decided within the strict definitions of a biomedical ideology.
BARBARA ROTHMAN, PROFESSOR OF SOCIOLOGY AND AUTHOR

Assumed unsafe until proven safe (precautionary)
Assumed safe until proven unsafe (anti-precautionary)
OPPOSING PRINCIPLES OF MEDICAL PRACTICE

Two weeks before Ms. S is due to give birth, she and her husband leave their three young children with their grandmother and go to the local hospital in their small town. The year is 1999. Ms. S is having occasional contractions, and they want to find out what's going on, though they are not overly concerned. Ms. S has had three normal births, with no cesarean sections, and considers herself a childbirth veteran.

At the hospital, a nurse examines Ms. S and determines that the contractions are too infrequent and irregular for her to be in active labor. The nurse calls Ms. S's obstetrician, Dr. K. The obstetrician orders that Ms. S be admitted to the hospital, though she has expressed a strong desire to go home. Four hours later, Ms. S still badly wants to go home. The nurse calls her doctor again and asks if it's okay for her to go, but it appears the obstetrician has a plan, as he orders that she be kept in the hospital.

Three hours later Dr. K arrives, examines Ms. S, and finds that she is indeed not in active labor. He inserts twenty-five micrograms of Cytotec into her vagina to induce labor. Ms. S is aware that something has been inserted, but the obstetrician does not tell her what or even that his goal is to induce labor. Nor does he tell her that the drug he put inside her is not approved by the FDA for use in inducing labor and has serious risks.

Ms. S is put to bed and an electronic fetal monitor (EFM) is hooked up. Though continuous monitoring with EFM is not necessary for a normal labor, it is important when inducing labor with a powerful drug known to have serious risks, such as Cytotec. In Ms. S's case, however, the EFM is left off much of the time

Dr. K visits again four hours later. He gives Ms. S another dose of Cytotec. The monitor is now on, and within an hour it shows that Ms. S's uterus is contracting far too rapidly for the baby to get a good supply of oxygen—a condition known as uterine tachysystole or uterine hyperstimulation. Nurses' notes state how rapidly the uterus is contracting, but there is no mention of hyperstimulation or any other indication that the nurses recognize that the situation is potentially hazardous to Ms. S and her baby.

Four hours after the second dose of Cytotec is administered, the monitor shows both rapid uterine contractions and a dangerous change in the baby's heart rate. Nevertheless, Dr. K, who is not there to check his patient, orders over the phone that Ms. S be given Pitocin, another drug used to induce labor. Although it is not unusual for an obstetrician to add Pitocin when inducing with Cytotec if the labor is not progressing, it is dangerous to do it when the patient is already experiencing continuous rapid contractions, as it seriously increases the risks.

When the obstetrician returns, he ruptures Ms. S's bag of waters, or amniotic sac membranes. A few minutes later all hell breaks loose. The baby's heart rate becomes so slow that it is obvious that the baby is in extreme distress. Dr. K tries to help the baby by stretching Ms. S's cervix to look for the umbilical cord. Meanwhile, Ms. S begins to complain of shortness of breath and chest discomfort. The obstetrician tells her to push, while a nurse tries to tell him that Ms. S is in no shape to push, as she is gasping for air and turning blue.

Dr. K, however, is not focused on the woman; he is focused on the baby. He applies forceps and, after three pulls, gets the baby out and hands it off to a waiting pediatrician. He then turns to the mother, but at this point she is unresponsive and can't be aroused. It has been twenty minutes since both Ms. S and her baby went into severe distress and shock. Dr. K gives Ms. S CPR and oxygen, but there is no response. He calls "code blue," an emergency signal that tells hospital personnel to come immediately. But there is nothing more that can be done. Ms. S is dead.

Meanwhile, the baby is not breathing and has an extremely slow heart rate. An hour and a half after the baby is born, a call is made to a larger regional hospital that, unlike this hospital, has a neonatal intensive care unit. For some reason, instead of sending the baby to the larger hospital by ambulance, a one-hour ride, hospital staff keeps the baby at the smaller hospital while the larger hospital sends an ambulance to pick the baby up, wasting precious time. The baby is having seizures and still needs help to breathe. Later the baby is found to have severe brain damage with cerebral palsy due to lack of oxygen during labor and birth.

The autopsy of Ms. S showed amniotic fluid embolism (AFE), a condition that can occur when amniotic fluid (the water in the sac surrounding the fetus) leaks into the mother's bloodstream. Debris that has collected in the fluid during the pregnancy—baby's skin cells and hair—blocks the small air sacks in the mother's lungs, leading to shock and a collapse of heart and lung functions. For amniotic fluid to leak into the bloodstream and produce blockage, there must be a break in the normal anatomical barrier that keeps the fluid separate from the mother's blood vessels. Overly strong uterine contractions can break this barrier and cause microscopic lacerations in the uterus or cervix. Cytotec causes unusually strong contractions. AFE has a high mortality rate, about 80 percent, and is one of the known risks of using Cytotec on a pregnant woman.

In another case, an eighteen-year-old African American woman we'll call Ms. Q was expecting her first child. She received her prenatal care in a local health clinic, some distance from her home in a rural area in the South. She was assigned to a young, newly trained obstetrician, who decided to induce her with Cytotec because it was one week beyond her due date, though, as I will explain later in this chapter, this is not a valid indication for inducing labor unless the baby is in trouble, and tests showed that her baby was doing just fine.

Ms. Q arrived at the hospital and was given Cytotec. Within an hour she started having contractions and within two hours she was having contractions too frequently—hyperstimulation, which can cause fetal hypoxia (lack of oxygen). Four hours after admission, she was given more Cytotec, which was dangerous since her contractions were already too frequent. Eleven hours after admission, she was given even more of the drug. By then she had been having excessively rapid uterine contractions for several hours, and there were dangerous changes in the baby's heart rate, indicating severe fetal distress. Later the doctor gave Ms. Q Pitocin, stimulating her uterus even further, in effect whipping a nearly dead horse.

During the last hour before birth, after what was now more than twenty-four hours of uterine hyperstimulation, which blocks oxygen from getting to the baby, the monitor showed that the baby was in extreme distress. The baby was moribund (that is, unresponsive and dying) at birth and died thirty-five minutes later.

A few minutes after the birth, Ms. Q began to bleed profusely from her vagina. The hemorrhage could not be stopped, and as she was going into shock she was given a blood transfusion. Her uterus had become completely floppy, which is a disaster because when the placenta detaches from the inside of the uterus after birth and comes out the vagina, there's an open wound inside the uterus where it had been attached. Normally, the uterus contracts down to stop the bleeding, but if the uterus does not contract, the bleeding becomes severe. Hospital staff massaged Ms. Q's uterus and gave her more powerful drugs to try to make her uterus contract, but to no avail. Tragically, Ms. Q died a few hours after giving birth. As with Ms. S, the autopsy gave the cause of death as AFE. Between 1997 and 2004, nineteen cases of AFE after Cytotec induction were reported to the FDA.[1] I personally know of more than twenty-five cases in the United States in the past ten years in which a woman has died at or shortly after childbirth after labor was induced with Cytotec, and in all these cases the official cause of death was AFE.

Were these deaths preventable? There is general consensus that a significant proportion of cases of maternal mortality are preventable, as they result from bad obstetric care. A crucial question in Ms. Q's case is why her uterus was floppy, leading to the hemorrhage. In *Williams Obstetrics,* a leading obstetric textbook, the following sentence is in bold type: "The uterus that contracts with unusual vigor before delivery is likely to be hypotonic [floppy] after delivery, with hemorrhage from the placental implantation site as the consequence."[2] More than twenty-four hours of severe uterine hyperstimulation definitely qualifies as "contracting with unusual vigor," so the decision to induce labor using Cytotec must certainly be implicated in the hemorrhage. *Williams Obstetrics* also states that vigorous contractions in a woman having her first baby can lead to circumstances in which AFE is likely to develop.[3]

The rate of women dying around the time of birth has been increasing in the United States for twenty-five years. What about the rate of AFE cases? Evidence suggests that AFE-related deaths are increasing as well.[4] It is clear that the increase in AFE cases in the United States is connected with the increasing use of uterine stimulant drugs, such as Cytotec, for labor induction.[5] Another possible reason for the increasing rates of AFE deaths is that this diagnosis is being used by doctors who are trying to cover up their mistakes. This possibility will be discussed in chapter 7, on obstetric litigation.

Chapter 1 began with a real-life Cytotec induction story, about a family in Oregon. In that case, the baby died, and the woman's uterus ruptured and was removed, so she can have no more children. So here we have three innocent families whose injuries will never heal. How did this happen?

Given that a fundamental principle of medical practice is "First, do no harm," new drugs and other interventions must not be used until they have been adequately tested for safety. However, when we study the history of obstetrics in the United States, we find ethics that are anti-precautionary and more akin to the Wild West or what might be called "vigilante medicine." American obstetricians consistently use new interventions without waiting for the judge, claiming that to wait for adequate research on safety takes too long and impedes "progress." But the idea of progress in obstetrics is to a great extent a myth. The maternal mortality rate in the United States is not going down, it is going up, and the slight fall in the rate of babies who die around the time of birth (perinatal mortality) in the past ten years is due not to a decrease in the percentage of babies who die before they are born, but rather to a slight decrease in the rate of babies who die shortly after birth, which can be attributed to neonatal intensive care, not obstetric care. There has been no improvement in the past twenty years in the rate of babies born who are too small—a major cause of neurological handicap—and in 2004 the rate went up. Nor has there been any lowering of the rate of babies who develop cerebral palsy.

Meanwhile, we have one iatrogenic (doctor-caused) obstetric tragedy after another. The 1930s saw routine X-ray of the woman's pelvis during pregnancy before research proved that it causes cancer in the baby. In the 1950s, the drug diethylstilbestrol (DES) was widely used during pregnancy in the hope that it might stop vaginal bleeding (it didn't), before research proved that it causes defects in the baby's reproductive organs. In the 1970s, doctors used thalidomide on pregnant women, again in the hope that it might stop vaginal bleeding, before studies showed that it causes deformities of the arms and legs in babies. There seems to be a new tragedy every twenty years, and in the 1990s, right on schedule, we had Cytotec being used to induce labor. It seems that the only thing we ever learn from obstetric history is that we never learn.

Before we go any further, let's take a look at how this most recent case of vigilante obstetrics got started. In the late 1980s, a drug with the generic name misoprostol (given the brand name Cytotec by its manufacturer, Searle Pharmaceutical, Inc., now a division of Pfizer) was approved by the FDA for use on adults with stomach ulcers. The manufacturer was well aware that one possible side effect of the drug was severe uterine contractions, so it stated on the label that it should *never be given to pregnant women*. There is even a silhouette of a pregnant women with a slanted line through it on the label. However, soon after the drug hit the market, obstetricians discovered that, because it causes uterine contractions, Cytotec can be used to induce or augment (speed up) labor. Completely disregarding the warning on the label, they began using it on pregnant women. In doing so, obstetricians are taking advantage of a significant loophole in our drug regulatory system. Once a drug is approved by the FDA for a specific medical indication and put on the market, there is no law preventing a doctor from using the drug for any purpose he chooses, in any dose he chooses, on any patient he chooses. Since the drug label includes those indications that are approved by the FDA, using the drug for purposes not shown on the label is called "off-label" use.[6]

When obstetricians who use Cytotec for labor induction are confronted with the fact that they are unwilling to wait for the scientific evidence that will tell them whether or not the drug is safe, they invariably answer, "But we use drugs off-label all the time." This answer has several serious problems. The most fundamental one is that obstetricians who say this are expressing a cavalier disregard for the safety of women and babies as well as a lack of faith in the drug regulatory system. But beyond this obvious flaw, it is important to recognize that using Cytotec to induce labor is not just "off-label," it is "against label"—that is, the label states that this use is contraindicated (medically harmful). Given that drug companies have no incentive to limit the use of their products unnecessarily, we have to assume that if the Cytotec label explicitly states that the drug should not be given to pregnant women, there must be data that suggest possible serious risks involved in such use. So using a drug "against label" must be considered a higher level of risk than using a drug under conditions that are not mentioned on the label at all.

Another reason to be concerned with this standard response is that it lumps together all off-label drug use as though the risks involved were all equal. In Cytotec cases such as the three recounted in this book, in which the outcomes include death and severe disabilities, when the obstetrician offers the excuse, "But we use drugs off-label all the time," we can compare the obstetrician to a driver who goes one hundred miles per hour in a twenty-five-mile-per-hour zone. Imagine that the speeding driver causes a fatal car accident and then says, "Traffic laws are disobeyed all the time. Just last week there were dozens of parking tickets given out in this city." You can't compare the risks of speeding with the risks of illegal parking. And you can't compare the risks of using Cytotec for labor induction with the risks of giving other drugs to pregnant women off-label.

A survey of pregnant women conducted in the 1990s revealed that ten drugs were given to them off-label.[7] Nine of the drugs mentioned in the survey carried very little risk. Only the tenth drug, prostaglandin E2, a close relative of Cytotec that was popular for labor induction before Cytotec came along, had serious risks.

When obstetricians found that they could use Cytotec to induce labor, they began using it more and more, playing around with the dosage and experimenting with how and when to administer it. For the most part, they did this without telling their patients that they were participating in an experiment, essentially treating their patients and their patient's babies as guinea pigs and lab rats rather than as human research subjects. The results of these informal experiments were then passed on to other doctors by word of mouth—informal chats in the doctors' lounge or the cafeteria. Incredibly, in my experience short conversations with other doctors are the most common way doctors learn about new drugs or techniques. Sadly, reading the results of scientific studies in medical journals or hearing reports of studies at professional meetings are not typically part of most obstetricians' practice.

With the advent of the Internet, doctors found another convenient way to exchange medical information, though for the most part it has not meant more safeguards as to the validity of that information. In the early 1990s, while surfing around in Internet chat rooms frequented by doctors, I began to read more and more about the use of Cytotec for induction of labor. One doctor wrote, "I must say I have heard some great things about Cytotec myself. Just be careful. The stuff turns the cervix to complete MUSHIE."

That's when I went to the *Physicians' Desk Reference* and found that using Cytotec for induction of labor was "against-label-contraindicated." I went on to check obstetric journals and textbooks, and found that the only published research into inducing labor with this drug involved far too few women to draw reliable conclusions about risks. I got a cold feeling in the pit of my stomach as I sensed that this drug would result in another widespread obstetric tragedy—and it has.

In the years that followed, when I gave lectures to obstetricians around the country, more and more doctors told me that they were trying Cytotec, and I had the disturbing experience of seeing how rapidly "trying it out" solidified into accepted dogma. I remember one obstetrician in Sioux Falls, South Dakota, who proudly told me over lunch that he was the first doctor in his community to use Cytotec for labor induction and that he now urges other doctors to use it. He justified his actions by saying, "If we wait for the bureaucrats at the FDA to approve drugs, we'll wait forever. We must try them out ourselves if we want progress." He admitted that he doesn't tell the women to whom he gives the drug that it is not approved for the purpose, nor does he ask for their consent. He scoffed at my observation that he is experimenting on women without their knowledge, much less their informed consent.

In 1995, when I was lecturing in Oregon, the Oregon State Health Department told me that Cytotec was the most common way of inducing labor in that state and was being used on thousands of laboring women. Around this time, a few more studies of Cytotec induction began to appear in obstetric journals, but all were still far too small to scientifically evaluate the level of risks.[8] The studies did report risk tendencies, however, such as the possibility that the drug could make the uterus contract too fast (uterine hyperstimulation); cause signs of fetal distress (such as the fetus passing meconium or a change in the baby's heart rate); and, for a few women, cause uterine rupture. In 1999, a review of the scientific evidence for using Cytotec for labor induction was published by the Cochrane Library. The review concluded that because of the lack of sufficient scientific evaluation and the reports of serious side effects, Cytotec "cannot be recommended for routine use at this stage."[9]

These worrisome studies had no apparent effect on the spread of the drug. It can be reliably estimated, using annual total U.S. births and induction rates, that during the five years 1995 through 1999, more than a half-million women in the United States had labor induced with this drug that was (and is) *not* approved

by the FDA,

by the drug regulatory agency of any other industrialized country,

by the pharmaceutical company that makes it,

by reliable and valid scientific evidence (the Cochrane database), or

by the British Royal College of Obstetricians and Gynaecologists.

According to the Centers for Disease Control and Prevention (CDC), the rate of drug-induced labor induction in U.S. births doubled from 10 percent to 20 percent of births in the 1990s, an increase almost certainly due to the rampant use of Cytotec.[10] A survey in 2002 showed that 44 percent of all births are induced with uterine stimulant drugs.[11] Furthermore, data from the CDC tell us that much of this induction was done for convenience, as it parallels an increasing trend during the 1990s for vaginal births to take place Monday through Friday during daylight hours. So doctors' convenience has led to unnecessary labor induction, which has led to women's deaths.

The convenience factor is strong motivation for obstetricians to induce labor. Scheduling a labor induction, like scheduling a C-section, is a godsend to a busy, often sleep-deprived doctor. It offers the hope of practicing "daylight obstetrics." Many doctors have told me with satisfaction that when they bring a woman to the hospital in the evening and induce her with Cytotec (weekday evenings only, never on weekends), she will typically give birth by late the next afternoon, so the obstetrician can be home in time for dinner.

Induction of labor is an important convenience not only for obstetricians but also for hospitals, as it allows hospitals to organize an induction assembly line, with slots into which doctors can fit their patients. This assembly-line approach is confirmed by the printed protocol in a large hospital in Florida, "Scheduling Induction for Labor."[12]

In about 10 percent of all births there is a medical reason to induce labor with drugs, and before 1990, 10 percent was the rate of induction in most industrialized countries. Pitocin, which is a synthetic version of the naturally occurring hormone oxytocin, has been used to induce labor for decades. It has been approved by the FDA for this purpose after adequate, careful scientific assessment of its efficacy and risks, and we know a great deal about how best to use it.

Given that there is already a well-tested drug that can be used for induction, why did obstetricians start using Cytotec? There are several reasons. One is that Pitocin is administered with an intravenous drip (IV), whereas Cytotec doesn't require an IV, so it's easier to administer. It is in pill form and is given orally or inserted into the vagina. However, the form of the drug presents special difficulties when used for labor induction. Because Cytotec is made for patients with stomach ulcers and was never intended for use on pregnant women, it comes only in 100 and 200 microgram tablets. After a decade of unauthorized experimenting, 25 micrograms has emerged as the usual dose for labor induction. Have you ever tried to break a tablet that does not have a line down the middle or used a razor blade to cut it in half and then into quarters? Needless to say, the size of each quarter is never exact. Nevertheless, this is what some hospital pharmacies all over the country are doing. (Other hospitals find this unacceptable and do not allow induction with Cytotec because their pharmacies refuse to dispense inaccurate dosages.)

The convenience of using Cytotec is also a liability in that the drug is quickly absorbed and stays in the body for hours. Whereas a Pitocin IV can be pulled if any adverse effects arise, thus stopping the effect of the drug in seconds, when problems develop with Cytotec, there is very little that can be done to reverse its effects.

Another benefit of Cytotec that is frequently discussed among doctors is that it costs less than other drugs used for labor induction. It is surprising to hear doctors talk about saving money since, unless they have a financial interest in the hospital or clinic where they practice, it is not really their money. Cytotec is indeed far cheaper than other drugs used for induction of labor, but the question is, why is it so cheap? It is cheap because the pharmaceutical company has not spent the money on experimental clinical trials that would be required by the FDA to test the drugs' safety for labor induction. In other words, it is cheap because we don't know whether it's safe, and it is women on whom it is used who are paying the price. Of course, hospitals love to save money, but they must also realize that they are taking a huge financial risk when Cytotec is used to induce labor because they may well lose much more in litigation after a single bad outcome than they can save in years of using the cheaper drug.

In 1998, after Cytotec had been used for induction on millions of women in the United States, a paper was published about an experimental trial in which the drug was used for labor induction in women who had previously had C-sections who were having vaginal births after cesarean (VBACs). The study had to be stopped midway because too many women attempting VBACs with Cytotec induction ended up with ruptured uteruses, a catastrophic obstetric emergency that almost always means that the woman will not be able to have more children and that has a high risk of mortality for both the woman and the baby.[13] When the paper was published, I called ACOG and asked if the organization was aware of the sweeping use of Cytotec for induction. They replied that, yes, of course they were aware of it. I then asked why they were not doing anything about it. They replied that since it was off-label use and they had no position on off-label use, they

TABLE 5. CYTOTEC INDUCTION IN THE UNITED STATES, 1994–99

Total Cytotec induction in United States, 1994–99

Births per year (CDC)	4,000,000
On average, 15 percent are induced each year (CDC)	600,000
25 percent of inductions use Cytotec each year (ACOG)	150,000
Total Cytotec inductions in five years	750,000

Cytotec inductions with previous cesarean section in the United States, 1994–99*

Out of 4,000,000 births each year (CDC):

15 percent with previous C-sections (CDC)	600,000
25 percent try VBAC (ACOG)	150,000
on average, 7 percent of VBACs are induced (CDC) (VBAC induction rate is assumed to be half the overall induction rate)	10,500
25 percent of VBAC inductions use Cytotec (ACOG)	2,625
4 percent of VBAC Cytotec inductions rupture (P&B)	105
25 percent of uterine ruptures result in baby's death (P&B)	26

Over the five-year period (1994–99):

VBAC Cytotec inductions	13,125
VBAC Cytotec inductions with uterine rupture	525
VBAC Cytotec inductions resulting in death of baby	130

In sum:

More than a half-million women had Cytotec induction.

More than 10,000 women had VBAC Cytotec induction.

More than 500 women with VBAC Cytotec induction had uterine rupture.

More than 100 women with VBAC Cytotec induction and uterine rupture had dead babies.

An unknown but significant number of Cytotec inductions resulted in hyper stimulation of the uterus or rupture leading to brain damage in the baby (anecdotal evidence).

An unknown but significant number—more than twenty—of Cytotec inductions resulted in the woman's death (anecdotal evidence from FDA and Searle).

* The ACOG recommendation against using Cytotec for labor induction in VBAC was issued in November 1999.

SOURCES: Sources of data appear in parentheses. Estimates are all conservative and are based on data from the CDC, ACOG, and two papers: M. Plaut, M. Schwartz, and S. Lubarsky, "Uterine Rupture Associated with the Use of Misoprostol in the Gravid Patient with a Previous Cesarean Section," *American Journal of Obstetrics and Gynecology* 180, no. 6 (1999): 1535–40; and H. Blanchette, S. Nayak, and S. Erasmus, "Comparison of the Safety and Efficacy of Intravaginal Misoprostol with Those of Dinoprostone for Cervical Ripening and Induction of Labor in a Community Hospital," *American Journal of Obstetrics and Gynecology* 180, no. 6 (1999): 1543–50.

were not prepared to take any position (thus turning their backs on this serious obstetric issue).

Then, in June 1999, two more papers appeared in the same issue of the *American Journal of Obstetrics and Gynecology*, reporting alarming rates of uterine rupture when Cytotec was used for induction in women with previous C-sections.[14] In one study, 5.6 percent of women having VBACs induced with Cytotec had uterine rupture, and in the other study the rate of rupture was 3.7 percent. This is a twenty-eight-fold increase in the rate of rupture over having a VBAC without Cytotec induction. Furthermore, for one-quarter of the women who had uterine rupture, this resulted in the deaths of their babies.

Several months after these papers were published, ACOG came out with a recommendation that Cytotec not be used for induction in women who had previously had C-sections—shutting the barn door after thousands of horses were gone. It can be estimated that during the five years before ACOG finally made its recommendation, more than 25,000 women in the United States who had previously had C-sections were given Cytotec induction (see table 5). We can further deduce that more than 1,000 of them suffered ruptured uteruses, and between 50 and 250 ended up with dead babies. Though we do not have hard data on the number of maternal deaths caused by giving Cytotec to women with previous C-sections, we know enough about uterine rupture to know that probably ten to twenty women died from uterine rupture caused by Cytotec induction.

Strangely, obstetricians in the United States remain in denial about the tragedy Cytotec induction represents. In chapter 2, I mentioned a *Dateline NBC* television program on Cytotec induction of labor that aired on November 4, 2001. Alisa Goldberg appeared as a guest on the program, among other guests. She had just completed her obstetric training at a reputable hospital and was working at the National Institutes of Health. She was also the senior author of a paper on Cytotec induction published in a prestigious journal.[15] The following dialogue took place between Dr. Goldberg and the interviewer:

Interviewer: *"Do you think five years ago [i.e., 1996] doctors knew enough about Cytotec?"*

Dr. Goldberg is unable to give any answer. She sits twisting in her chair and smiling.

Interviewer: *"Do we know enough now about Cytotec?"*

Dr. Goldberg: "We are still fine-tuning. I think there is still more to be learned. That's the way medicine evolves."

Interviewer: "But should we wait until after we learn it before we say it is safe?"

Dr. Goldberg: "It's a catch-22. If you don't use it, then you don't learn."[16]

Of course, Dr. Goldberg could not respond to the question about whether we knew enough about Cytotec five years earlier, because if she said that we did, she would have to address the fact that it was only since then that we learned that the drug must never be used on women with previous C-sections because of the extreme risk of uterine rupture and the certainty that Cytotec has caused women and babies to die. If she said that we did not know enough, she would be condemning hundreds of her fellow obstetricians who were using this drug for induction five years earlier.

In effect, this obstetrician freely admitted on television that a vast, uncontrolled experiment is taking place on unwitting women without their knowledge, much less their consent, and there was no indication she felt remorse about that fact. Apparently, she saw no problem with using women as guinea pigs, most of the time in an unscientific way, without telling them. When she said, "If you don't use it, then you don't learn" (a classic anti-precautionary position), it was as if she had never heard of officially approved, carefully designed, controlled experimental trials in which the women involved give their informed consent. In other words, it sounds as though in obstetrics, valid science is dead.

You can be sure that this obstetrician is by no means alone. In 2005, five obstetricians from a prestigious Ivy League university hospital in New England all testified in a lawsuit involving a Cytotec induction that resulted in the death of the mother. Every one of them demonstrated their anti-precautionary approach to obstetric practice by saying that unless there is data proving significant risks, it is okay to use a drug before it has been approved by the FDA for this use.

Table 6 shows reliable estimates of the risk of uterine rupture during labor. When ACOG published recommendations for labor induction saying that Cytotec should not be used on women having VBACs, the organization took an ambiguous and somewhat confusing position on whether to use the drug for vaginal birth without previous C-section, saying only that it works: "Prostaglandin E analogues [a category that includes Cytotec]

TABLE 6. ESTIMATES OF RISKS OF UTERINE RUPTURE DURING LABOR

Normal (unscarred) uterus	1 in 33,000 births
VBAC—no induction	1 in 200 births
VBAC—oxytocin (Pitocin) augmentation	1 in 100 births
VBAC—oxytocin induction	1 in 43 births
VBAC—Cytotec induction	1 in 20 births
Normal (unscarred) uterus with Cytotec induction	UNKNOWN*
Neurological injury or death of baby after uterine rupture	30 percent
Death of woman after uterine rupture	1–2 percent

*Best scientific opinion—all evidence currently available shows significantly increased risk of rupture of unscarred uterus with Cytotec induction but the exact level of risk is unknown due to inadequate sample size of studies.

SOURCES: Estimates are all conservative and based on data from the CDC, ACOG, and two papers: M. Plaut, M. Schwartz, and S. Lubarsky, "Uterine Rupture Associated with the Use of Misoprostol in the Gravid Patient with a Previous Cesarean Section," *American Journal of Obstetrics and Gynecology* 180, no. 6 (1999): 1535–40; and H. Blanchette, S. Nayak, and S. Erasmus, "Comparison of the Safety and Efficacy of Intravaginal Misoprostol with Those of Dinoprostone for Cervical Ripening and Induction of Labor in a Community Hospital," *American Journal of Obstetrics and Gynecology* 180, no. 6 (1999): 1543–50.

are effective in promoting cervical ripening and inducing labor." Of course the contentious issue is not whether Cytotec works, but whether it is safe, and ACOG neither addresses safety in the bulletin nor actually recommends that Cytotec be used for induction. Contrast this to what the organization says about Pitocin (oxytocin) in the same bulletin: "Women in whom induction of labor is indicated may be appropriately managed with either a low or high dose oxytocin regimen."[17]

ACOG's position on Cytotec induction is undoubtedly a case of politics at work. The organization does not wish to explicitly recommend the use of a drug that has known serious risks and is against label, as that could make it liable, but it does want to offer ACOG members who use the drug some wiggle room. The subtlety of the organization's approach, however, appears to be lost on some obstetricians, as my conversations with them demonstrate that many of them believe that the bulletin constitutes a recommendation by ACOG of the use of Cytotec for induction with no previous C-section.

There is now good scientific evidence that inducing labor with Cytotec frequently causes the uterus to contract too fast (uterine hyperstimulation), and there is considerable anecdotal evidence that uterine hyperstimulation during labor can lead to severe, permanent brain damage in the baby. (The only time the baby can get oxygen from the mother during labor is between uterine contractions, so if the uterus contracts too often, the baby cannot get enough oxygen.) So, in addition to the babies that have died from Cytotec induction, we know for certain that babies have suffered brain damage as a result of Cytotec induction, though we do not know how many.

Here is one real-life story. A young married couple in rural Idaho, Mr. and Ms. M, were having their first baby in 1998. They were excited, as were their family and friends in the small community where they lived. There were two obstetricians practicing in their town, a partnership, and Mr. and Ms. M signed on with them.

The pregnancy went smoothly, and when Ms. M was just about due, one of the obstetricians told her to come to the local hospital the following Monday evening. In the chart he wrote, "Cytotec induction," though there was no medical indication for inducing labor.

Ms. and Mr. M arrived at the hospital at 5 P.M., and at 6 P.M. the obstetrician came in, examined Ms. M, and ordered the nurses to "follow the Cytotec protocol." Neither the doctor nor the nurses told the parents what drug was being used and why, nor that the drug is not approved by the FDA, nor that serious risks were involved. In other words, there was no fully informed consent.

Over the next several hours, nurses gave Ms. M three doses of Cytotec. The electronic fetal monitor began to show that her uterus was contracting too fast and the baby's heartbeat was irregular, but the nurses continued "the protocol." Although the nurses telephoned the obstetrician once at 11 P.M. because they were concerned about the baby's irregular heartbeat, the doctor did not visit Ms. M again until the next morning, when he came in for his regular morning rounds. It had been twelve hours since he last saw her, and several hours since she had received an epidural block due to the pain of the extreme contractions.

In the morning, the monitor was still showing uterine hyperstimulation, but the obstetrician ordered Pitocin to further stimulate labor—adding insult to injury. Though the monitor's printout strip clearly shows many hours of uterine hyperstimulation, the condition was never recorded in the patient's chart. Every time staff looked at the electronic fetal monitor strip, they recorded the baby's heart rate, but never the other line on the strip, the uterine contractions.

That evening, the obstetrician came in, cut Ms. M's vagina open with an episiotomy, put a vacuum cup on top of the baby's head, and pulled the baby out. The baby came out completely floppy and didn't breathe for the first five minutes. The staff put the baby on a breathing machine. In the first few hours after birth, the baby developed seizures and had to be transferred to a larger hospital with an intensive care unit for newborns. There, specialists diagnosed severe brain damage due to lack of oxygen during labor and birth.

In spite of excellent care at the newborn intensive care unit and wonderful continuing care from a host of health care workers provided by the state of Idaho, the baby now has severe cerebral palsy and severe mental retardation. The family, with lots of support from the local community, provides loving care for this child, a twenty-four-hour-per-day effort. Because the family could not possibly pay for all the care required for this child, they sued the obstetrician and his partner. As is typical in Cytotec cases, they received a large settlement before the case ever came to trial. (See chapter 7.) It is clear that a jury would not be sympathetic to the defense after hearing that Ms. M was given a drug that says on the label that it should never be given to pregnant women, and then was not adequately monitored after the drug was administered.

This story has many elements that are common in Cytotec induction cases gone bad. The drug was used for convenience, not because of medical need. The parents were not adequately informed of the risks. The obstetrician was absent for many hours during the labor. The obstetrician and other staff failed to recognize when the uterus was hyperstimulated. The excessive painful contractions led to an epidural block. And then Pitocin was added to the mix. Finally, the baby was pulled out by vacuum extraction.

Another undesirable consequence of drug-induced labor is a higher chance that a C-section will be performed.[18] As we saw in chapter 3, all such "surgical" interventions have increased risks for both the woman and her baby. Scientific evidence has proven again and again that although careful, judicious, clearly medically indicated use of obstetric interventions saves a few women's lives, the increasing use of these interventions and technologies beyond this minimal optimal level is not saving more women's lives but is doing the opposite—leading to an increase in maternal mortality. The increasing induction rates in the United States partly explain the rising C-section rate, which, in turn, is partly responsible for the rising rate of maternal mortality.

One way obstetricians who use Cytotec for induction try to justify their choice is by quoting data that scientists know to be inadequate. The studies they quote have several fatal flaws in their methodology. However, as I've said, the single greatest weakness in the evidence they cite is that not one study is large enough to have sufficient statistical power in calculating the risk rate of less common but catastrophic occurrences such as uterine rupture and death. That is why the Cochrane Library still maintains today that we do not know enough about the risks of induction with Cytotec to recommend its use.

A brief look at the two papers some obstetricians cite as evidence that Cytotec induction is safe will illustrate that the data is being misinterpreted and that the heavy bias of the authors invalidates their conclusions. The first paper is a review by Goldberg and colleagues that was published in the *New England Journal of Medicine*. As a review, it is an attempt to survey other published reports on induction with Cytotec. The first problem is that the authors greatly confuse the reader by lumping together all uses of Cytotec during pregnancy, including its use in medical abortion early in pregnancy, its use for labor induction, and its use to treat postpartum hemorrhage (bleeding after the baby is born). When the review claims that it evaluates 200 studies involving a total of more than 16,000 women, it is falsely inflating the data.[19] Each of the situations just listed has different indications, benefits, and risks, and the data should never be combined.

Of the studies on using Cytotec to induce labor at the end of pregnancy, many are not randomized experimental trials (the most reliable scientific method for evaluating drugs) and all, including those that are trials, are far too small. With one or two exceptions, the studies all involve fewer than 1,000 women, and most of them involve fewer than 400 women, but it would take a sample of at least 3,000 women to reliably investigate the risk of an adverse outcome such as uterine rupture. After lumping together all Cytotec data, the review goes on to say that prescribing a medication for an off-label indication is common in the treatment of pregnant women, as if this were a justification, when it is actually an indictment of obstetric practice. Doing something often does not prove that it's a good idea—a lot of banks are robbed, but that doesn't make it a good idea. The authors try to justify ignoring the FDA by saying that off-label use (i.e., not FDA-approved use) is not considered experimental if based on sound scientific evidence. Essentially, what they are saying is that it's okay for obstetricians to experiment on women without their knowledge or consent if they have good scientific data that it's safe. But if doctors already have good data, they don't need to experiment on patients. Furthermore, if there were good scientific data, the drug would have been approved by the FDA. So this is catch-22 nonsense. The whole purpose of the FDA is to guarantee the consumer that on-label use of approved drugs is backed by sound scientific evidence. And the best scientific opinion has been saying for ten years that we still don't have "sound scientific evidence" on the risks of Cytotec induction.

The paper by Goldberg and colleagues goes on at length documenting the efficacy of induction with Cytotec, but, again, no one is debating whether the drug works. The debate is over the risks, and here the authors admit that the relative risk of rare adverse outcomes with the use of misoprostol (Cytotec) for labor induction *remains unknown.* So the authors themselves never say that this drug is safe for induction and they admit that we do not know enough about the risks. Then, in the very next paragraph, they go on to recommend its use for induction, having just admitted that the risk of "rare adverse outcomes" (meaning uterine rupture, AFE, and fetal and maternal death) is unknown. Incredible. The paper also uses the word *safe,* but if we don't know the risk of these tragic outcomes, what can we say about safety?

As discussed earlier, there are prominent groups, such as the Cochrane Library, that disagree with the authors' conclusion that it's okay to use Cytotec for induction of labor at the end of pregnancy. When experts disagree on the evidence, the prudent course for doctors is to follow the fundamental principle of all medical practice: first, do no harm.

A fundamental obstetric attitude is revealed in this paper by Goldberg and colleagues. Is a new drug or intervention considered unsafe until proven safe (precautionary approach) or, as clearly illustrated in this paper, considered safe until proven unsafe (anti-precautionary or vigilante approach)? These are two diametrically opposed approaches to the introduction of new interventions in medical practice. The Goldberg and colleagues review—and most of obstetric practice in the United States—clearly uses the anti-precautionary or vigilante approach of assuming that something is safe, calling it safe in published articles, and using it until something happens that proves it to be unsafe.

The precautionary principle used in science states: "When an activity raises threats of harm in human health, precautionary measures should be taken even if some cause-and-effect relationships are not fully established scientifically."[20] This means that the burden is on those introducing a new technology to prove it safe, not on the rest of us to prove it harmful. This principle is based on the same assumptions as in courts of law. Society balances a trial in favor of the defendant because convicting an innocent person is far worse than failing to convict someone who is guilty. In the same way, we should balance decisions on risks in favor of safety, especially where the damage, should it occur, is serious and irreparable.

And the anti-precautionary principle? According to Peter Saunders, a professor of mathematics at Kings College, London, and a pioneer in the precautionary principle, using the anti-precautionary principle means that when a new technology is being proposed, it must be permitted unless it can be shown beyond a reasonable doubt that it is dangerous. The burden of proof is not on the innovator, it is on the rest of us. Those who accept this anti-precautionary principle and pursue vigilante practices push forward with untested, inadequately researched technologies and insist that it is up to the rest of us to prove them dangerous before they can be stopped, and, furthermore, the perpetrators refuse to accept liability if the technology turns out to be hazardous.[21] Advocates of the anti-precautionary principle—such as Goldberg and colleagues—do not wait for a new drug or intervention to be proven safe through experimental trials; rather, they assume it is safe and continue to do so until someone proves it to be unsafe.

This is what happened with Cytotec induction of VBAC in the 1990s and with all the earlier obstetric tragedies mentioned in chapter 3. A concrete example illustrates that obstetricians—including an academic obstetrician in a prestigious university hospital—see no problem with the anti-precautionary approach, even when it results in tragedy. Yale–New Haven University Hospital was among the earliest to use Cytotec induction even when not part of formally approved research trials. In the mid-1990s, an assistant professor there was asked to develop a protocol for misoprostol (Cytotec) induction and he wrote such a protocol after talking with others around the country. He believed that it was okay to use a drug off-label based only on the experience of others and without experimental data—anti-precautionary.

Then in 1998, a woman at the Yale–New Haven hospital with a previous C-section died following Cytotec induction of labor. During a subsequent legal deposition, this same physician testified that if the data on the risks with VBAC had been available in 1998, obstetricians at the hospital would not have used misoprostol for induction, showing no apparent concern about using a drug when no data are yet available. He testified that there were no data out there in 1998 demonstrating that induction with misoprostol was more dangerous in VBAC than in other births. He then admitted that since that time, data have been published that show that it is more dangerous. He argued that since in 1998 there was nothing "out there" to suggest that misoprostol induction of VBAC was dangerous, it was okay to induce VBAC using it. He insisted that you must have a suspicion of a risk in order to study it—a classic anti-precautionary position.

This case, as well as many other examples discussed in this book, leaves no doubt that the anti-precautionary or vigilante principle is widely used and accepted in U.S. obstetrics today. But the fundamental principles of medical practice and of drug assessment operate on the precautionary approach—first, do no harm; assume a new drug may not be safe; and do not approve its use until it is proven safe. How did the obstetric profession come to follow the opposite principles?

The second paper some obstetricians rely on to justify Cytotec induction of labor is a meta-analysis by Sanchos-Ramos and colleagues.[22] First, even when adding up eight small trials, the combined sample size of experimental subjects is 966 (488 recipients of the drug and 478 controls). As indicated earlier, in order to have sufficient statistical power to determine the risk of rare but very serious adverse outcomes such as uterine rupture, AFE, perinatal mortality, and maternal mortality, the minimum sample size would have to be at least three times as large as this. Furthermore, some of the individual trials included in the analysis had extremely small sample sizes (four had a total sample size of less than one hundred), and these tiny trials cannot be expected to have a high level of individual validity.

An equally serious flaw in this meta-analysis is the wide variation in methodology among the eight trials on elements such as dose of the drug, dose interval, definition of controls, and indications for induction, which make it impossible to add the results together. What the authors of this meta-analysis have done is the equivalent of adding up apples, oranges, and bananas.

It appears that the authors do not understand the basic scientific flaws in this meta-analysis, as the paper concludes: "Published data confirm the safety and efficacy of intravaginal misoprostol as an agent for cervical ripening and labor induction."[23] The fact that some obstetricians accept this faulty study and that those who peer-reviewed the paper did not mention the problems with it is perhaps even more disappointing.

When I was a medical student and then a young practicing doctor, I believed that the highest quality of medical care was found in medical schools and university hospitals. Because research is conducted there, it seemed logical to assume that these institutions would have a serious investment in evidence-based practice. But the Yale–New Haven and UCLA hospitals were among the first to use Cytotec induction, and not as part of formally approved research trials. This is bad, because it demonstrates to medical students and doctors in training that it's okay to use drugs for conditions that are contraindicated on the label. It promotes vigilante medical practice among those who are most vulnerable to influence. In South Carolina in 2000, a woman died after Cytotec induction, and when the young obstetrician who had given it to her was asked why he did it, he replied that he had been taught to use Cytotec for induction just a year or two before while in training in obstetrics at the University of Maryland Hospital.

In August 2000, a Cytotec drama was played out that raised the situation to a new level of hypocrisy. By this time, the FDA and Searle Pharmaceutical had received so many reports of women and babies dying after induction with Cytotec that Searle, working closely with the FDA and with the FDA's encouragement, sent a letter of warning to all health care providers in the United States. After reminding doctors that giving the drug by any method to women who are pregnant is contraindicated, the letter went on to say, "Serious adverse events that have been reported following off-label use of Cytotec in pregnant women include maternal or fetal death, uterine hyperstimulation or rupture or perforation requiring uterine surgical repair, hysterectomy or salpingo-oophorectomy [surgical removal of the uterus or ovaries], amniotic fluid embolism, severe vaginal bleeding, retained placenta, shock, fetal bradycardia and severe pelvic pain." This is a horrendous list of risks, and ACOG, as well as the many obstetricians using Cytotec for induction of labor, were very upset with the letter. Instead of taking the message to heart, however, they launched a spin campaign. The letter put them in danger of severe criticism and great vulnerability to litigation. They had to neutralize it.

First, in October 2000, ACOG wrote a letter to the FDA (and sent a press release to the media) saying that the vast majority of adverse effects reported to Searle and the FDA were the result of the drug not being used correctly. The doses were too high or too frequent, or Pitocin was given too soon afterward, or the drug was given to women who had had too many babies or had had previous C-sections. Needless to say, ACOG did not present any data to back up this claim, as there is very little systematic data on the practice of induction of labor with Cytotec. ACOG did not indicate that the organization's leadership had seen the adverse reports sent to the FDA and Searle, nor did it acknowledge the many cases where there were bad outcomes that did not fit into a high-risk category (such as the case of Ms. S, recounted at the beginning of this chapter). Finally, their implication that Cytotec induction is safe if used correctly was not backed up with scientific evidence, as there has been no trial large enough to prove such a statement.

Then, in November 2000, ACOG sent a "citizen petition" to the FDA demanding that the FDA require Searle to withdraw its letter. In this petition, ACOG went so far as to imply that Searle's letter to doctors was motivated by something other than regard for the safety of women and babies, saying, "ACOG is concerned about the content, timing and tone of this [Searle's] letter." The petition went on to accuse Searle of being less concerned about the use of Cytotec for labor induction than its use together with RU-486 in medical abortion early in pregnancy. There was no evidence to support this accusation that Searle was playing abortion politics, and, in reality, it was ACOG that was introducing abortion into the discussion.

The FDA did not demand that Searle retract the letter, so the campaign continued. Two months later, in January 2001, ACOG wrote an editorial that was published in the same issue of the *New England Journal of Medicine* as the biased and flawed review of Cytotec induction by Goldberg and colleagues critiqued earlier. In its editorial, ACOG calls the article "an excellent review," further demonstrating the organization's inability to recognize faulty science, and then complains bitterly that Searle made its letter public without first consulting ACOG. The source of the organization's bitterness was that the Searle letter had the intended effect. As explained in the editorial, "The [Searle] letter did provoke a response from many hospital attorneys, administrators, and pharmacies—an automatic refusal to allow misoprostol (Cytotec) to be dispensed or used." Some hospitals (but certainly not all) stopped using Cytotec for induction out of fear of litigation. The editorial ends by begging Searle and the FDA to retract the Searle letter.[24]

Searle has never retracted its letter, but the use of Cytotec continued. In April 2002, the FDA made another effort to stem the tide and published a statement saying that of course it was aware that Cytotec was being used off-label for labor induction and, if you are to use it, for God's sake don't ever use it on certain extremely high-risk women.[25] This statement is not a form of FDA approval of Cytotec induction under any circumstances (high-risk or not), but, predictably, many obstetricians now claim that, with this statement, the FDA approved Cytotec induction.

As an example of how badly misinformed some prominent obstetricians are about Cytotec and how this can lead to false information getting to the public, on May 6, 2004, the CBS affiliate in San Francisco, on its evening news (I-Team) aired a segment on Cytotec. While preparing the segment, CBS interviewed Dr. Ben Sachs, chief of obstetrics at Beth Israel Hospital in Boston, who said that Cytotec had been approved for induction of labor at term by the FDA in 2002. Because I already had been interviewed for the same program and had told the journalist that the drug was not approved by the FDA for this purpose, CBS contacted the FDA and was told that Cytotec had never been approved by the FDA for labor induction. So the news segment begins with Dr. Sachs saying that Cytotec is approved by the FDA, and then a few minutes later in the same segment, Dr. Sachs is told that the FDA had just told CBS that it is not approved and the journalist then asks Dr. Sachs if he still thinks it is approved and he responds: "As far as I know, that is the case." He won't back down on camera even when presented with the facts. The public should never receive such misinformation.

Because such a misunderstanding appears to be common among obstetricians, a meeting was held at the FDA offices in late 2004 (which I attended) to discuss methods the FDA might employ to more clearly inform both doctors and the public that the FDA does not approve Cytotec induction. As a result of this meeting, the FDA put an item on its Web site in May 2005 clearly explaining that it has not approved Cytotec for the induction of labor and urging any physician who uses Cytotec on a pregnant woman to fully inform her of the risks, including uterine rupture.

Try to imagine how many hours and how much money ACOG has spent trying to get the FDA to approve Cytotec for labor induction. If the FDA would only approve it, ACOG could finally recommend it and satisfy its members. All this effort, and yet there has been no carefully controlled study showing that it saves lives. On the contrary, the FDA and Searle continue to receive reports of women and babies dying from Cytotec induction. ACOG's campaign to win approval for the use of Cytotec for induction is baffling, but at least it does serve the organization's primary purpose, protecting the interests of members. (It certainly does *not* serve ACOG's secondary purpose, promoting better health for women and babies.) What is even more baffling, however, is why obstetricians would *want* to use this drug for induction. For those cases where there is a solid medical reason for inducing labor, there are several other drugs that have been adequately studied and are FDA-approved for that use. There is no urgent need to use Cytotec, and yet doctors want to use it, so ACOG must campaign to get it approved for this use.

An often overlooked issue with Cytotec induction cases that precipitate litigation is whether or not the woman has been told the whole truth about the drug and asked to give her consent before it is administered. In the sixteen cases with which I am familiar where Cytotec induction led to an adverse outcome and litigation—cases where the outcomes included brain-damaged babies, dead babies, dead mothers, or a combination of these—the day the family discovered that the drug was not approved by the FDA for labor induction was the day they picked up the phone and called a lawyer.[26]

On the *Dateline NBC* television program on Cytotec that aired in November 2001, when the obstetrician representing ACOG was asked: "Does the doctor tell the pregnant woman [getting the drug for induction] 'just so you know, this drug is not FDA-approved for this purpose'?" he replied, "A doctor has to exercise his or her own discretion in deciding just how much the patient needs to know about specific approval by the FDA." This attitude is patronizing—as your doctor, I will decide what you, the patient, need to know. This is not fully informed choice but "selective informed choice." Legislation in nearly every state requires that informed choice in medical practice be inclusive of all known facts, and the FDA strongly recommends that patients receiving drugs be fully informed.

The decision to induce labor is not one that should be taken lightly. To quote a highly respected obstetric textbook: "*The decision to bring pregnancy to an end is one of the most drastic ways of intervening in the natural process of pregnancy and childbirth* [emphasis mine]. The reasons given for elective delivery (which may be achieved either by inducing labor or by elective cesarean section) range from the life-saving to the trivial. There has been very little methodologically sound research on the indications for elective delivery."[27]

There are certain specific conditions under which inducing labor has been shown to save lives—serious intrauterine growth retardation (the baby is too small for its gestational age), documented placental malfunction (the placenta is losing its ability to adequately nourish the fetus), and deteriorating preeclampsia (a serious condition with rising blood pressure).[28]

"Macrosomia" (the baby is too big) has also been used as an excuse for induction, but data do not support this. Instead, research shows that more C-sections are performed when labor is induced in cases of macrosomia, with no improvement in perinatal outcomes. Indeed, induction in this situation is contraindicated, as trying to hammer out a too large baby can harm the baby.[29]

Having the bag of waters break before labor begins means that the baby and the womb are no longer protected from germs and infection may occur (a condition known as premature rupture of membranes or PROM), but there is disagreement about how long it is safe to wait for spontaneous labor once the waters have broken. The consensus used to be twelve hours, then twenty-four hours, and now studies show that under certain conditions, it is safe to go forty-eight hours or longer if there are no signs of infection. (Several prospective studies have shown that practicing "expectant management"—that is, administering antibiotics immediately and waiting for labor to begin spontaneously—does not increase the risk of infection.)[30] However, even if we add PROM to the list of indications for inducing labor, the indications still apply to only a small percentage of pregnancies.

The big debate today regarding inducing labor surrounds "post-term" pregnancies, or rather the point at which we can say that a pregnancy has gone too far beyond the normal due date of forty weeks' gestation. Of course, birth can never be predicted down to a specific day. Rather, an estimate is made of the expected due date (EDD), based on the last menstrual period and/or ultrasound scans during the pregnancy, and the expectation is that the birth will happen *around* that time. Spontaneous birth between thirty-eight weeks and forty-two weeks is a perfectly normal variation. There is normal variation found with all biological events. In the case of human childbirth, the normal variation is two weeks on either side of the EDD, and babies born in this time period have no increased risks.

A study published in 1963, using data from 1958, found that the number of babies who died in the uterus before birth increased slightly after forty-two weeks and then increased significantly after forty-three weeks.[31] After this study, there was a trend toward inducing labor if a pregnancy went more than forty-two weeks. However, only about 3 percent of pregnancies go beyond forty-two weeks. If we add "post-term" pregnancies to the list, that brings the total of scientifically valid medical indications for labor induction up to around 10 percent. Interestingly, that is just about what the rate was in the United States until about fifteen years ago, and it is also what the induction rate is now in many industrialized countries with excellent birth outcomes.

Induction is a good example of an unfortunate characteristic of obstetric practice—a bandwagon effect whereby doctors jump on and the wagon gets going faster and faster, until everyone is afraid to get off. In 1982 and again in 1989, sound research was published that found no significant increase in neonatal mortality rates after forty-two weeks and only a slight increase after forty-three weeks, but the induction bandwagon didn't slow down at all, it just kept going faster and faster.[32]

In 1996, a valid study was published that looked at 1,800 postdate pregnancies (pregnancies that went beyond forty-two weeks) and found no increase in baby deaths as well as no increase in complications compared with births of babies born "on time" at between thirty-eight and forty-two weeks.[33] But the bandwagon kept right on rolling. Small studies that show that inducing postdate pregnancies, rather than simply waiting for labor to begin spontaneously, resulted in slightly fewer C-sections are frequently quoted as a reason to induce, but these studies do not show that induction reduces the numbers of dead or damaged babies, only that it lowers the C-section rate slightly. (The risks of induction are generally understood to be less than the risks of C-section, so these studies are used to justify induction.)

Induction reveals another characteristic of obstetric practice as well—a fear factor that often leads to a creeping overreaction in obstetricians. There seems to be a belief that if a little bit helps, a whole lot is even better. Induction was first done only at forty-three weeks' gestation, but before long it was being done at forty-two weeks, and now it is creeping to forty-one weeks. Now we're in big trouble, because forty-one weeks is entirely within normal pregnancy limits, and when we start inducing at forty-one weeks, we put large numbers of normal pregnancies at risk with an unnecessary procedure. At this point we have a situation in which the treatment is worse than the disease.

The truth is that only about 10 percent of babies at more than forty-three weeks' gestation get into trouble, but instead of treating these cases appropriately, we now induce labor long before the pregnancy gets to forty-three weeks with a powerful drug that has serious risks for both the woman and the baby. In investigating litigated cases of a baby or a woman dying as a result of an induction, it is common to find "postdate" on the woman's chart as the indication for induction. When we look more closely at the chart, however, it is common to discover that the pregnancy was not postdate at all but was only at 41 ½ weeks or even 40 ½ weeks. Claiming that the pregnancy was postdate allowed the doctor to do the induction he almost certainly wanted to do anyway for his own convenience.

When an obstetrician sets out to convince a pregnant woman to consent to an induction, he is almost always successful. All he has to do is communicate his own fears by conveying directly and indirectly all that might go wrong with a natural birth. The baby might suddenly die in the uterus. The baby's heart might suddenly stop. All these tests we're doing are to make sure that the baby is okay. When the woman is finally asked to sign an informed consent form, the form is likely to list every disaster that might happen if the induction is *not* done, but it does not list every disaster that could result from doing the induction.

So when the doctor suggests induction, the idea is appealing to the woman because it appears to end a dangerous situation for the baby—remaining in the womb. Women are rarely told that every day the baby remains in the uterus, it grows bigger and stronger and becomes less likely to develop complications during the birth. They are rarely told that a woman's body knows when the baby is ready. Women are not told that only 3 percent of pregnancies, if left alone, will go beyond forty-two weeks and that only 10 percent of those babies past forty-three weeks get into trouble—10 percent of 3 percent = 0.3 percent of babies will get into trouble.

Yet in the United States we are inducing labor in more than 40 percent of all pregnancies. It's like taking a baseball bat to a mosquito. The obstetrician's fear that a pregnancy will have trouble if it goes "too long" dovetails nicely with the great convenience of being able to schedule an induction.

As mentioned earlier, a Maternity Center Association survey found that in 2004 we were inducing labor in 44 percent of births. If we add to this the 16 percent of cases in which drugs are used to stimulate or speed up a labor that has already started (augmentation), the total number of pregnancies in which powerful and dangerous drugs are used is 60 percent, or nearly two-thirds of all births.[34] It is ridiculous to think that two-thirds of American women have such lousy uteruses that they must be whipped into shape with drugs in order to have babies.

The widespread use of Cytotec for labor induction without adequate evaluation appears to be impervious to the usual methods of quality control in health care. The FDA, the pharmaceutical industry, scientific opinion, and peer review have all failed to significantly slow down, much less stop the Cytotec epidemic. That leaves two last methods of quality control—educating the public and litigation.

At this stage, it is very important to discuss Cytotec induction in the media. Women and families need to know the truth about this drug, so they can "just say no" when an obstetrician offers it.[35] But there has been little or no information made available to the public, in large part owing to "tribal loyalties" among doctors. Many obstetricians are aware of the problems with Cytotec, but they will not speak out in public. Most give journalists the "party line" about how good the drug is. Investigative reporting has become essential in protecting women and babies from dangerous obstetric practices. Already one national television network in the United States has done a program on induction with Cytotec, as has a national

Canadian network, and several regional affiliates have reported on the issue. Highly critical newspaper, magazine, and Internet articles have appeared as well.[36] Let's hope that our media will continue to spread the word and that eventually their efforts will result in changes.

Litigation can also have an effect on the Cytotec problem, but almost all Cytotec cases are settled out of court and the settlements include gag orders, so the public never hears about them. Of course, insurance companies, hospitals, and pharmaceutical companies do hear about the big settlements. Their initial response is to rush to their political friends and try to lobby the government to cap malpractice awards or limit the right of patients and families to sue. But it is only a matter of time before hospitals and insurance companies will begin to put pressure on doctors not to use a drug that is not approved by the FDA and could end up costing them lots of money in litigation. In chapter 7 we will look further at the important role "drug regulation by litigation" plays in our society.

In the United States, many obstetricians have no faith in democratic institutions such as the FDA. They express disdain for the public realm and contempt for any attempts to monitor, much less regulate, their practices. Their attitude reveals a desire to go it alone that, when combined with decades of a reactionary approach to medical care, undermines the social contract between doctor and patient. It is an underlying problem that touches many areas of American reproductive life.

Most obstetricians are also gynecologists, and the hot new field in gynecology—artificial reproduction (in vitro fertilization, etc.)—is also full of hype, false promises, and malpractice.[37] Every other industrialized country has found it necessary to develop government regulations around artificial reproductive services. But in the United States, after congressional hearings, regulations were adopted for the laboratories used by the reproductive services, but the clinical part of the practice, the part that involves gynecologists, was left unregulated, even though that is where malpractice is rampant.

American medical practice overall has far and away the least amount of regulation of any country in the world—making it fertile ground for vigilante practice. Not only do many of our doctors lack faith in democratic institutions, so do many of their patients—the American public. Health care consumers in the United States are generally timid and have been quick to acquiesce to doctors' complaints of encroachment by HMOs and government, allowing the tyranny of an obstetric monopoly to continue. They put physicians on a pedestal because they need to believe that doctors can help them when they're sick, and as a result, doctors believe that they are above the law. These attitudes create an environment where vigilante practice is possible, and nowhere is this more apparent than in the use of drugs and technology by American obstetricians.

In the United States, the obstetric establishment is powerful and the government regulatory bureaucracy is too weak to stand up to pressure from the pharmaceutical industry, the insurance industry, and the medical industry (doctors and hospitals). The results are underregulated drugs, a lack of safety studies and studies of questionable quality, seduced or sleepy media, and underinformed women and families. We must do all we can to turn this around. On a grassroots level, there are encouraging signs, such as several Internet support groups formed by women who have suffered from uterine rupture and survived. One has more than 350 members.[38] The question now is: How many women and babies will have to die or be damaged before the tragic practice of inducing labor unnecessarily is ended?

FIVE **HUNTING WITCHES:** MIDWIFERY IN AMERICA

Because the midwives feared God, they did not do as commanded by the king.
EXODUS 1:17

A midwife is lectured at by committees, scolded by matrons, sworn at by surgeons, bullied by surgical dressers, talked flippantly to if middle aged and good humored, seduced if young.
"THE TIMES," LONDON, 1857

After working as a practicing physician for several years, I became a perinatologist and perinatal scientist, as well as a full-time faculty member at the Schools of Medicine and Public Health at UCLA. Then I became a director of maternal and child health for the California State Health Department. In that capacity, I learned that in the rural town of Madera, California, doctors had decided that they no longer wanted to attend births in the Madera County hospital. They complained that it took too much of their time and didn't pay enough. So in 1968, two out-of-state midwives were recruited by the county to fill the gap. After two years of midwifery practice at the hospital, the rate of babies dying around the time of birth in the Madera County hospital was cut in half. Alarmed that their style of maternity care was being made to look bad, the doctors in town agreed that they would once again attend births in the hospital if the two midwives were fired. The hospital fired the midwives, the doctors returned, and soon the rate of babies dying around birth rose to its earlier higher levels.[1]

This natural experiment comparing the safety of doctors and midwives left me confused and full of questions, because, in spite of my years of experience as a physician, I had no real knowledge of midwifery. Who are these midwives? How are they trained? Could it be that, as seen in Madera County, they are generally safer birth attendants than doctors? Through no fault of their own, Americans, including obstetricians, have little understanding of midwifery. In the early years of the twentieth century, a witch-hunt against midwives in the United States and Canada resulted in the elimination of midwifery as a legitimate health profession. The profession has gained ground in the last two decades, but most people today have no personal experience with midwives and have been exposed to considerable misinformation about midwifery.

From California I left for Europe, where I joined the staff of the World Health Organization (WHO). There I was exposed to the essential role midwives play in maternity care in other highly industrialized countries and in developing countries. I also learned much about the profession, including the fact that in every other highly industrialized country, midwives are highly valued health care professionals.

Throughout history, there have always been women in the community to whom other women can turn for support with women's concerns—not just reproductive health care but also issues such as spousal abuse. The word *midwife* is early English for "with woman." The French word for midwife, *sage femme* (wise woman), goes back thousands of years, as do the words in Danish, *jordmor* (earth mother), and in Icelandic, *ljosmodir* (mother of light).

Hippocrates formalized a midwifery training program in Greece in the fifth century BC. Phaenarete, the mother of Socrates, was a midwife. In the Bible, the Book of Exodus recognized the strength and independence of midwives who defied the Pharaoh's command that they kill all sons born to Hebrew women. The first law to regulate midwifery in Europe was passed in Germany in 1452 and required a midwife to be in attendance at all births. Since then, every little girl in Europe has grown up with the understanding that if she has a baby, she will have a midwife to assist her.

When Europeans migrated to the New World, midwives were among them. In the mid-1600s, the king of France commissioned midwives and sent them to practice in New France (now Canada). The British government also paid for the services of midwives in the New World, including in the American colonies. Midwives were a valued part of the developing health care system in colonial times and by the mid-1880s they were teaching medical students in at least one university.[2]

As the number of physicians increased in the United States, medical doctors attempted to monopolize health care through state medical practice acts that defined health care parameters, including who can practice.

By the end of the nineteenth century, it was common for midwives to be accused of witchcraft and tried in court, and midwifery practice began to disappear. The case of Hanna Porn was one of the most famous and had far-reaching consequences. In Gardner, Massachusetts, in 1909, a judge sentenced forty-eight-year-old Hanna to three months in the House of Corrections. Her crime? She was a practicing midwife.[3] An immigrant from Finland, Hanna Porn served primarily Finnish and Swedish laborers' wives. Fewer than half as many of the babies whose births she attended died as babies whose births were attended by local physicians. But the Massachusetts Supreme Judicial Court used her case to rule that midwifery was illegal in Massachusetts, based on the testimony of physicians who said that midwives were incompetent. In 1910, an attempt was made to reestablish midwifery by opening a school of midwifery in Massachusetts, but the idea was defeated by opposition from nurses as well as physicians. Other states quickly followed suit and made midwifery illegal, and it remained illegal in nearly all states for more than fifty years, until nurse-midwifery began to be legalized.

What is it about the practice of midwifery that attracts so much hostility and criticism? There are several excellent books that explore this question.[4] The overarching issue is simply that midwives have always been at the center of the "woman's world"—that part of life and society that women have some control over, and from which men tend to be excluded, including, until recently, pregnancy and childbirth. The profession has always attracted strong, independent women in the community, woman who are difficult for men to control and whom some men come to fear. If men wish to control their women, they must find a way to control midwives. When physicians (who until fifty years ago were almost all men) began to practice maternity care, they found themselves competing directly with midwives for pregnant clients. Even nurses (who until recently were all women) supported the medical domination of maternity care, because nurses have always been controlled by doctors and they believed that their jobs depended on keeping doctors happy.

Despite this attempt to dismantle the profession in the United States and Canada, midwifery continued to thrive in Europe and other parts of the world. And while the profession was severely hampered in the United States for decades, it was not stamped out. Throughout history, every attempt at ending the practice of midwifery has failed. It seems that there will always be women who want to be midwives and women who want midwives to attend them when they give birth.

When officially sanctioned midwifery was attacked in the United States, midwives went underground. Women who became known as "granny midwives" (because they tended to be older) continued to practice, especially in poor communities. In the 1920s, Mary Breckenridge, a public health nurse, decided first to get training in midwifery and then to form the Frontier Nursing Service to serve families in the Appalachian region of Eastern Kentucky. She wanted to improve the lives of poor children by providing maternity care to families in rural areas where there were no doctors. The organization included a central hospital with one physician and several nursing outposts and featured nurses on horseback, who were able to reach remote locations in all kinds of weather. Within five years, the Frontier Nursing Service provided care to more than one thousand families over seven hundred square miles. The staff formed the organization that later became the American Association of Nurse-Midwives, as well as the Frontier School of Midwifery and Family Nursing, which trained hundreds of women in what became a new profession in America, nurse-midwifery.

The number of nurse-midwives grew slowly but surely, and by 1977 the profession was licensed in every state. After nursing school, a nurse can elect to go on to midwifery school, a kind of graduate school, for about two years and become a nurse-midwife. This is not the same as becoming a labor and delivery nurse, a nursing specialization that has no training requirement and usually involves about six weeks of on-the-job training.

Women who want to be midwives and do not want to become nurses first can train as "direct-entry" midwives—that is, women who go directly to midwifery school without training first in nursing—a group that has also grown steadily in numbers and recognition. In 2006, the practice of direct-entry midwifery was legal in twenty-four states, "alegal" (that is, direct-entry midwives were allowed to practice without legal interference) in seventeen states, and explicitly illegal in only nine states. In the last decade, more and more states have been legalizing direct-entry midwifery, so the number of states in which direct-entry midwifery is legal can be expected to increase. The U.S. federal government recognizes the training for both nurse-midwives and direct-entry midwives and has authorized the Midwifery Education Accreditation Council to accredit midwifery schools and programs.

Despite the current renaissance of midwifery in the United States, the fact that midwives were harshly persecuted for more than a century has left the profession with a legacy of public reticence and confusion that must be overcome. Many myths surround midwives, myths that are often reinforced by obstetricians who view them as competition. One is that mid-wives are not trained but are "hippy-dippy" lay women who attend only home births. Another is that midwives are religious zealots or witches who use magical potions. That nurse-midwives attend births only in hospitals is a common misconception, as is the idea that a midwife is a second-class doctor for women who can't afford a real obstetrician. None of these ideas is remotely true. There are two excellent books by nurse-midwives that describe their home birth practices, and several organizations are working to educate the public about midwifery practice.[5] Scientific data (which will be discussed later in this chapter) have proven that for attending low-risk births (that is, births without complications), midwives are not second-class obstetricians, but rather obstetricians are second-class midwives.

Many American obstetricians are confused about midwives, as I was before I joined the WHO. During a recent panel discussion on a popular American television talk show, a practicing obstetrician said, "Midwives are obstetrician's assistants," another common myth. As a fellow panel member, I tried to correct his misperception. Because American obstetricians have always had nurses to do their bidding, including labor and delivery nurses, many of them believe that midwives are working for them. Even today, many obstetricians just don't get it. They try to boss midwives around, inviting them to join their practices and then cavalierly firing them, pushing them off of hospital staffs, accusing them of practicing medicine without a license, and so on. To avoid getting in the middle of this professional turf struggle, a pregnant woman must be prepared to do her own research, ask questions, and form her own opinions. One way to measure a particular doctor's openness and attitude toward women in general is simply to ask about the doctor's opinion of midwifery.

In reality, a nurse-midwife or direct-entry midwife transferring a laboring woman to an obstetrician is analogous to a family physician referring a patient to a specialist, such as a cardiologist. It does not mean that the family physician is the cardiologist's assistant or somehow less competent, only that the cardiologist has a different expertise than the family physician—an expertise in handling certain complications. It is no more appropriate for an obstetrician to give orders to a midwife than it is for a cardiologist to give orders to a family physician. The relationship should be an active collaboration based on mutual respect between health professionals of equal standing. In New Zealand, a midwife has the same rights and privileges as a family physician and receives the same flat fee for attending a birth that a doctor receives.

Though styles of practice vary among individuals, there are several general differences among the practices of nursing, midwifery, and medicine. Nursing means assisting doctors (and taking orders from doctors), though a nurse's focus is on caring for the needs of the patient rather than on medical diagnosis and treatment.

The scope of a midwife's practice is often defined by the setting or institution in which she practices. Midwifery can be limited to maternity care or it can be practiced more broadly as primary health care for women—that is, providing all basic health services related to a woman's gender, such as family planning, screening for cervical cancer, and treatment of reproductive tract infections.

That midwifery is much more than just catching babies was brought home to me when I visited Povungnituk, a tiny Inuit village on the far northern shore of Hudson Bay in Canada. For many years, the government of Canada had flown pregnant Inuit women a thousand miles south to give birth in a large hospital. This practice was destroying the Inuit culture, as it meant that the role of Inuit midwives was severely reduced and no babies were born on Inuit land. The Inuit people demanded to have their babies born in the far north, and finally their demand was met. The government sent two direct-entry midwives to Povungnituk to train Inuit women as midwives. When I visited a year later, the training midwives told me that although they were teaching only care during pregnancy and birth, the women of the village were spontaneously seeking out the Inuit midwives for help with all kinds of "women's problems," such as abusive husbands. They were once more the "wise women" of the village.

Generally speaking, a fundamental difference between midwifery care and physician care at birth has to do with control. Childbirth is a complicated physiological process regulated by the woman's nervous system. Childbirth is not under the conscious control of the woman giving birth, but rather is directed by hormones and neurological feedback systems that neither the woman nor someone assisting her can control. Labor is controlled by the parasympathetic portion of the autonomic nervous system, which is not under conscious control (intestinal mobility and sexual orgasm are other examples of physiological functions controlled by the parasympathetic nervous system). Anything that causes fear or alarm shuts down the parasympathetic system and fires up the sympathetic nervous system (adrenalin). Fear and anxiety stop intestinal mobility, stop any chance of orgasm, and stop labor. Any intervention that increases a laboring woman's fear or anxiety will interfere with, slow down, or even stop the birth processes.

A wise birth assistant, be it midwife, nurse, or doctor, knows how to facilitate these autonomic responses and not interfere with them. The key elements in the midwifery model of birth are normality, facilitation of natural processes (with minimal intervention, all evidence-based), and the empowerment of the birthing woman. Taking on the role of facilitator, midwives will typically reassure, calm, and encourage birthing women. Obstetricians, on the other hand, typically try to get the birth under their own control by overriding the natural processes with drugs and medical procedures and giving orders. The medical model and the midwifery model are essentially different paradigms or ways of looking at women and birth. Doctors "deliver" babies and believe that having a baby is something that *happens to* a woman. Midwives assist at birth and believe that giving birth is something that a woman *does.*

Midwives tend to believe that a woman giving birth needs to be the one making decisions about her birth experience. The woman giving birth needs to believe in her own body and feel responsible for her body, while at the same time letting go of the need to control what is happening, since she cannot. However, though a woman has decision-making authority when she hires a midwife, her authority may be challenged within a hospital setting. I know a midwife who puts a doorstop under the door when she is attending a client in a hospital. When a member of the hospital staff comes to the door, they find that the door won't open. The midwife calls, "Who is it?" and when the person outside the door—be it doctor, nurse, medical student, nursing student, or lab tech—identifies him- or herself, the midwife asks the birthing woman if she wants the person to come in. It is interesting that a two-dollar rubber doorstop can change who is in control of the situation, at least temporarily.

In reality, I have never seen a hospital where, on a day-to-day basis, the patient is truly "in control" or has final decision-making authority. At the end of the day, the doctor and the hospital will decide what will happen to the woman unless the woman is willing to insist on having some control and is willing to fight for it. (See chapter 7 for a discussion of patient rights.) Yes, by law, doctors must get their patients' informed consent before doing procedures, but there is a difference between giving consent and having control. Consent means that the patient accedes to what the doctor wants. That is not control. If an obstetrician tells a woman that, if she chooses, she may walk around early in her labor, that is not putting the woman in control, it is simply giving the woman permission to do what the doctor chooses. The doctor remains in control. A hospital is doctor territory and doctors will always fight to be in control, regardless of what they may tell their patients.

Another fundamental difference between midwives and doctors is how they view pregnancy and birth. Midwives understand that pregnancy is not an illness. They typically call the women in their care "clients," not "patients," since they are not sick and are not getting medical treatment. Though midwives know what can go wrong during pregnancy and birth and know how to identify problems early and to cooperate with doctors in managing complications, their focus is on birth as a life-enhancing experience. Although they believe it is essential to have medical assistance available when needed, they are trained to go beyond medical care and empower women to achieve their goals for themselves and their babies.

Obstetricians, on the other hand, tend to focus on what can go wrong during pregnancy and birth. All doctors have been trained to look for trouble (diagnose a problem) and decide what to do about it (decide on a treatment), and that is what comes naturally to obstetricians. In prenatal care they take the same approach, focusing on what can go wrong and ordering numerous testing and screening procedures. This attitude casts a shadow over the maternity care a woman receives. When an obstetrician runs a test or gives a preemptive treatment, it is an unspoken vote of no confidence in the woman's body. Although the occasional test is a good idea and sometimes a treatment is necessary, we've seen in earlier chapters that much of what obstetricians do to pregnant and birthing women is unnecessary and serves only to calm the doctor's own fears.

Midwives trust in women's bodies and their capacity to give birth successfully with little or no intervention in most cases. They are trained to express confidence in every way possible, thus modeling a positive attitude that is passed on to the woman herself and often results in an empowering birth experience. Since a birthing woman will be faced with the daunting task of rearing a child for the next twenty years, having confidence in herself and her abilities is vital.

Another important difference between midwife-attended low-risk birth and obstetrician-attended low-risk birth is the quality of the experience for the woman. Many surveys have shown that women who have midwives as their attendants have far higher levels of satisfaction with their birth experience than women who have obstetricians attending their births.[6] This is not hard to understand. Midwives give great attention to building close relationships with their clients and their clients' families. They spend an average of twenty-four minutes with a woman during each prenatal visit, compared with obstetricians, who spend ten minutes per visit on average.[7] If a woman decides to have a midwife as her birth attendant at a planned out-of-hospital birth, or selects one of the unusual midwives who works in the hospital but is not on an eight-hour shift, her attendant will probably be there continuously from the beginning of her labor until after the birth. If she has an obstetrician as her primary attendant, the doctor will pop in only from time to time—usually once every few hours. Between doctor visits, she'll have brief visits from one or more labor and delivery nurses (whom she probably has never met before), but again only from time to time.

Generally speaking, midwives are direct, open, and honest in their dealings with clients and take an egalitarian, intimate, woman-to-woman approach. Midwives do not guarantee a good outcome, and their honesty about their role and its limitations contributes to the level of satisfaction women feel with their services. On the other hand, in a doctor-patient relationship, there is no egalitarian tradition. Rather the doctor's superior knowledge and status are for the most part unquestioned and there is a belief (or hope) that the doctor can perform miracles.

After experiencing both the obstetric and the midwifery worlds for some years, I see a sharp contrast. Go to an obstetric meeting and you'll see serious faces, hierarchical maneuvering, obsequious behavior by lower-ranking medical students, interns, and obstetric residents, and condescension and occasional strutting by doctors in the higher ranks. It is not an exaggeration to describe most obstetric meetings as a celebration of self-importance and success. Casual talk runs to cars, boats, private planes, the evils of interference from managed-care organizations or government agencies, greedy lawyers, and how to make more money to pay for high malpractice premiums. Words that come to mind in such a setting are *hard, competitive, elitist, aggressive,* and *a man's world.* It's amazing to me that there are doctors who survive in this world and remain open and caring.

Go to a midwifery meeting, and you'll see women breast-feeding babies, kids running around, lots of laughter and warmth—a celebration of life, family, and birth. Casual talk runs to child rearing, long-suffering husbands, tricks of the trade, how obstetricians interfere with midwifery, and how to make enough money to pay the mortgage. Words that come to mind in that setting are *humble, warm, cooperative, we're all in the same leaky boat together,* and *a woman's world.*

Midwives, like doctors, are human. They have bad days and they make mistakes. Science now tells us, however, that overall midwives are safer than doctors for low-risk births. Of course, American obstetricians have worked hard to convince the public that they are the "safest" kind of professional to assist at *all* births, but the evidence simply does not support their position. A large study, published in 1998, looked at all births in the United States in one year—more than four million births. Because doctors really do need to manage the few births that develop serious complications (around 10 percent), the study eliminated these high-risk births, and looked only at low-risk births. Compared with physician-attended low-risk births, midwife-attended low-risk births have 33 percent fewer newborn infant deaths. Furthermore, midwife-attended low-risk births have 31 percent fewer babies born too small, which means fewer brain-damaged infants.[8] So if a woman is among the 80 to 90 percent of all women who have normal pregnancies, the safest attendant for her hospital birth is not a doctor but a midwife. In chapter 6, we will look closely at the scientific evidence on planned out-of-hospital births attended by midwives.

One of the primary reasons midwives are safer than doctors is that they use far fewer unnecessary interventions.[9] Obstetricians are surgeons, and their training leads them to turn birth into a surgical procedure. In earlier chapters I discussed some of the problems with the practice of putting a birthing woman on her back in a bed. High-tech birthing beds are really nothing more than modified surgical tables, where the surgical patient (a woman in labor) has her legs up in surgical stirrups. In this position, the baby's head compresses the woman's main blood vessel (aorta), reducing the blood and oxygen going to the womb and to the baby. When a woman is in a vertical position (sitting, squatting, or standing), more blood and oxygen gets to the baby, the woman's pelvis is more open to let the baby out, and the woman is giving birth downhill instead of uphill against gravity.[10] We've known for more than twenty-five years that a horizontal position is the worst possible position for a woman giving birth, but with obstetricians controlling maternity care, the practice continues. I've been telling women for years that an easy way to tell whether a hospital is practicing modern, evidence-based maternity care is simply to find out what position women are put in to give birth. If the hospital is still putting women on their backs (and elevating the head and shoulders does not make a difference), they are ignoring the scientific data, and it is a sign that the hospital is pretending that birth is a surgical procedure.

Another sign that American obstetricians have turned birth into a surgical event is the simple fact that between 60 and 80 percent of American births involve actual medical procedures—whether it's drugs to start or speed up labor, cutting the genitals to widen the vaginal opening, using metal forceps or a vacuum extractor to pull the baby out, or performing a cesarean section.[11] There is a need for these procedures in no more than 20 percent of all births, and in births where the midwife is the primary assistant they occur no more than 20 percent of the time.[12] And, as discussed in previous chapters, since all medical procedures carry risks, the high rate of unnecessary medical procedures in physician-attended births means more dead and damaged babies and women.

Midwives have good hands, and they know how to sit on them. Midwives use fewer interventions because they tend to trust women's bodies, favor low-tech assistance (such as skilled use of their hands), and pursue normalcy, while obstetricians in general trust drugs and machines more than bodies, use high-tech assistance, and focus on abnormality. One simple example: midwifery considers breech birth (cases where the baby's head is not first coming out of the vagina) a variation of normal, whereas obstetricians consider it an abnormality.

In the past two decades we've seen a renaissance of midwifery in the United States. Each year, the number of births attended by midwives increases. According to the CDC, in 2004, 10 percent of all births in the United States had a midwife as primary birth attendant, and in New Mexico it was 30 percent of all births.[13] Several large HMOs are hiring more midwives and some now have more midwives than obstetricians on staff.

Another group that has been attacked by doctors and hospital administrators who have very little understanding of what they do is doulas. Doulas are woman who provide support to birthing women. They receive professional training for this (like midwives, they are trained by apprenticeship and must pass an examination) and have knowledge of common birth procedures, as well as of problems that can come up. But doulas do not pretend to be nurses or midwives or doctors. They do not serve as the primary attendant at a birth. Their role is to offer loving support and practical help. Doulas work primarily in hospitals, although some also provide postpartum home care. As we've seen in earlier chapters, many labor and delivery wards in the United States are not particularly supportive places for women. Overworked nurses cannot provide continuous support, and when the birth attendant is supposed to be an obstetrician (as is the case in about 90 percent of births), and there is likely to be no one around, a doula can be a godsend. In fact, research clearly shows that the presence of a doula at a birth shortens the length of labor and reduces the number of complications.[14]

Nevertheless, by now I'm sure it will not surprise you to hear that many obstetricians don't like having doulas around. One of the things a doula does is to advocate for the laboring mother, who may be in pain and may not have the ability to ensure that her wishes are honored. For example, when a woman employs a doula, she will usually develop a written birth plan. The doula will be familiar with the plan, so when the obstetrician comes with scissors to do an episiotomy, it may be the doula who reminds the doctor that the birth plan specifies "no episiotomy." Although doulas are not generally legally persecuted, they must have thick skins, as doctors have been known to throw them out of the delivery room. Sadly, some hospitals forbid doulas from entering the hospital at all or develop protocols that doulas must follow that severely limit their role. Doulas must walk a fine line between supporting and protecting a woman giving birth and offending the hospital staff. Good luck.

The more the practice of midwifery grows and succeeds, the more threatening midwives are to the obstetric monopoly, so, predictably, there has been an obstetric backlash. Now, a hundred years after Hanna Porn was persecuted, we have another American witch-hunt against midwives. In many states, doctors are reporting midwives to various authorities as dangerous. In 1995, I wrote an article about this published in a prestigious medical journal, titled "A Global Witch Hunt," and the hunt is still on. No one knows how many midwives have actually been charged, but in 1995, I was aware of legal altercations involving more than 145 out-of-hospital midwives in thirty-six states.[15] In the past ten years, at least that many more midwives have been charged.[16]

The challenge faced by nurse-midwives, most of whom work in obstetricians' offices or in hospitals, is somewhat different but also daunting. During the latter part of the twentieth century, nurse-midwives were the first midwives to be recognized and accepted in the United States. In the beginning, they were tolerated by obstetricians because they were providing care in areas where no obstetrician wanted to go, such as Appalachia. Later they were seen as handy helpers who would do an obstetrician's bidding. Historically, accommodating obstetricians has been a central strategy for nurse-midwives. They are trying to live in a doctor's world and survive. But as more nurse-midwives are hassled by obstetricians, obstetric residents, and so on, and often eventually fired, they are beginning to realize the need to assert their independence.

In the past five years, most of the nurse-midwives in Austin and San Antonio, Texas, and most of the nurse-midwives in Cleveland, Ohio, were summarily fired—for no apparent reason other than that the hospitals where they worked said they needed to save money. This reason is hard to accept, given that midwives cost much less than obstetricians. One of the largest hospitals in New York City, Columbia Presbyterian, recently disallowed its midwives from attending births, and one of the largest hospitals in Washington, D.C., Georgetown University Hospital, recently fired all its nurse-midwives, again claiming it was for financial reasons. None of the nurse-midwives who were let go had been accused of malpractice or anything else. They were simply getting in the way of the obstetric monopoly.

Over time, the presence of nurse-midwives in hospitals has had both a positive and a negative influence on the midwifery profession. The good news is that they can provide midwifery care to women giving birth in hospitals, which is where most childbirth in America takes place. The bad news is that hospital-based nurse-midwives must struggle daily to practice real midwifery and to resist pressure from doctors to become "medwives" who accept the medical model of birth. Many nurse-midwives and labor and delivery nurses tell me that they prefer to work nights and weekends, because they feel they can give their patients better care when the doctors are not around.

Nurse-midwives are often victims of hospital politics, and those politics can become quite vicious. Here is a real-life illustration. A nurse-midwife was in independent practice in a large suburban private hospital in Washington State. A number of private practicing obstetricians worked in the same hospital. Many of these obstetricians had high intervention rates; several had 50 percent C-section rates, and one had a combined C-section plus forceps delivery plus vacuum extraction rate of 80 percent. By contrast, the nurse-midwife's practice was low-intervention, with less than 15 percent of births involving forceps, vacuum, or C-section. She had a good reputation in the community, and her practice was growing rapidly. The obstetricians in the hospital asked her to cut down on her practice, giving no reason although it was apparently out of fear of competition. She did not comply with their wishes.

Then a baby died under the nurse-midwife's care. In view of her large practice and the number of births she had attended—and in view of the usual perinatal mortality rate in that hospital and state—this was not unexpected. Ordinarily, a perinatal death in this hospital resulted in an internal review by a perinatal committee to determine if any serious mistakes had been made. But in this case, the nurse-midwife was immediately reported by the hospital to the state's Nursing Care Quality Assurance Commission.

There are three major issues with this referral to the state. First, the referral was made before the hospital had conducted an investigation—the nurse-midwife was considered guilty until proven innocent. Second, there were several perinatal deaths attended by obstetricians in this hospital the same year, and the obstetricians were not reported to the state, so it appeared to be a case of doctors and hospital administrators using selective reporting to the state for professional and personal gain. Finally, in Washington State, nurse-midwifery practice is monitored by nurses, not by nurse-midwives or other midwives, and there were no midwives on the Nursing Commission.

After making its report to the state Nursing Commission, the hospital searched through the nurse-midwife's patient charts looking for something with which to accuse her. As someone who has practiced medicine for many years, I know that no doctor, midwife, or nurse can survive such a fishing expedition unscathed.

Then two events took place further indicating that the hospital's complaint to the Nursing Commission was motivated by doctors' fear of competition. Before the hospital's investigation was completed, the obstetricians who had been providing backup to the nurse-midwife announced that they were withdrawing their backup. (As I have pointed out elsewhere, withdrawing backup is one of the most common ways obstetricians successfully eliminate competition from midwives.)[17] Then a new hospital brochure for the public was published before any investigation of the midwife had been completed that listed the maternity services staff, and the nurse-midwife's name had mysteriously disappeared.

Although the hospital completed its investigation of the nurse-midwife and found no malpractice, the hospital report nevertheless demanded that she get psychotherapy and stipulated that the hospital must have the opportunity to tell the therapist what was wrong with her. Her problem, in their view, was her insistence that she be treated as an equal. The doctors felt that this revealed her "inability to be a team player," a euphemism for not doing what she was told. (Many doctors love a team as long as they are the team leader.) Careful reading of the case makes it clear that there were two real problems: doctors who were afraid of the competition and a hospital staff that did not understand the role of nurse-midwives in maternity services. In the doctors' view, the nurse-midwife was not subservient and compliant enough, when in truth she correctly saw herself as a professional equal. She was practicing midwifery, which is not the practice of medicine.

In her practice, when nurses or doctors, misunderstanding what she was doing, had tried to prevent her from using her midwifery skills, she put the needs of the woman first and occasionally asserted her authority as the principle caregiver in a case. Long before the death and the legal case, the nurse-midwife had repeatedly expressed concern that the staff was not familiar enough with midwifery practice and had suggested staff training on the appropriate roles of maternity care professionals to improve their understanding, but no action was taken. Instead, she was told she needed psychotherapy. Labeling someone emotionally unbalanced and using psychotherapy as a tool to force compliance was a method used in the former Soviet Union. Even after years of experience in medicine, I was startled to find such draconian tactics in an American hospital.

In one of my papers on the midwife witch-hunt, I pointed out that in the United States, hospital and state quality assurance systems are increasingly used to punish deviance from the style of practice preferred by those in authority.[18] I suggested that abuses of the system can be identified by asking two questions: Is the complaint evidence-based? (That is, is it about a practice that has been determined to be faulty by scientific studies?) And are there clear professional (or nonprofessional) gains to be had by those making the complaint? In this case, the complaint was in no way evidence-based. Furthermore, the obstetricians in the hospital clearly had something to gain by complaining—a chance to maintain their monopoly in maternity services and a chance to maintain their hierarchical system among hospital staff. And, in this case, the obstetricians succeeded: the nurse-midwife was driven out. The nurse-midwife resigned and opened a home birth practice in the community with an obstetrician who was not practicing at her former hospital providing backup.

The nurse-midwife's decision to leave the hospital was a predictable outcome. I know of quite a few nurse-midwives who have gotten tired of the prejudice they face in hospitals and have moved into out-of-hospital practices, either working in a free-standing birth center or attending home births. However, even moving out of the hospital does not always mean that a midwife can escape persecution. In New Jersey, an obstetrician filed a complaint with the state medical board against a nurse-midwife attending home births, a practice of which he did not approve.[19] The board searched through her home birth cases trying to find evidence of incompetence. The board pulled several cases and asked a nurse-midwife with no experience in home birth to review them. The reviewer, a "medwife" in her opinions, aggressively attacked some of the home birth practices. Fortunately, the nurse-midwife under investigation was able to get other midwives with considerable home birth experience to evaluate the same cases, and they reported no evidence of incompetence. The board found no cause for alarm, but still asked that all of this nurse-midwife's home birth cases be reviewed by another nurse-midwife with home birth experience for one year. At the end of this year of observation, the nurse-midwife was again free to practice home birth, but this unjustified attack caused her much anxiety and emotional distress.

It is more difficult for obstetricians to control direct-entry midwives, as most have independent out-of-hospital practices in the community, either attending home births or serving in a birth center—which explains why doctors resort to witch-hunt tactics. One tactic is to pretend that they don't exist. As recently as 2006, ACOG issued a policy statement titled "Lay Midwifery," stating: "While ACOG supports women having a choice in determining their providers of care, ACOG does not support the provision of care by lay midwives or other midwives who are not certified by the AMCB [American Midwifery Certification Board]." The AMCB certifies nurse-midwives and certified midwives (CMs), the latter trained under a program approved by nurse-midwives. So ACOG completely ignores the thousands of qualified direct-entry certified professional midwives with proven track records (see the Johnson and Daviss study discussed in chapter 6) and their highly developed training program, approved by the federal government, and characterizes them with the pejorative descriptor *lay*. Such a public statement makes ACOG look foolish: first it says that it supports women having a choice of providers of care and then it tries to eliminate certified professional midwives, a legitimate choice of provider.[20]

These direct-entry midwives are trained professionals who offer safe, empowering care to women giving birth in the United States. Yet they are often treated with unbelievable harshness. In 1995, a direct-entry midwife with a home birth practice in upstate New York received a phone call from a couple saying that they wanted to plan a home birth with the midwife. The couple made an appointment and came to the midwife's home, where arrangements were made for the management of the pregnancy and home birth. Several days later, a police car showed up at the midwife's home. The midwife was put in handcuffs and hauled off to the police station. Her house was searched and her client records confiscated. It turns out that the home birth "couple" were undercover police officers who had taped their call to the midwife and were wired for the visit—entrapment. Obstetric cops and robbers. Her crime? She was a direct-entry midwife assisting at home births. The state had a new midwifery law and it was unclear whether direct-entry midwives were legal under the new law. She was to be a test case. A long series of hearings and trials followed, and eventually the midwife found it necessary to move to a nearby state. New York's loss was the neighbor state's gain.[21]

Nearly identical scenarios have been played out in California, Illinois, Connecticut, and many other states. Home birth is not against the law in any state—in our democracy, families clearly have the freedom to choose where the births of their children will take place. But there is a variety of state midwifery laws that attempt to limit the practice of midwives, and these are frequently tested through complaints to the state.

Even though it is not against the law for a midwife to attend a planned home birth, doctors often wait for a home birth to be transferred to the hospital, and then complain to the state. Some of the most common complaints: the midwife was practicing medicine without a license, the midwife made a mistake that resulted in transfer to the hospital, the midwife is not properly trained, and so on. After an investigation, the midwives are usually cleared, but the harassment is nevertheless traumatic for them and will put the fear of God into other home-birth midwives practicing in that state. So while home birth is not against the law, in many parts of the country it is difficult for a family to find someone to attend a planned home birth, since doctors are threatening midwives and are no longer willing to attend home births themselves.

In many cases, these attacks on midwives are simply attempts by doctors to eliminate the competition. Current legal challenges of midwifery practice across the United States are similar to the persecution of the midwife Hanna Porn, who was accused not of malpractice but just of practicing midwifery. Cases against midwives are, with very rare exceptions, not initiated by the families the midwives serve, as is typical of litigation against obstetricians. Instead they are initiated by physicians. Typically a doctor, a group of doctors, or a hospital reports the midwife to the state agency that regulates midwifery, accusing her of practicing medicine without a license, a charge that may simply be a demonstration of the doctor's ignorance. In a few states, such as New Mexico and Oregon, if the complaint is against a direct-entry midwife, it will go to a board that specifically has the task of reviewing midwifery cases. However, in other states, such as California, the complaint will go to the general medical board, on which no midwives serve, only doctors. If the complaint is made against a nurse-midwife, it goes to the state nursing board, where, as in the story told earlier, there are often no midwives serving, only nurses. These cases often draw a lot of attention from the media, which usually take a negative view of midwifery and home birth, as journalists (with some exceptions) tend to believe whatever doctors say. This negative publicity is exactly what the accusing physicians are after. The midwives who are charged, however, usually receive a lot of support from other midwives, local clients, and women's groups.[22]

Recently in Las Vegas, Nevada, a low-income Hispanic family decided that they wanted to plan a home birth, and they secured the services of a midwife.[23] The pregnancy was normal, as was the birth, until, when the baby came out, the midwife noticed a small amount of meconium present on the baby's skin (meconium is fecal material that accumulates in the baby's intestines during pregnancy and is occasionally discharged at or near the time of birth). Although the baby was fine, since the midwife knew that occasionally a baby can aspirate meconium and develop pneumonia, she wisely decided to be very cautious and take the baby to the hospital for a checkup. Since the baby was not in acute distress, the midwife insisted that the mother stay home, as she was exhausted after her labor and birth.

When the father with his baby and the midwife arrived at the ER, the father explained to the nurse that the baby had been born at home. The nurse screamed, grabbed the baby, and ran out of the room. The father was given no support or reassurance. Instead he had to witness the doctors and nurses treat the midwife with open hostility. The father and midwife searched and found the baby in the neonatal intensive care unit, where a neonatologist proceeded to lecture the father about all the terrible things that might now happen to the baby because he had irresponsibly permitted the baby to be born at home. Contrary to the neonatologist's dire predictions, however, the baby was just fine, and was soon discharged from the hospital.

Happy ending? No, the trouble was just beginning. The hospital staff reported the family to the local social services agency as a case of child abuse, and the family was investigated and interrogated—for no other reason than that they had chosen a home birth. Where did the doctors get such a bizarre idea? Perhaps it was from two of the past presidents of the American College of Obstetrics and Gynecology, who made public statements equating planned home birth with child abuse.[24]

Then the authorities began an investigation of the midwife, which led to an outcry from the midwifery community across the country. Letters from scientists, women's organizations, midwives, and clients poured in and were published in the Las Vegas press. The public discussion that took place in the press recognized that the central issue was not the safety of the baby, since the baby was fine and there is no law against home birth in Nevada and no scientific data proving home birth to be dangerous. The protesting citizens were concerned about the freedom and sanctity of the family. Eventually, the social services investigation was ended and the case was closed. The obstetricians and neonatologists of Las Vegas took a gamble and lost. But the emotional toll on the family and on the midwife was considerable.

Similar attempts to put midwives out of business go on all over the United States. Another common tactic is to question a midwife's qualifications. It is common to hear direct-entry midwives called "lay" midwives when they are being attacked, a clearly pejorative label that implies that they are not trained. Ironically, direct-entry midwives aren't even eligible to take the standardized national midwifery examination until they have attended at least fifty births, but there is no requirement for a labor and delivery nurse to have experience as a birth attendant before a hospital assigns her to monitor women in labor, and doctors who do not become obstetricians often finish medical school having attended, if they are lucky, maybe one or two births, but any M.D. is licensed to attend births.

In 1995, in Connecticut, a direct-entry midwife attending home births was arrested for practicing medicine without a license—a test case that ended up in a state hearing at which a hearing officer would decide whether or not she should be able to practice.[25] At the hearing, the director of the state's health department insisted that this midwife should not be allowed to practice because she was a "lay" midwife, trained in an apprenticeship.

When it was my turn to testify, I said that I have a license to practice medicine in California even though by the director's definition, I am a "lay" doctor. I explained: My first two years in medical school at UCLA, I was not required to attend classes; I just had to show up for and pass examinations. The next two years in medical school, I was rotating on various hospital wards and clinics where my teaching was "bedside" teaching, that is, an apprenticeship. My internship was pure apprenticeship—there was no classroom teaching and there weren't even examinations to pass. And my specialty training in neonatology and obstetrics was an apprenticeship with no classes, as all I had to do was pass the final specialty examination. So I pointed out that my training as a physician was also by apprenticeship and examination, just like the midwife's.

In the United States, we tend to believe that the "formal" classroom is the only legitimate place to learn. But for one hundred years, the apprenticeship model has been the foundation of all medical education. Direct-entry midwifery training uses the apprenticeship model as well, with midwives gaining experience in prenatal care and assisting births together with a midwife mentor. Then, after documenting the minimum experience required, midwives take standard examinations. This training has now been officially approved by the U.S. Department of Education.[26]

The renaissance of direct-entry midwifery in the United States over the past two decades is largely due to the development of the North American Registry of Midwives (NARM) standardized national examination required for the certified professional midwife (CPM) training and certification process. Educators see the NARM examination and the CPM certification process as exemplary, progressive programs because they combine apprenticeship and distance learning, an approach most see as the wave of the future for educating health professionals.

The WHO's definition of a midwife is one who has successfully completed the educational program recognized by the government that licenses the midwife to practice. The definition does not specify the length or type of education or training or mention specific academic degrees, as these matters are decided by individual governments. In the United States, most of those states that license direct-entry midwives use CPM certification as the official definition.

Some American obstetricians believe that they are responsible for supervising midwives (a belief that has been used to keep midwives from practicing freely). But this is a misunderstanding. Midwives are not supervised by doctors. A midwife is an independent professional, separate from other maternity care providers. Note that the WHO's definition of midwifery does not contain the words *nurse, obstetrician,* or *supervision,* because in most of the world midwives are not trained first as nurses and they are not supervised by obstetricians.

The evaluation and standardization of the NARM examination has been extremely thorough—perhaps even more thorough than most medical or nursing examinations. There can be no doubt that someone who passes the NARM examination and is a CPM is competent to assist during normal births and can carry out all necessary procedures, including administering oxygen or drugs, performing neonatal resuscitation, and so on. An apprenticeship includes formal and informal instruction in all scientific and clinical topics necessary to practice competent midwifery.

In recent years, around half of the states have passed legislation legalizing direct-entry midwives to attend planned out-of-hospital birth. In approximately sixteen states, the legislation refers to the NARM examination and CPM certification. In several states that have such legislation, when it was up for consideration in the state legislatures, medical and obstetrical societies testified against it in an attempt to protect their monopoly. They usually took the position that midwives and planned out-of-hospital births are "not safe," but, as there are no data to back up such claims, after careful consideration of the scientific evidence, every one of the legislatures determined that these are safe options for their citizens, and the laws were passed.

In the Connecticut case, the hearing officer ruled that the practice of midwifery is not the same as the practice of nurse-midwifery, and that the direct-entry midwife was legally providing midwifery services. The hearing officer further advised the Department of Public Health in Connecticut that if it wanted to regulate the practice of midwifery, it would have to pursue it through the legislature.

The Connecticut Department of Health has yet to do so, but, six years later, in 2002, it again attacked direct-entry midwives who had passed the NARM exam and were CPMs.[27] First, the Department of Health sued two CPMs who refused to release the records of a client who did not want her records disclosed. The client had had a home birth the previous year that ended in a timely transfer to a hospital when medical assistance appeared to be needed. The woman and baby recovered with no problems, but the state Department of Public Health threatened to charge the two CPMs with practicing "outside the scope of their nursing licenses" or "practicing nurse-midwifery without a license" if they did not release the records— rehashing the arguments that were thrown out in the hearing six years earlier.

Around the same time, two Connecticut CPMs were charged with "practicing medicine without a license"—again, because they had transferred their home birth client to the hospital.[28] In this case as well, the woman and the baby were fine. It is important to note that, in both cases, the birthing families were pleased with their care and felt that the transfer from midwifery care to medical care was appropriate. Both families continue to support their midwives and have had no part in instigating the charges brought against them, so it is likely that the charges were brought by the hospital. These cases illustrate again that it is doctors and their allies, not families, who go after midwives in legal cases, whereas when obstetricians are sued, it is usually by families who are looking for answers.

Another common strategy in the witch-hunt (which was used in all three Connecticut cases) is to accuse a midwife of practicing medicine without a license, a charge that reveals a fundamental misunderstanding of midwifery. Midwifery is not the practice of medicine; it is a professional practice in its own right. The cases in Connecticut are similar to other cases in Vermont and Kansas in the 1980s and 1990s in which a legal determination was made that practicing midwifery is not the same as practicing medicine.[29] In December 1999, the same charge was raised in California. In the decision, J. R. Roman, an administrative law judge on California's Medical Quality Hearing Panel, wrote:

> Unlike physicians, physicians' assistants, physician assistant midwives, registered nurses or certified nurse midwives who practice within the context of a medical model, licensed midwives practice within the context of a midwifery model. Physicians and surgeons and certified nurse midwives will not, within the context of the medical model, undertake the delivery of children at home. Midwives, in contrast, within the context of the midwifery model, will. Were this tribunal to employ the medical model on licensed midwifery, as the Complainant urges, no home birth could be competently assisted. . . .
>
> Sufficient evidence has been provided this tribunal to competently conclude that properly conducted midwife-led home births are as safe as births conducted by physicians in hospitals when effected within standards of practice. Accordingly, without dismissing either model or deferring to either model, protection of the public can be effected, and the licensure of professional lay midwives promoted, by this tribunal's adoption of the midwifery model of practice to licensed midwives. . . .
>
> No physician and surgeon in the State of California for reasons primarily (and sadly) born of liability or restrictions imposed by their insurance carriers, will supervise a licensed midwife who conducts home births. . . . In an effort to practice their art, virtually all of California's 109 licensed midwives have, with the cooperation of physicians sympathetic to their plight and who seek to expand the options available to patients, *developed a relationship that involves collegial referral and assistance, collaboration, and emergent assistance* [what is commonly referred to as a "backup" physician] *without direct or accountable physician and surgeon supervision of licensed midwives* [my emphasis].[30]

But the witch-hunt continues. In the last several years in many states, including Illinois, Utah, California, Vermont, Virginia, Nevada, Oregon, Indiana, and Ohio, police have arrested direct-entry midwives for practicing nursing or medicine without a license.

One can't help but wonder why someone would choose a career as a midwife or a doula. Midwives and doulas are harassed by doctors, nurses, hospitals, and sometimes even local newspapers. They're on call 24/7, and when a client goes into labor they may be away from home, attending the birthing woman, for hours or days. The pay is not good and often uncertain. To choose that life, someone must really want it. When I talk to midwives and doulas, there is no doubt in my mind that it is more than a job, it is a vocation—for some, even a "calling." Midwives and doulas love the one-on-one with women, the hands-on experience of assisting at many (beautiful) births. For some, it is an ideal career to start later in life, after raising children. Most important, a midwife or doula knows that she is playing a part in the historical struggle for equality for women.

To understand the source of a midwife's deep commitment, it helps to observe or read about home births. Juliana van Olphen-Fehr, the director of the School of Midwifery at the University of Shenandoah in Virginia and the author of *Diary of a Midwife,* wrote of her own home birth: "This was my strength . . . if I could have a baby on my own and with all my dignity, I could do anything in the world. . . . No one could take away my competence, my knowledge, my compassion and my integrity as a midwife."[31]

Maternity care in the United States is changing, and one of the most important changes still in progress involves who will catch the three and a half million babies a year whose mothers have had normal pregnancies. That is, who will be the primary birth attendant for low-risk births? In the past decade, the percentage of births attended by midwives has gone from 5 percent to 10 percent, and, as mentioned earlier, there are a few places where it is closer to 25 percent. HMOs are hiring more and more midwives. Kaiser Permanente, one of the largest HMOs in the country, has many midwives on its staff and the largest HMO in New Mexico has more staff midwives than staff obstetricians. There are several reasons for the growth of midwifery in the United States, and a big one is money.

Midwifery is far cheaper than obstetrics for two reasons. On average, obstetricians take home a *net* income in the neighborhood of two hundred thousand dollars a year, whereas midwives earn about one-quarter of that. Equally important, the cost of the obstetric interventions, such as induction and C-section, performed *unnecessarily* can easily be cut in half by having midwives, rather than obstetricians, assist at normal births. Health care in the United States is very much driven by the bottom line, and slowly but surely the insurance companies, managed health care organizations, HMOs, and even state and federal government agencies are realizing that the obstetric monopoly is wasting enormous amounts of money. The day that truth fully sinks in will be the day the obstetric monopoly is on its way out. For a detailed discussion of cost saving by using midwives, see chapter 9.

As midwifery becomes better established in the United States, it becomes more difficult for the obstetric establishment to perpetuate the myth that midwives are not as safe as doctors. Pushing the "safety" issue has backfired as a way for obstetricians to protect their territory. Because there is such a campaign by American obstetricians to convince the public that planned home births attended by midwives are dangerous, it is necessary to carefully review the scientific evidence. This is done in chapter 6, where a review of the research leaves no doubt that a planned home birth attended by a nurse-midwife or direct-entry midwife is a perfectly safe option for the 80 to 90 percent of women who have had normal pregnancies. As more state legislatures look carefully at the data and realize that they have been denying families a safe maternity care option, momentum will grow and laws that support and protect midwives will spread to other states.

Another reason midwifery is going to grow: Americans believe in a free market economy with open competition. Obstetricians and midwives both offer primary maternity care. They compete for clients. In those states where doctors are still regulating midwives, we can expect that eventually a midwife who has had her license revoked will sue the state medical board for restraint of trade as it becomes clear that doctors are using their power unlawfully to eliminate their competition.

Finally, midwifery will continue to grow as more women come to appreciate that maternity care is not primarily a health issue but a women's issue. Midwifery plays an important role in strengthening women's control over their own bodies and reproductive systems. The following story illustrates the degree to which fundamental human rights are now at stake in the realm of maternity care.

A woman in northern Florida we will call Ms. P had a normal vaginal birth with her first pregnancy.[32] Her second birth, however, ended with a C-section that she believed was unnecessary, so when she got pregnant a third time, she sought a local midwife and signed on for a planned home birth.

Ms. P had a normal pregnancy, and when she went into labor, her midwife came to her home to attend the birth. The labor progressed nicely, but after some hours Ms. P was having a hard time keeping fluids down. Since the local hospital was only a couple of blocks away, her midwife suggested that they go over to the emergency room for a short time to get an intravenous drip (IV) to hydrate her, and then return home.

In the ER, Ms. P told the staff that she was giving birth at home and would like an IV for a short time. She was put in a room and told to wait for a doctor. When the doctor arrived, he asked if she had had a previous

C-section, and when she replied yes, the doctor said that he wanted to admit her for an immediate C-section. Ms. P said, "No thank you, I just want the IV, and then I'm going home." The doctor became adamant, telling her that she "must" have a C-section, and said that he would consent to give her the IV only if she consented to the C-section. When she refused his attempt to coerce her, the doctor said that if she did not consent to the C-section, the hospital would get a court order to do the C-section. The doctor then asked her to wait, and left the room.

As is typical in any hospital, word of what was going on in the ER spread among the staff. After a few minutes, a nurse ducked into the room where Ms. P was waiting and whispered, "If you don't want to have a cesarean section by force, you better get out of here quick. There is a back entrance to the ER if you go out and turn right."

Ms. P escaped by the back entrance and went home, where she continued her labor without the benefit of an IV. (Note that the hospital never offered Ms. P the option of having a vaginal birth in the hospital with a staff doctor handy.)

Meanwhile, the chief of obstetrics called an emergency meeting with the hospital administrator and told him that the woman's baby was in grave danger of dying due to a ruptured uterus if an emergency C-section was not done quickly. What he said is not true. Studies have shown that Ms. P's C-section meant that she had a slightly higher chance of uterine rupture than a woman who had never had a cesarean, but the risk was still small—especially since labor was not being induced with drugs—and the chance that the baby would die was even smaller. The hospital administrator, however, was not an obstetrician and had no idea whether or not the information was accurate. He called a local judge and told him to rush over, as it was a life-and-death situation. The judge came to the hospital and was told the same story by the obstetrician. He signed a court order for an immediate C-section—by force, if necessary.

Ms. P was continuing her labor at home when there was a knock on the door. She opened the door to the local sheriff, who was a friend of hers and a member of her church. The sheriff said, "I'm really terribly sorry, Ms. P, but I have here a warrant for your arrest." Shocked, Ms. P said, "What on earth for?" The sheriff answered, "I'm terribly sorry. I don't know what the hell is going on. My orders are to take you to the hospital, in handcuffs if necessary."

Against her wishes and the repeated objections of her husband, Ms. P was taken to the hospital, taken to the surgery ward, tied down on an operating table, and given a forced C-section. The story doesn't end here. Ms. P and her husband sued the doctors and the hospital. However, in Florida a judge must decide if a case deserves to go to trial, and another local judge decided that Ms. P's case was not worthy of proceeding, so her case never went to trial—a shocking miscarriage of justice, given the serious violation of Ms. P's basic rights. Since then, Ms. P has had another baby, born vaginally at home with no problems. Needless to say, there was no visit to the hospital during the labor.

It is important that women in this country become aware of the danger to birthing women and join the movement to protect them. Ms. P's family's wishes were not honored, and her body was invaded against her will. Her human rights were violated. In another recent case, a woman in Utah who refused a C-section and had a stillborn was accused by the district attorney of murder. She was able to avoid the homicide charge by pleading guilty to lesser child endangerment charges, but the case raises important and troubling issues regarding the autonomy rights of pregnant women and whether a disparity exists between the rights of pregnant women and other persons.[33] Treating pregnant women in this manner goes against the Nuremberg Code and the Helsinki Accord, which explicitly state an individual has absolute rights over her or his own body and no medical treatment can ever be forced. Cases like this indicate a dangerous trend in U.S. maternity care toward totalitarian control of a woman's reproductive life by doctors.

Midwives have been fighting to protect the rights of birthing women for a long time. They have not always presented a united front, however, and the divisions among them have hurt the cause. Midwives of every stripe have been oppressed in the United States for more than a hundred years, and, as often happens in oppressed cultures, the oppressed fight among themselves rather than taking on the oppressor. In the 1960s and 1970s, nurse-midwives were the only midwives practicing in the United States, with the exception of a small number of underground home birth midwives. As direct-entry midwifery began to flourish in the 1980s and 1990s, a tragic struggle evolved. In some states, when legislation to legalize direct-entry midwifery was proposed, nurse-midwifery organizations joined with medical and nursing associations and testified against it. In the 1990s in New York, a new state midwifery board was formed, but only nurse-midwives were included on the board, and when the police came to arrest the direct-entry midwife in upstate New York in the story recounted earlier in this chapter, the state midwifery board took no action to stop it.

Early in the 1990s, a group of certified nurse-midwives (CNMs) who had roots in direct-entry midwifery and home birth formed a "bridge club" with the goal of bridging the gap between CNMs and direct-entry midwives in the United States. Some dialogue took place, but after a short effort, the discussions ended badly. Now change is in the air. Younger graduates of nurse-midwifery schools have a better understanding of direct-entry midwifery and are more willing to work with their counterparts in that profession. In states such as Virginia and California, state nurse-midwifery organizations have worked to pass legislation to legalize direct-entry midwifery.

This increasing unity among midwives is at least partly due to the fact that although direct-entry midwives were the original victims of the witch-hunt, more nurse-midwives have felt the heat in recent years. Earlier in this chapter we saw that in the past several years, groups of nurse-midwives in Texas, Ohio, New York, and Washington, D.C., have been fired. American midwives now understand that unity is critical in their fight to expand and legitimize midwifery as the primary health profession for normal pregnancy and birth.

Another key strategy for midwives must be to push for autonomy— recognition that midwifery is an independent health care profession with its own certification, licensure, and state boards—and for an egalitarian relationship with doctors. From the beginning, nurse-midwives elected to join the nursing and physician camps in order to survive, though midwifery is not the practice of nursing or medicine. They did survive, so they can't be faulted, but now they're faced with the hard task of extricating themselves from both camps. Direct-entry midwives have taken a lot more heat for being out-of-hospital independent practitioners, but, in their position, achieving autonomy, though not easy, is less difficult.

One of the strongest tools available to all midwives as they work toward autonomy is scientific evidence. The data are in: midwives are safe, midwifery practice is far closer to evidence-based practice than obstetric practice is, and midwives don't need "supervision" any more than other primary care workers, such as family physicians, need supervision. For this reason, it would behoove midwives to insist on accountability and transparency in maternity care. Their results are excellent, with very low rates of mortality for both women and babies, even though they often work with families who are at higher risk, such as families living in poverty. Fortunately, transparency and accountability are becoming ever more popular in the United States, in all areas, from education to business to health care.

SIX WHERE TO BE BORN: HERE COME THE OBSTETRIC POLICE

Home birth is child abuse in its earliest form.
KEITH RUSSELL, PAST PRESIDENT OF THE AMERICAN COLLEGE OF OBSTETRICIANS AND GYNECOLOGISTS, 1992

Discussions of home birth usually generate much more heat than light.
WORLD HEALTH ORGANIZATION, 1985

Women in the United States have the right to choose who they want to attend the birth of their child, and they also have a choice regarding where the birth will take place—in a hospital, in an alternative birth center, or at home. These are two different choices, though if an American woman chooses a doctor as her birth attendant, she cannot choose a home birth, since doctors in the United States no longer attend home births. Home births are attended only by midwives, and since that represents a loss of business for doctors, doctors attack home births with zeal.

In chapter 5, I told a story about a direct-entry midwife in upstate New York who was entrapped by the "obstetric police" masquerading as a couple expecting a baby. The midwife was fully trained and had experience, and there was no evidence of malpractice. She could have been licensed in many states without difficulty, but it was unclear whether she was licensed in New York State because it had an ambiguous new midwifery law. A passionate turf battle has been taking place in New York State since the 1980s between direct-entry midwives and obstetricians, with most nurse-midwives taking the side of obstetricians. This particular midwife was caught in the middle.

Such battles are by no means limited to New York State. A California midwife, Ms. S, was at home with two of her three children, ages five and eleven, when she heard loud banging at the front door and someone shouting "Open up! Police!"[1] Before she could get to the door, six armed policemen burst in (the door was unlocked), one of them wearing a bulletproof vest. They ordered the midwife and her children to stay in the living room while they ransacked the house. Ms. S was not permitted to leave the living room to see what the police were doing.

"Why?" she asked.

"Because you might have a gun," the man in charge replied.

While this was going on, the midwife's nine-year-old son arrived home from school and was upset to find armed police going through his home. The three children became hysterical. Ms. S told the policeman in charge that she intended to phone her mother to come and get the children. She was prevented from doing so. In time the police got tired of the sound of screaming children, however, and relented. When the grandmother arrived, the police demanded to see her I.D. before "turning over" the children to her. The midwife told the police, "These are not your children, they're mine. This is my house." She won that round; the children left with their grandmother.

The police spent three hours searching and packed up thirty-eight boxes of Ms. S's possessions—a strange miscellany that included not only midwifery equipment and client records, but also books and magazines about childcare, toiletries, even a hair curling iron. The items were impounded and turned over to the district attorney. Imagine some young assistant district attorney painstakingly sorting through the boxes, scratching his head and wondering what the devil that curling iron was used for—possibly a baby born with straight hair?

This midwife's only crime was that she had attended home births. There had been no adverse outcomes to precipitate a malpractice complaint. A local obstetrician who was against home birth simply reported her to the California State Board of Medical Quality Assurance because he "thought she might be dangerous." He offered no specific charges, and no charges were needed. The board was willing to investigate. As part of the investigation, the board wanted to search the midwife's patient charts for possible malpractice, and, without providing a shred of evidence beyond the obstetrician's vague complaint, they were awarded a search warrant.

One hundred of Ms. S's friends and supporters, many of them families whose births she had attended, rallied to her defense in a demonstration at the state capitol. The demonstration received considerable media coverage. One TV channel ran a call-in poll on whether home birth midwifery should be legal. The poll recorded 88 percent in favor. Ultimately, no charges were brought against Ms. S.

In another case, the California State Board of Medical Quality Assurance instigated an entrapment operation that led to local police arresting a breast-feeding midwife. They took away her infant and threw the midwife in jail—for no other reason than that a young obstetrician practicing in the same area accused her of practicing medicine without a license. (He was trying to build his practice and the midwife was formidable competition.) This midwife had had no bad outcomes from her home births that might have raised concern among doctors.

California midwives were outraged. They raised money, secured an excellent lawyer, and located outside medical experts to testify. Then, suddenly, just as the court case got started, the district attorney dropped the charges. Perhaps he had not expected such serious opposition. In any case, the suit had already achieved its purpose: the midwife had been harassed.

In another California case, a midwife's thirteen-year-old daughter was held on the floor at gunpoint while the police searched their home for evidence.

Nurse-midwives in California have not escaped police either. Three nurse-midwives were handcuffed and jailed after a home birth.

Although it is usually a doctor or hospital who makes the original complaint against a midwife, it is medical boards that initiate and pursue these cases and order police investigations, and a representative of the board usually accompanies the police. These aggressive police actions—bursting through the door, holding a child down on the floor, handcuffing, taking midwives off to jail—are inexplicable. None of these women resisted arrest. No one can think there was any real danger of life and limb. The only reasonable explanation is police harassment.

The "obstetric police" (state medical boards that order police investigations) don't limit their harassment to midwives; they also do everything they can to intimidate home birth families. In New York State, an orthodox Jewish family had a home birth with a midwife. The state medical board got wind of it and started an investigation. When the authorities asked the family who the midwife was, the family replied that the birth of their child was guided by religious customs and was no business of the government. The parents were summoned before a grand jury and told that if they didn't name the midwife, they would be found in contempt of court and could go to jail. They refused.

One final real-life story from the obstetric police files: In 2002, a woman in California having her fourth baby in a planned home birth developed a possible minor problem during labor, and her midwife transferred her to a large HMO hospital. The hospital staff attempted to scare the woman by telling her that she had put the life of her baby in serious jeopardy by attempting a home birth. They irresponsibly told her that research has found that twice as many babies die in home births as in hospital births, mentioning a study in Washington State that, as we will see later in this chapter, has been discredited for gross misclassification. The birth proceeded normally, and after both mother and newborn had been checked by a doctor and found to be fine, the woman asked to be discharged. The pediatrician said no, terrified that a baby born after the mother had labored at home might develop serious medical problems. When the mother insisted, the pediatrician called the police to file a complaint to force her and her baby to stay in the hospital until he said that it was okay to go home.

These stories, like the story in chapter 5 of a woman having a home birth who was taken to the hospital against her will and given a forced C-section, illustrate human rights abuses that we might expect to see in a police state but not in our free country.[2] Why is it happening? Where does all this medical anger toward planned home birth come from? Let's trace it back.

The technological era that followed World War II touched all aspects of life in the United States, including medicine and health care, and shaped our attitudes in profound and subtle ways. If we can put a man on the moon, the thinking went, then surely we can make sure that every baby is born healthy: the answer is to have all women give birth in hospitals, where the latest technology is available. There were no studies done to investigate the validity of this thinking. It was simply assumed that hospitals were safer for births, whether or not the birth involved complications. Inside the hospitals, the practice of using interventions in maternity care and assuming that they were safe before any scientific evaluation became the norm. As far as most health care professionals were concerned, high-tech birth was the wave of the future.

In 1975, the American College of Obstetricians and Gynecologists (ACOG) made its position official and published a recommendation against home birth: "Labor and delivery, while a physiological process, clearly presents potential hazards to both mother and fetus before and after birth. These hazards require standards of safety which are provided in the hospital setting and cannot be matched in the home situation."[3] ACOG cited no studies to back up this statement, apparently assuming that everyone would simply take the organization's word.

At that time, what little research had been done on out-of-hospital birth failed to separate planned and unplanned out-of-hospital births. But then scientists showed that the findings in these studies were seriously faulty. There were more babies dying in out-of-hospital births because the studies put all out-of-hospital births in one category. When out-of-hospital births were separated into two categories—planned home births and unplanned out-of-hospital births (those that never made it to the hospital and took place, for example, in a taxi cab)—then the rate of babies dying in planned home births was no higher than the rate of babies dying in hospital births, while the mortality rate in unplanned out-of-hospital births was fifty times higher.[4]

In the quarter century since this separation and clarification, ACOG has never changed its policy against home birth. In fact, in 2002 it reissued its recommendation against home birth—still with no references to back up its position.[5]

Over time, other events contributed to the mounting distrust of high-tech hospital birth. Doctors insisted that moving birth to the hospital was the reason for the falling rate of perinatal mortality (babies dying around the time of birth) in the United States in the 1950s to 1990s. But epidemiologists corrected them, explaining that this perspective was a case of two things happening at the same time and falsely assuming cause and effect. Gradually an understanding evolved in the scientific community that the fall in perinatal mortality was due largely to social factors, such as better housing, better nutrition, and family planning. To the extent that doctors and hospitals played a role in saving babies, it was the introduction of general medical advances such as antibiotics and safe blood transfusion that were responsible, not women giving birth in hospitals or any of the high-tech interventions. Then, in the 1950s and 1970s, two of the drugs that were frequently given to pregnant women, thalidomide and diethylstilbestrol (DES), were found to cause birth defects. The women's movement became aware of how doctors were imposing their will on women's reproductive lives and maternity care, and a reaction against the medicalization and dehumanization of birth began.

In the 1980s, two quite different approaches to maternity care evolved: the medical model advocated by doctors, and the social or humanized model advocated by most midwives, perinatal scientists, and many public health professionals and women's groups. Humanized birth means putting the woman giving birth in the center and in control so that she, not the doctors or anyone else, makes all the decisions about what will happen.

Humanized birth means that the focus of maternity services is community-based (out-of-hospital) primary care, not hospital-based tertiary (specialist) care, with midwives, nurses, and doctors all working together in harmony as equals. Humanized birth means maternity services that are based on good scientific evidence, including evidence-based use of technology and drugs.[6]

In the 1980s, the scientific evaluation of maternity services began in earnest. Many studies revealed startling truths about technology, such as that routine use of electronic fetal monitoring on every birthing woman does not lower the perinatal mortality rate, but sharply increases the rate of C-sections. This led to a fundamental shift away from peer standards of practice, in which the standard of practice in a given community is whatever the physicians in that community do, to evidence-based standards of practice, and as more studies have been done, the findings continue to support the need to expand the medical model of birth to include the social or humanized model and give women the choice of a planned out-of-hospital birth.

The maternity care establishment in the United States has been seriously challenged by the trend toward evidence-based practice in medicine. Control, status, and, for many obstetricians, financial benefits have been threatened. The struggle is on, and place of birth has become a central issue. Why do obstetricians get so emotional about home birth? My own experience as a physician may shed some light on the situation.

The first time I attended a home birth, I was shocked. I had been a practicing physician for years, but this was the first time I had witnessed the full power of a woman in control of her own body. Believe me, it's a scary experience for a man. It took me a long time to come to grips with the truth: we men are afraid of women, whether consciously or unconsciously. We're afraid of unleashed nature, we're afraid of childbirth. We've all heard Freud's theory of "penis envy," but it isn't necessary to be an adherent of psychoanalytic theory to believe that many male obstetricians experience "womb envy," a term introduced by a German psychoanalyst, Karen Horney, to refer to an abiding sense of male inadequacy in the face of women's unique childbearing gift.[7]

Put simply, men are outsiders at birth—always have been, always will be. So watch out. Hell hath no fury like a man marginalized. When men are afraid and angry at being afraid, they cope through denial of their fear and through controlling whatever they're afraid of.[8] In light of this theory, it makes sense that the male-dominated obstetric profession would try to control birth—though it is an impossible task, given that labor is a function of the autonomic nervous system, something even the woman herself has no control over. The only way to control the birth process is to override normal uterine function—introducing drugs to start or accelerate labor, inhibiting the normal physiology of labor with epidural block, and turning birth into a surgical event by pulling or cutting the baby out. And the only way to use these interventions is to have birth in hospitals. Hospitals are doctor territory, the only place where doctors have nearly absolute control. Doctors fear out-of-hospital birth because they are afraid of birth and because they have no control outside the hospital.

With few exceptions, obstetricians in the United States are against out-of-hospital birth, even though they have never seen a planned birth in a home or in a freestanding birth center, and are unwilling even to look at the evidence on the matter. I believe this is due to a dire need to control women and birth and a deep fear of childbirth. It's easy to see what I'm talking about. Just ask an obstetrician to tell you about the risks of childbirth or about all the women and babies he has pulled back from the precipice of death during childbirth. So what we have is an obstetrician's basic conviction that childbirth is dangerous dovetailing with the fact that if a birth takes place in a freestanding birth center or a home, he has lost control, power, and money.

Obstetricians campaign against out-of-hospital birth with a variety of strategies. As discussed in chapter 5, in many places obstetricians have fought to make it a requirement that nurse-midwives have an obstetrician "supervisor" and licensed direct-entry midwives have an obstetrician "consultant." Obstetricians want to supervise or consult for midwives in order to control them. But, as a result, obstetricians now claim that insurance companies may charge higher premiums for an obstetrician who provides backup for out-of-hospital births and that, at least in theory, they are liable if something goes wrong.[9] So now obstetricians (even those who have never provided backup to midwives) complain that if a birth takes place outside of a hospital, a doctor is still responsible if something goes wrong and is therefore liable. In other words, obstetricians fight for control, and then when they win these fights and get control, they complain because with the control comes responsibility and liability.

Almost everywhere in the world outside of the United States, obstetricians do not "supervise" midwives and are not liable for what midwives do or don't do. Even in the United States, some judges do not see the relationship between an obstetrician and midwife as one of supervision, control, and liability, but rather as a collegial relationship. Judicial opinions like the one by Judge J. R. Roman in California (see chapter 5) make it clear that obstetric groups in the United States could rather quickly change the present system so that they are no longer responsible or liable for midwives. But they don't want to change the system. They don't want to give up control of midwives. They would rather use their high insurance premiums to gain sympathy from politicians and get them to pass laws that make obstetricians sue-proof and their practices beyond the reach of regulation and litigation.

With all the frightening propaganda about how dangerous birth is, even women who want the freedom to control their own birth experience sometimes feel that they need the "security" of an institution. These days for such women there is a way to have it all. A woman can choose to be assisted by a midwife, control her birth experience, and still feel protected by an institution by choosing an alternative birth center (ABC) that is "freestanding" (i.e., not in a hospital) and staffed by midwives.

That an ABC is free of control by a hospital is essential. Some hospitals have something called a birth center in their maternity wards, but a hospital claiming to have a "birth center" is like a bakery claiming to sell "home-baked" bread. In a real birth center, a birthing woman always has the final say about everything that happens to her, and that is unlikely ever to happen in a hospital unless she fights for it. It is also essential that an ABC be staffed by midwives who use protocols or standard procedures that have been established by midwives, not doctors.

The type of care provided in an ABC is different from the care provided in a hospital in significant ways. In a hospital an obstetrician is in control, whereas in an ABC the birthing woman is in control. In a hospital the emphasis is on routines, whereas in an ABC the emphasis is on individuality, education, and informed choice. Hospital protocols are designed with all the possible complications in mind and are then applied to all women across the board, whereas in an ABC, protocols focus on normality, screening, observation, and when to transfer. In hospitals, pain is defined as an evil to be stamped out with drugs, whereas in the ABC it is understood that labor pain has a physiological function and can be relieved with scientifically proven, nonpharmacological methods such as immersion in water, changing positions, massage, the presence of family, and the continuous presence of the same birth attendant.

In a hospital, labor is frequently induced or stimulated using powerful drugs that increase labor pain and have many risks. In an ABC, labor is very rarely induced, but may be stimulated using nonpharmacological methods such as walking around and various types of sexual stimulation such as massaging the nipples. In a hospital, there is intermittent attendance by the doctor, with nurses changing shifts every eight hours. In an ABC, the woman's midwife is present for the entire labor and birth. In a hospital, the family does not know the staff, whereas in an ABC, the family knows the staff. In many hospitals, new babies are often taken away from their mothers for various reasons, for example to allow a doctor to perform a newborn examination, whereas in ABCs, babies are never taken from their mothers. In the hospital, when a woman and her baby are discharged, there is no follow-up at the family's home, only a visit to the doctor's office six weeks later. After an ABC birth, in contrast, there are follow-up visits in the ABC or in the family's home.

ABCs are naturally a threat to doctors and hospitals, as well as to the manufacturers of obstetric technologies. Because medicalized birth is so expensive (with a costly hospital stay and highly paid obstetricians using costly high-tech interventions), physicians and hospitals try to convince the public and those who control funding for health services that giving birth in a hospital is the only safe option.

Are ABCs a safe place for a woman to give birth if she has had no complications during the pregnancy? Let's look at the scientific evidence.[10] In the 1970s and 1980s, a number of descriptive studies of ABCs were done. Then, in 1989, a seminal paper was published reporting results of the U.S. National Birth Center Study, which looked at eighty-four ABCs and 11,814 births.[11]

Regarding safety, there were no maternal deaths at all in the U.S. National Birth Center Study. The rate of perinatal deaths (1.3 per 1,000 live births) is comparable to the rates among low-risk hospital births. Sixteen percent of ABC births were transferred to the hospital due to complications, a rate that compares favorably to the number of planned hospital births that are transferred from a labor ward to a surgical suite due to complications. The intention to treat analysis was used (if the intention was to have the birth in the ABC, then all subsequent events such as hospital transfer are recorded in the ABC category), so that all complications, interventions, and outcomes from ABC births that were transferred to a hospital are included in the ABC statistics. The results of this study are clear: ABCs are perfectly safe for the vast majority of pregnant women who have had no serious complications during pregnancy.

Around the same time, several other studies compared ABC birth with hospital birth, one of which was a randomized, experimental trial.[12] These additional studies confirmed the safety of ABCs. In these studies, the outcomes of ABC births were as good or better than the outcomes of low-risk hospitals births. These studies also went beyond safety and found that 99 percent of the women who chose an ABC birth said that they would recommend an ABC birth to their friends, and 94 percent said that they would return to the ABC for future births. These studies found significantly increased rates of successful breast-feeding among women who gave birth in ABCs. And one study found that 63 percent of women who gave birth in ABCs experienced an increase in self-esteem, whereas only 18 percent of women who gave birth in hospitals experienced an increase in self-esteem.

When rates of specific obstetrical interventions in the U.S. National Birth Center Study are compared with rates in hospitals in Illinois, 99 percent of ABC births were spontaneous vaginal births, compared to 55 percent of hospital births.[13] Less than 4 percent of ABC births involved induction or augmentation of labor, with artificial rupture of membranes and/or use of oxytocin (Pitocin), compared to 40 percent of hospital births. Only 8 percent of ABC births involved routine use of electronic fetal monitors (i.e., used without a specific indication on all birthing women), whereas monitors were used routinely in 95 percent of hospital births. Anesthesia (including epidural block) was used in 13 percent of ABC births and 42 percent of hospital births. Forceps or a vacuum extractor were used in less than 1 percent of ABC births compared to 10 percent of hospital births. Because any births transferred from an ABC to a hospital were counted in the ABC group, studies were able to compare the percentage of ABC births that ended in C-sections (5 percent) and the percentage of low-risk hospital births that ended in C-sections (21 percent). When we see these results side by side, the logical question is not whether an ABC birth is safe, but whether a hospital birth is safe.

As the good news spreads, more and more ABCs are being established around the world. Between 1990 and 2000, Germany went from having one ABC to having more than seventy.[14] In Japan, in the first half of the twentieth century there was a network of midwife-run "birth houses" that provided a significant percentage of maternity services in the country. But during the American occupation after World War II, U.S. Army doctors and nurses put pressure on the Japanese to close the birth houses and move birth to hospitals. Now, there is a resurgence of birth houses in Japan. Located in the homes of local midwives, these birth houses are not only places to give birth, but also places where women can meet other women in the neighborhood and get restored and revitalized as women. They receive midwifery care during pregnancy and at the birth, which takes place at a birth house. All the women in the neighborhood receive information on pregnancy, birth, and other women's health concerns and also discuss women's issues and personal problems.[15]

In the United States, in spite of the scientific evidence showing that ABCs are a perfectly safe choice for most women, the aggressive obstetric campaign against out-of-hospital birth has taken a toll. In Illinois, ABCs are outlawed, and repeated efforts made by women's groups to change the law have failed. At a meeting of the Illinois Medical Society in Chicago (the Illinois chapter of ACOG), hospital organizations testified that ABCs are dangerous. They had no scientific data to back up their statements, just testimonials that they know ABCs are dangerous. When a bill on ABCs comes up, these organizations also testify before the Illinois state legislature. In collusion with these hospital and doctor organizations, the Illinois State Health Department insists that all ABCs must meet the same regulations as hospitals, a nonsensical strategy designed to keep ABCs out.

Fear-mongering and nonscientific public statements against ABCs have not been limited to Illinois. In 2001, the Texas State Board of Midwifery was considering rule changes for midwives working in ABCs. A neonatologist in Austin sent an unsolicited e-mail message to the board of midwifery expressing his opinion that out-of-hospital birth with midwives is dangerous. To prove his point, he described a recent birth in an Austin birth center in which the newborn baby had difficulty breathing—difficulty that was almost certainly due to a genetic blood disorder, the presence of which the birth center had nothing to do with. His description of the case (with which he had absolutely nothing to do) was wildly inaccurate, beginning with his statement that the baby had died, when, in fact, the baby is very much alive. He also said the baby was Hispanic, which it is not, and that the pregnancy was high-risk, which it was not. He also said that putting a woman in labor in a warm bath is dangerous, which it is not.

In fact, when the board investigated, they found that it was a midwife from the ABC who noticed the baby's breathing difficulty (which was not present when the baby left the ABC) during a visit to the family's home the day after the birth and urged the family to seek medical attention. Ironically, rather than illustrating that ABCs are dangerous, the case illustrates the value of midwifery and the value of the close follow-up provided by the ABC. So the doctor's e-mail message had an effect opposite to what he intended—it drew to the board's attention the value of the ABC's care.

The neonatologist's e-mail message to the board of midwifery is an example of the way local doctors talk to one another behind closed doors whenever an out-of-hospital birth is transferred to the hospital, condemning the midwife and the family before they know the facts. The director of the ABC wrote to the board that the neonatologist "knowingly distorted this situation in order to block the new midwifery rules" and that he "considered the ABC an easy target which could be attacked to accomplish the blockage of any rules which he perceives give midwives greater power."[16]

This ABC has every right to be offended by someone spreading false information about its practice. Using families, health professionals, and health facilities for political gain and to promote selfish territorial concerns is inexcusable. In addition, such tactics invade the family's privacy by broadly disseminating inaccurate information in a message in which their child is easily identifiable.

In chapter 2, I described how obstetricians in Iowa managed to close down an ABC that they feared would take their patients away by seeing that no physician in the area would provide backup. These are just a few examples. Yet, in the face of all this obstetric aggression, American women continue to support birth centers. There are now 160 freestanding ABCs in the United States, and there is a National Association of Childbearing Centers that is working to promote ABCs as a real choice for birthing women.[17] There is even talk of a new ABC opening in the same city in Iowa.

If anything, the propaganda campaign against planned home birth is even more aggressive than the one against birth centers, and for the most part, the media have been happy to assist with coverage that is sensationalist, to say the least. There's something about the drama of a woman giving birth in her own home that the media just love. An article in the *New York Times* quoted a top public health official in Connecticut: "While home births are legal in Connecticut, women do not have an absolute right to one, in the absence of a licensed nurse-midwife or doctor, 'any more than they have a right to have brain surgery at home,' said Stanley K. Peck, the Department of Public Health's director of medical quality assurance."[18] Vivid but misleading quotations such as this make good copy.

Once it was firmly established in the scientific community in the 1970s that any study of home birth must make the distinction between planned and unplanned births, study results have continued to show that home birth is a safe alternative for women. In the 1980s and 1990s, a number of small studies were conducted in Kentucky, Missouri, South Carolina, Tennessee, and California that prove that midwives are fully competent to assist at home births, and an excellent review and meta-analysis of these studies, published in 1997, concluded that planned home birth, when attended by either a nurse-midwife or a direct-entry midwife, is safe.[19]

Then in late 2001 and early 2002, two new studies of home birth were presented within a few months of each other. One was presented at the annual meeting of ACOG and the other was presented at the annual meeting of the American Public Health Association. It is no accident that these two studies, which were presented to two very different groups of health professionals, had opposite methodologies and came to opposite conclusions. So it behooves us to take a closer look.

The first study, presented to ACOG by J. Pang and colleagues, is titled "Outcomes of Planned Home Births in Washington State: 1989–1996."[20] Though the title uses the phrase *planned home birth,* the methodology used makes it impossible to tell if any of the home births were actually planned or intended. The study relies solely on birth certificate data that indicates actual place of birth but does not indicate the planned or intended place of birth. The only way these data could be valid is if researchers were able to follow up on individual cases to determine the intended place of birth, but in this study they could not do that because their research was approved only for "birth certificate data from unidentified participants."

In the study, the researchers attempted to "minimize misclassification of intended location of delivery," but they freely admit "the potential for misclassifying unplanned home births as planned home births." Finally, they say, "Since we tried to minimize misclassification, but had no possibility to eliminate it, there remains potential for a significant amount of misclassification of accidental or unplanned home births as planned home births." In other words, the authors of this study did not heed the legacy of scientists that came before them and repeated earlier mistakes by failing to make the essential distinction between planned home birth and unplanned home birth.

It's interesting to look at the kinds of cases that were counted as "planned" home births. In one example, there was a precipitous (unplanned) home birth of a full-term baby. Then the family went to a hospital to have the woman and baby checked. While at the hospital, a midwife, nurse, or physician certified on the birth certificate that the birth had occurred at home. For the study, the birth was counted as a *planned* home birth, because it satisfied the study's definition of a planned home birth: "those singleton newborns of at least 34 weeks gestation who were delivered at home and who had a midwife, nurse, or physician listed as either the birth attendant *or certifier* on the birth certificate." In Washington State, attending home birth is not within the scope of practice of registered nurses, and the Midwives Association of Washington State knows of no physicians in the state who attend planned home births.[21] Therefore, home births certified by a nurse or doctor are most likely not planned home births. By including these cases in the planned home birth group, the researchers increased rather than minimized the misclassification of unplanned home births as planned home births.

Hospital transfers were another source of misclassification in this study. The researchers identified hospital births that started as home births and were transferred to the hospital and placed them in the home birth group. This would be correct methodology, except that the researchers had no way of knowing if the birth started at home because that was the plan or because the family was delayed in getting to the hospital.

Finally, yet another source of error is simply the high rate of inaccurate data on birth certificates, especially with out-of-hospital births. The authors of the study acknowledged, "A study done by Meyers et al. showed that birth certificate data correctly identified attendant type for out-of-hospital births 30 percent of the time."[22]

The authors of the study go on to admit that "misclassification of any unplanned home births as planned home births in this study would result in inflated risk estimates of neonatal mortality." This is because, as the authors also point out, "in previous studies, neonatal mortality among unplanned home births was high (73 of 1,000 to 120 of 1,000 live births)."[23] Thus, because the neonatal mortality rate of unplanned home birth has been shown to be fifty times higher than with planned home birth, only a small number of misclassified cases would bring more cases of neonatal mortality into the home birth group. In fact, misclassifying only eight cases of neonatal mortality as planned home births that were really unplanned home births would lead to identical neonatal mortality rates in the home and hospital groups. With half as many misclassified cases, any significant statistical difference in neonatal mortality between home and hospital groups would disappear.

This is probably what happened in this study—cases of unplanned home births were counted as planned home births, resulting in inflated neonatal mortality rates in the home birth group. The most important conclusion is that it is impossible to know if this is what happened or if the authors are correct in concluding that there was higher neonatal mortality in the home birth group. The data in this study do not prove either case, and this study cannot be used as evidence of the safety or lack of safety of planned home birth.

The paper goes on to say that 40 percent of the neonatal deaths in the home birth group were due to congenital malformation, but the authors do not mention that previous research shows a higher rate of major malformations in newborns born to women receiving prenatal care from midwives in Washington State.[24] This higher rate of malformations is probably due to the fact that the women going to midwives for care are less likely to terminate pregnancy. This could also have an effect on the rate of newborn babies dying in the home birth group.

The paper also reports more postpartum bleeding and more prolonged labor in the home birth group, but these "problems" are defined and managed differently by midwives and doctors, so this difference is most likely a difference in the definition of these problems, not in their rate. Furthermore, neither "problem" is an issue unless it is so severe as to lead to other consequences for which the researchers have no data, so it is inappropriate to conclude, as the authors did, that "This study suggests that planned home birth had greater maternal risks."[25]

In the process of "trying to minimize misclassification," the researchers eliminated several subcategories of low-risk births. To qualify for the study, a birth must be near term, not low-birth-weight, only singleton, and have no pregnancy complications. This narrows the definition of low-risk birth to the point where births in the study's home birth group and in the hospital birth group may be compared, but the groups cannot be compared with other studies. The neonatal mortality rate in the hospital group is very low, lower than reported in other studies of low-risk hospital birth, and is so devoid of risk and removed from reality as to be of little or no use in research on low-risk birth.

Rather than attempting a balanced reporting of facts about home birth, the paper by Pang and colleagues contains a clear bias favoring hospital birth. It is essential that those doing research have no bias that can influence study results. In this study, there were no home birth providers among the researchers, who are like geographers trying to map a country that they have never seen because they believe it too dangerous to go there.

One kind of bias begins with the incorrect use of the phrase *planned home birth* in the title. Throughout the text, *planned home birth* and *intended home birth* are used in situations where intention is not known but is based on assumption, approximation, or an educated guess. Assumptions are clearly weighted toward results that put hospital birth in a positive light.

Other language choices reveal bias in other ways. For example, the statement, "The risk of neonatal death was almost twice as high for infants born to women intending to deliver at home," sounds rather dramatic until one realizes that the increased risk amounted to only one more death in every one thousand births.

The choice of outcomes to study or not to study also reflects a bias in favor of hospital birth. For example, the same birth certificate data would have allowed comparisons between the home birth group and the hospital birth group regarding interventions such as induction of labor, forceps, vacuum extraction, and C-section. But these interventions were not analyzed. Had they been, it is likely there would have been findings favorable to home birth, since previous research shows significantly lower rates of interventions in planned out-of-hospital birth. The paper does, however, mention advantages of hospital birth, such as the early identification of congenital heart disease.

The literature review in this paper also is slanted to favor hospital birth. It mentions several studies that are small and use questionable methodology and are interpreted to show better outcomes with hospital birth than with home birth. But it does not mention the scientifically valid meta-analysis of home birth studies by Olsen, which showed no increased risks with planned home births.[26] The meta-analysis is in the reference list in the paper, but is conspicuously absent from the review of literature.

The final sentence in the paper is: "Future observational studies using a study design that accurately assesses the intention to deliver at home are needed."[27] This conclusion is ironic, as it is both an admission that their study did not accurately assess the intention to deliver at home and a plea that such research be done so we can learn the facts about the safety of planned home birth.

The question must be asked: How did this paper ever get published? An editorial in the *New York Times* makes the point that coauthors of scientific papers must carry a "big share of responsibility" for the contents of a paper and are "the first line of defense against fraud."[28] Where were the five coauthors when the paper was given a fraudulent and misleading title that includes the phrase *planned home births?* At least one of the coauthors is said to be connected with the federal Centers for Disease Control and Prevention and should have recognized that this was false science. Before publication, the paper was presented at a large ACOG meeting. One might hope that at least a few scientists had been present who could point out the serious methodological flaws, but that was not the case. And how did the flawed paper get by the journal reviewers at *Gynecology and Obstetrics* when there is such hype about the importance of peer review before accepting papers for publication? The same *New York Times* editorial, speaking about another paper published in another prestigious journal, says: "The journal that published the fraudulent papers also needs to raise its guard. Their expert reviewers deemed the findings important enough to publish but somehow missed the fraud underlying them." The senior author of the paper, Dr. Jenny Pang, told me that before being accepted for publication, the paper had to be revised and resubmitted, so it seems that someone was trying to review it carefully, but, again, missed the basic flaws in the study's design. In the end, a whole system of checks and balances failed to uncover the fundamental flaws in the methodology of this paper.

The other study on home birth, presented to the American Public Health Association in 2001 and published in the *British Medical Journal* in 2005, coincidentally does precisely what the Pang study concluded needed to be done.[29] In October 2001, Dr. Kenneth Johnson, an epidemiologist, and Betty-Anne Daviss, a midwife, presented a prospective study of planned home births attended by certified professional midwives (CPMs) in North America. There are many differences between this study and the Pang study, but one crucial difference is simply that it is a prospective study, whereas the Pang study looked back on births retrospectively. The subjects in the Johnson and Daviss study were identified and recruited into the study as pregnant women, before the birth, so it is possible to clearly determine whether a home birth was intended or planned. The woman could also be followed prospectively, so valid data were available on the outcome of each planned home birth. In addition, there was no mixing of planned and unplanned births as there was in the study by Pang and colleagues.

The study population consisted entirely of clients of CPMs in the United States and Canada who planned home births to take place in the year 2000. For the CPMs, participation in this study was mandatory for re-certification. Procedures to validate the reliability of the data were built into the study from the start, including having all pregnant women sign a consent form that included contact information so they could be contacted later. All forms were sent to the study office before the planned home birth. At three to nine months postpartum, study center personnel phoned the women to get information on the birth to validate the information earlier sent by the attending midwife. Data forms were received from 534 practicing CPMs, covering 7,214 births.

In 6.6 percent of the cases, risk factors during pregnancy ruled out home birth. Of the sample population, 12.5 percent discontinued care with the CPM for a variety of reasons including miscarriage, complications, client moved, changed midwife, and chose hospital birth. As a result, at the time of birth, of the original 7,214 women recruited, 5,358 women (83 percent) intended to give birth at home, 651 women (10 percent) intended to give birth at a birth center, and 431 women (7 percent) intended to give birth in a hospital. All data analysis used the "intention to treat" method in which all cases, including their intervention rates and birth outcome rates, are placed in three categories: intended home birth, intended birth center birth, and intended hospital birth. There were 448 women (7 percent) who had previous C-sections.

Of the home birth cases, 11.7 percent were transferred to a hospital, and of those, 3.5 percent were considered urgent. Time of transfer included 2.1 percent at first assessment, 7.3 percent during the first stage of labor, 2.6 percent during the second stage of labor, 0.4 percent during the third stage of labor, and 1.3 percent postpartum.

The intervention rates were as follows: 2.2 percent of the women giving birth at home received episiotomies. Of cases transferred to a hospital, 0.4 percent involved forceps, 0.3 percent involved vacuum extraction, and 3.7 percent ended in C-section.

There were 5,358 intended home births at initiation of labor. In this group, there were three fatal birth defects, six intrapartum deaths (death occurring during labor or delivery), and eight neonatal deaths, resulting in an intrapartum plus neonatal death rate of 2.6 per 1,000 intended home births. There were no maternal deaths.

In summary, this prospective, highly reliable study, which followed the course of more than seven thousand pregnant women planning home births attended by CPMs, collected data on more than five thousand women who intended home birth at initiation of labor. Among these women, the obstetric intervention rates were far below the rates reported in low-risk hospital births. The combined intrapartum/neonatal death rate (babies dying during labor, birth, or shortly following birth) was as low or lower than rates reported for low-risk hospital births. And the maternal mortality rate was zero. This study is by far the largest scientifically valid study of planned home birth ever conducted. We now have good, solid scientific evidence that makes clear that planned home birth attended by a midwife is a perfectly safe option for the 80 to 90 percent of women who have had normal pregnancies.

In addition to the scientific research on home birth, there is other evidence that home birth is a safe option. Whenever I discuss home birth with obstetricians in the United States, I need only ask, "What about the Netherlands?" to see their faces fall. The Netherlands has a long tradition of planned home birth. As recently as thirty years ago, *half* of all births in the Netherlands were planned home births. The percentage fell to one-third in the 1980s, but the rate has been climbing for the last ten years and is now more than one-third—36 percent. The Dutch do not have significantly more women and babies dying around the time of birth than other Western European countries, and they have lower mortality rates than the United States does.

Obstetricians can be very creative when they try to explain away the Dutch experience. It would be amusing if it weren't so pathetic. I have heard many U.S. doctors say that the Dutch success with home birth is due to the fact that they have a homogeneous population. To this I have two responses. First, it is simply not true. There are many "minority" groups in the Netherlands. For example, the percentage of Netherlands citizens with Southeast Asia backgrounds is comparable to the percentage of African Americans in the United States. Second, think about what these doctors are saying. This statement reveals a subtle racist arrogance that I find offensive. Their implication is that the United States has more dead babies than other countries because there are minority groups in the United States. But if maternal and infant mortality rates are higher among minority women and babies in the United States, why isn't the obstetric establishment working to change that, for example by campaigning for federal and state legislation guaranteeing all pregnant women in the United States prenatal care and care during birth regardless of ability to pay, such as European countries have? It gives the perhaps partly unfair but nevertheless bad impression that obstetricians would rather use minority groups as an excuse for their high failure rates than take responsibility for improving.

I have also heard U.S. obstetricians try to explain away the Dutch success with home birth by saying that Dutch women have bigger pelvises than American women and their babies are smaller. I've asked to see the data to back up these remarkable statements, but as yet they have not materialized.

I have also heard another explanation for the success of home births in the Netherlands—the idea that distances between a woman's home and the hospital are shorter there. But, based on extensive experience, the Dutch have established thirty minutes as a maximum transport time from home to hospital for a safe home birth. So, when I hear this excuse from an American obstetrician, I ask, "How many homes in your state are more than thirty minutes from a hospital?" Common sense tells us that very few homes in the United States are more than thirty minutes from a hospital.

Finally, obstetricians in the United States seem to have the idea that obstetricians in the Netherlands do not believe in their home birth system. I have visited the Netherlands dozens of times and have lectured at many large Dutch conferences. I have spoken to hundreds of Dutch obstetricians. I know for a fact that the vast majority of Dutch obstetricians believe firmly in their present system. The Dutch track record with planned home birth is an enormous thorn in the side of American obstetricians.

I've asked myself why obstetricians in the United States find it so hard to believe that a country where one out of every three babies is born at home has a lower infant mortality rate than the United States does. In my view, it goes back to their fear of birth and their belief that without obstetric technology and expertise, babies will die. When confronted with the scientific evidence and the Dutch track record, most obstetricians reply, "But what if there is an out-of-hospital birth and something happens?" This "what if" question reveals several false assumptions worth examining.

The first assumption is that during birth things happen fast. In fact, with very few exceptions, things happen slowly during labor and birth and a true emergency when seconds count is extremely rare. Have you ever spent time in a hospital labor and delivery ward? The atmosphere is not like the ER but rather, for the most part, quiet and peaceful. Regardless of what is seen in movies and television, nobody is running around. It's also important to remember that if trouble does develop, a trained midwife who is providing constant one-on-one care to the birthing woman has a better chance of anticipating it or recognizing it quickly than a labor and delivery nurse or a doctor in a hospital who is responsible for several women in labor and can look in only occasionally.

The second false assumption is that when trouble does develop, there is nothing an out-of-hospital midwife can do. This assumption can be made only by someone who has never observed midwives at out-of-hospital births. Again, with few exceptions, an out-of-hospital midwife can do everything that can be done in the hospital, including giving the women oxygen. The condition known as shoulder dystocia (when the baby's head comes out but the shoulders get stuck) is another example. The only way to solve the problem is to maneuver the woman and baby, and that can be done just as well by a midwife in an ABC or home as it can in a hospital. The most successful maneuver for shoulder dystocia that's been reported in the obstetric literature, by the way, is the Gaskin maneuver, named after the home birth midwife who first described it, Ina May Gaskin.[30]

The third false assumption revealed in the "what if" question is that if there's a problem, there will be faster action in a hospital. That might be true if the doctor happened to be in the room, but the doctor is not even in the hospital most of the time. If there's a problem, a nurse has to call the doctor, and the doctor's "transport time" to the hospital is usually as long as the woman's "transport time" to the hospital if she is in a birth center or at home.

Within a hospital, even when an emergency C-section is indicated, it takes thirty minutes, on average, for the hospital to set up for the surgery, locate the anesthesiologist, and the like. In one study that looked at 117 hospital births where there were emergency C-sections for fetal distress, in 52 percent of the cases the time between the obstetrician's decision to do a C-section and the time the actual incision was made into the woman's belly was more than thirty minutes.[31] So, when there is the need, during this thirty minutes, the out-of-hospital obstetrician or the out-of-hospital birthing woman—or both—can be in transit to the hospital. Again, this is why it is important that an out-of-hospital midwife have a good collaborative relationship with the hospital, so when she calls to inform the hospital that she is transporting a birthing woman, hospital staff will waste no time in making arrangements.

Unfortunately, hospitals are often not open to developing this kind of relationship. Because of the irrational fear and anger many doctors and nurses have around home birth, too often there is little or no communication between home birth midwives and hospital staff. When a midwife calls and says that she is coming in, if hospital staff are resistant to home birth, they may fail to prepare for the woman and baby in a timely way. If the hospital staff don't see the midwife as a trained professional who can contribute greatly because she has been the woman's primary maternity care provider, when the midwife arrives at the hospital with the woman and the baby, all information about the pregnancy and what happened during the birth is lost. Since hospital staff are often abusive to both the midwife and the parents who have chosen a home birth, midwives may hesitate to call for advice or to transport a woman to the hospital when signs of trouble first appear. Thus, unnecessary delays in treatment are one of the tragic effects of the marginalization of midwives and false assumptions about home birth in the United States

An irrational fear of out-of-hospital birth can also blind obstetricians and neonatologists to what is really going on in a particular case. I've seen it happen many times. In one case, in Florida, a woman planned an out-of-hospital birth and had a normal pregnancy, labor, and birth. However, the baby, though nice and pink at birth with a good heart rate, was not breathing well. The baby was resuscitated by the midwife and rushed to the hospital.

Resuscitation continued in the hospital. A pediatrician did a thorough examination and then transferred the baby to another hospital that had a neonatal intensive care unit. The resuscitation continued in the intensive care unit, where a neonatologist did another thorough examination. Both examining doctors wrote in the chart that the baby was born in a planned out-of-hospital birth and that their initial diagnosis was brain damage from lack of oxygen during labor and birth. The diagnosis was not questioned through many months of subsequent hospitalizations due to severe neurological problems.

The family was urged to sue the midwife by doctors who said that the baby's tragic disability must be a result of the out-of-hospital birth. The lawyer for the midwife asked me to look at the records to see if there was evidence of malpractice on her part, and I made an amazing discovery. Both the pediatrician who examined the baby when it was first transported to hospital and the neonatologist who examined the baby a couple of hours later in the neonatal intensive care unit had measured and recorded the baby's head circumference. The two head measurements were identical, and both revealed a significantly smaller than normal head size.

Suddenly, it was obvious what had happened. The cause of this child's neurological problems is microcephaly (a brain too small), which takes weeks to develop in the uterus. The baby's episodes of apnea (not breathing) were the result of the intrauterine brain damage, not the cause of it. My experience is that many neonatologists are just as adamantly opposed to planned home birth as obstetricians. Two different doctors, both baby specialists, were so blinded by the knowledge that this baby had not been born in a hospital that they didn't recognize the significance of their own measurements, missed the diagnosis, and repeatedly spoke to the parents about their terrible mistake in choosing to give birth outside the hospital.

With the scientific evidence and the Dutch experience, it is clear that it is safe for a low-risk woman to give birth in an ABC or at home. The real issue, then, is not safety; the issues are freedom and the sanctity of the family. A woman must have the freedom to control her own body and her own reproductive system. She must have access to accurate, complete information about her choices for pregnancy and birth. To limit the information she receives or prevent her in any way from freely choosing the kind of childbirth she wants is to go down the road toward totalitarian control of women's reproductive lives by doctors.

Some people say that an obstetrician must protect the interests of the fetus by overriding a woman's choice if that choice is not approved by orthodox obstetricians. However, to accept the principle of family sanctity is to understand that, unless there is solid evidence of abuse, a family has the right to decide what will happen to their child. When two former presidents of ACOG called home birth child abuse, they were not only ignoring the scientific evidence, but also letting their own self-interested bias and irrational fears interfere with their professional opinions, and using the influence of their positions to deny women and families their human rights.[32]

As a physician who firmly believes in individual freedom and family sanctity, I am grateful to the orthodox Jewish family in upstate New York for holding firm in their position that the birth of their baby was the business of the family, not the government. I am grateful to the woman in California, discussed in chapter 1, who wanted a natural birth and, when she got an unnecessary high-tech, invasive birth instead, decided to sue the obstetrician who deceived her for his own convenience. And I am grateful to the woman in Florida who fled out the back door of the hospital when she heard that doctors were going to give her a forced C-section. These strong, independent, courageous women and their families may not always have gotten what they wanted, but they gave it their best shot and are heroes in today's movement toward humanized birth.

A common scare tactic used by obstetricians is to say that every out-of-hospital birth transported to the hospital is a "train wreck." The answer to this point is, "Of course." A competent out-of-hospital midwife will transport only those rare cases where there is a serious problem requiring surgical interventions not available in the home or birth center. For those obstetricians who have never attended a home birth (which is to say nearly all obstetricians), these out-of-hospital cases with problems are their only experience, so they erroneously assume they represent all out-of-hospital births. That is why it is essential that doctors experience out-of-hospital birth firsthand.

The shocking stories at the beginning of this chapter are hard to understand until one understands that calling in the cops is merely a heavy-handed attempt by doctors, medical organizations, and government boards to intimidate women and midwives and to steer them away from out-of-hospital birth. These tactics are scary, no doubt about it. But it's fascinating to me that in many of these cases, the intimidators have somehow managed to pick on the wrong midwife. They attacked strong, gutsy midwives who were not about to knuckle under, who were willing to fight for their clients' right to choose the kind of birth they want. The midwives have succeeded: a planned birth in an ABC or at home is an option for most women in the United States, though exercising that option can be a challenge.

As I discussed in chapter 2, it is possible for a group of obstetricians in a given community to actually close down an ABC by discouraging and perhaps threatening any physician who agrees to provide backup. Arranging backup for a home birth practice can also be an enormous challenge, as one nurse-midwife, Juliana van Olphen-Fehr, wrote in *Diary of a Midwife:* "Because I covered a wide geographical area, I was always searching for more backup physicians. Because of the restrictions on nurse-midwives, I was forced into begging doctors to work with me. I developed a schedule for myself so I could tolerate this degrading and emotionally exhausting exercise. After initiating one meeting with a doctor, I would give myself a three-week break before initiating another one. This would give me ample breaks between doctors and their rejections."[33] Midwife Fehr is an intelligent, highly educated, highly trained, and caring professional, now the coordinator of the School of Midwifery at the University of Shenandoah in Virginia. It is a sad day when such a highly qualified professional must go with hat in hand to obstetricians and beg for collaboration.

Another story recounted in *Diary of Midwife* further illustrates the vicious nature of obstetric politics (for the long, exciting version, read the book).[34] During a planned home birth, Midwife Fehr transferred to the hospital a woman who was bleeding during labor. The ambulance squad that arrived at the home couldn't take the woman to the hospital where the midwife's backup physician was on staff because the ambulance was authorized only to take patients to another hospital and therefore took her to this other hospital. Midwife Fehr and her client arrived at the hospital at midnight. The staff contacted the obstetrician on call, Dr. G, who did not come in but gave a few orders over the phone. Midwife Fehr stayed with the woman in the hospital until her bleeding stopped a couple of hours later. When the obstetrician came in the next morning, long after the bleeding had stopped, "he admonished the woman for having a home birth. He fiercely massaged her uterus, barked discharge orders to the nurse, and left."

A few days later, Dr. G called Midwife Fehr at home. "I'm calling the Board of Health on you," he screamed. "I think what you're doing is illegal. I'm going to find out the rules about home birth. I bet you're breaking them. I'll make sure you don't practice anymore." Several weeks later, the state board of health called Midwife Fehr to say that Dr. G had filed a complaint and there would be an investigation.

Several months later, Midwife Fehr attended a board meeting of a state maternity care system committee where another obstetrician (not Dr. G) said, "Midwives are dangerous. I have a letter here that an obstetrician sent to the board of health about a nurse-midwife in the Winchester area who dumped a lady hemorrhaging after a home birth, leaving him to save her life." This obstetrician on the committee was not on the board of health, and should never have seen the letter, but not surprisingly the letter was passed around among the obstetricians and brought out to justify their prejudice.

When Midwife Fehr was completely cleared of any charges by the state board of health, the state board of medicine decided to go after Midwife Fehr's backup physician, who hadn't even been involved in the case. There was an investigation, but thankfully, the physician remained completely supportive of the midwife and was also completely cleared. This episode of harassment took its toll on Midwife Fehr as well as on the rest of the home birth midwives and their backup physicians in Virginia.

Those who hope to eliminate out-of-hospital birth also use the media to scare women. When the study by Pang and colleagues came out, ACOG issued a news release to tell the world how dangerous home birth had proved to be.[35] ACOG either didn't recognize the serious methodological faults that rendered the study valueless or didn't care about them. Finally, after thirty years of saying that home birth is dangerous without any evidence to support the statement, ACOG had a study to quote and it wasn't going to hold back. The Reuters News Service came out with a report that started, "Twice as many infant deaths occurred during home births as with hospital deliveries," and the *New York Times* had its own article parroting Reuters and ACOG.[36]

In sharp contrast, in 2005, when the Johnson and Daviss paper, using impeccable scientific methodology, was published in the *British Medical Journal (BMJ)*, a prestigious medical journal, clearly showing the safety of planned home birth attended by midwives, there was no news release from ACOG, no media coverage, and no ACOG letter to the *BMJ*. Readers may respond to *BMJ* articles with online "rapid response" letters, which are immediately posted on an online list of responses. My rapid response letter, sent a month after publication and titled "Silence of the Lions" reads in part:

> When a study is published with scientifically valid evidence against an
> important position of a clinical group, clinicians have two common reac-

tions: ignore the study and hope it goes away; torture the data until it confesses to what they want it to say.

It is instructive to observe who has and who has not responded to date to the study of planned home birth by Johnson and Daviss. The largest group of responders consists of midwives and other supporters of the demedicalization of birth. This group recognizes the excellence of the methodology, the importance of the findings, and the consistency with the existing weight of evidence. The second largest group of responders is primary care physicians, some of whom are generally positive about the findings while others try to torture the data to justify running away from the heresy of agreeing to health care which is not in some kind of medical setting: "this information does not change my practice."

Then we have the silence of the lions: why are the obstetricians not responding? With one possible exception, there are no obstetrician responders to a study with major implications for obstetric practice. And the one physician responder, who may or may not be an obstetrician, rejects supporting planned home birth, even if safe, because of the "pernicious legal system." Fear of litigation is a highly selective excuse used by some obstetricians when there is something which is not obstetrician-friendly such as planned home birth (over which they have no control and no profit). . . .

It is doubtful there will be obstetrician responders to this study because of their hope that by ignoring it, this study will go away. . . . And their silence in the face of the present outstanding study by Johnson and Daviss of the safety of home birth is to be expected.[37]

Meanwhile, woman are telling another story, as e-mail messages fly among midwives, women's groups, and consumer groups exposing the ways the medical world is trying to limit a woman's legitimate choice of place of birth and birth attendant. And the Johnson and Daviss paper makes the Hit Parade in the *BMJ*. The *BMJ* released its 2005 annual top ten list of articles receiving the most attention on the Web. This paper on home birth was the second most popular among several hundred papers, having been accessed on-line in some form almost forty thousand times since publication.

So, in spite of all the strategies reviewed here—from calling in the obstetric police to lying to legislators to withholding insurance or physician backup to the media blitz—women continue to give birth outside of hospitals. In fact, every year the National Center for Health Statistics reports an increase in home births attended by midwives.[38] Freedom, family sanctity, the woman's choice, and human rights should dictate place of birth, not autocratic attempts at control made by the medical establishment.

SEVEN

RIGHTS AND WRONGS: THE "MALPRACTICE CRISIS," LEGAL
PROTECTIONS FOR PREGNANT WOMEN, AND REGULATION BY LITIGATION

Democracies die behind closed doors.
JUDGE DAMON KEITH, U.S. COURT OF APPEALS

THE LITIGATION "CRISIS"

On the same day in May 2002, I learned two related pieces of information. At a press conference on "the malpractice crisis" called by the American College of Obstetricians and Gynecologists (ACOG), obstetricians were complaining bitterly about the expensive malpractice insurance premiums they have to pay. Later that day, I got a phone call from a lawyer telling me that a case against two small-town obstetricians practicing in Idaho (discussed in chapter 4) had been settled. The doctors' insurance company would now have to pay millions of dollars to a family whose son was severely brain-damaged because labor had been unnecessarily induced with Cytotec. Putting these two pieces of information together, I asked myself why ACOG continues to promote a drug for inducing labor that has not been approved by the FDA, when the drug has caused the damage and death of women and babies and has resulted in lots of legal cases that end in big settlements and drive up malpractice premiums.[1]

Obstetricians are sued more than physicians in any other specialty. In the United States, a member of ACOG can expect to be sued 2.53 times over the course of his career, and in 1999, 76 percent of ACOG fellows reported that they had been sued at least once so far.[2] Obstetrics-gynecology is considered a "high-risk" specialty by malpractice insurers, and in 2000, obstetricians were listed first by the Physicians Insurance Association of America among twenty-eight specialty groups in the number of claims reported against them.[3]

As a result, fear of litigation has a profound influence on all aspects of American obstetrics. It affects attitudes and policies in obstetric organizations and hospitals, and it affects the behavior and judgment of individual obstetricians. After years as a practicing physician, I can say that fear of litigation is a factor for many doctors when they decide on a care plan for a patient. So it was no surprise when a Harris survey found that three-quarters of physicians "feel their ability to provide quality care has been hurt by concerns over liability cases."[4]

When obstetricians in the United States are asked why there is such a gap between the way scientific evidence says they should be practicing (regarding interventions) and the way they are actually practicing, they frequently defend their actions by saying that interventions are necessary to protect themselves from litigation. In effect, what these doctors are saying is that they view themselves as victims of the legal system and they feel that this justifies making treatment choices that have nothing to do with the patient or the patient's condition. This is a striking admission.

Obstetricians spend a great deal of energy acting out their victim role and bemoaning what they've labeled "the litigation crisis." At professional meetings it is always a popular topic, and I can assure you that the emotions can become very intense. At a recent UCLA medical alumni meeting, I listened to discussions where angry doctors railed against "mercenary attorneys" and the "stupid families" they recruit.

Yes, most American obstetricians have been sued, and yes, there are high insurance premiums, but I don't believe these two realities are enough to explain obstetricians' extreme attitude. It is obvious to me that obstetricians have an enormous fear of ending up in court. Court horror stories circulate frequently among doctors, and the theme of many of these stories is that a doctor in court is not in control, out of his element. Furthermore, as discussed in chapter 2, doctors don't admit that they make mistakes, and the whole point of litigation is to identify and prove that a doctor indeed made a mistake. This is humiliating and shatters an obstetrician's inflated sense of security. In an obstetrician's daily world, everyone with whom he comes in contact looks up to him and follows his orders. In a courtroom, an obstetrician may even be looked down on. In chapter 2, I stated my view that being an obstetrician in the obstetric world is like living as an animal with no natural predators. A courtroom is not in the obstetric world. Predators lurk in the courtroom.

This means that when an obstetrician provides prenatal care to a woman or "attends" a birth, the possibility that the patient could end up suing if something goes wrong is never far from his mind. This can only contribute to the antagonistic "us versus them" mentality discussed in chapter 2 and hamper the doctor's ability to be compassionate with a birthing woman under his care.

The constant threat of litigation also means that many obstetricians in the United States go about their practice with a defensive mindset. The decision to do a C-section, which we might call the ultimate intervention, is often based not on medical need but on a desire to avoid litigation. There is a widespread belief among obstetricians that if a C-section is not done and the baby is not perfect, the doctor takes the risk that he will be accused of not doing "everything possible" to address complications or potential complications. Conversely, when a C-section is done, it appears that the doctor made every effort to safeguard the health of the woman and baby. Doing a C-section has become a kind of insurance against litigation. This is because, in our society, surgery is perceived as a definitive cure. Regardless of what an obstetrician may or may not do during a women's labor (such as performing interventions that put the mother and baby at risk), performing a C-section negates possible criticism. The perception that surgery represents the ultimate human effort exists despite the fact that, as we saw in chapter 3, when an obstetrician performs a C-section unnecessarily, he puts the mother and baby at risk.

On a more subtle level, an electronic fetal monitor (EFM) is often used defensively as well. Using a machine to monitor contractions and the fetal heartbeat may seem harmless enough, but using an EFM routinely on every woman in labor interferes with the woman's ability to move (stand up, sit, walk, etc.), and a lack of movement increases the risk that her labor will slow or even stop. Furthermore, studies have shown that routine use of an EFM does not increase the chance of a healthy baby but *does* increase the chance that invasive interventions such as C-section, which carry significant risks for both the woman and her baby, will be done unnecessarily. However, for many doctors, routine use of an EFM is perceived as protection. If there is a bad outcome and a doctor is sued, he can bring the EFM printout to court and say, "See, the machine says the baby was fine," or conversely, "See, the machine says the baby was in distress, so the C-section was necessary."

There are several serious problems with defensive obstetrics—that is, doctors choosing practices that they believe will help them avoid negligence claims. A fundamental principle of medical practice is that whatever the doctor does must be done first and foremost for the benefit of the patient. If a doctor picks up a scalpel and cuts open a pregnant woman's belly because the doctor is afraid of being sued or afraid of rising insurance costs, that doctor is not practicing medicine. He is practicing fear and greed.

Defensive thinking has spread to every part of obstetrics practice. In chapter 4, I discussed how obstetricians use a false diagnosis to protect themselves from litigation. In cases where a woman and/or her baby are harmed by the use of Cytotec for inducing labor, it is common to find the diagnosis "postdate" in the patient's chart as the reason for the induction, and then, on closer examination, to discover that the baby had not been late after all.

In chapter 3, I described a case in which a doctor's defensive attitude was behind a poorly conceived study that led to a baby's death. An obstetrician decided to look at using a prostaglandin to induce labor in women who'd had previous C-sections, though the drug's label specifically says that it should not be used in this way. The study was a disaster, and the obstetrician later admitted that one of the primary reasons for undertaking it was that he and other doctors in his hospital wanted to use the drug, had in fact already been using it, and hoped their research would produce "evidence" of its safety that would protect them from litigation.

Following is another story of what happens when research is conducted to protect doctors from litigation. In chapter 4, I told of a woman who died following a Cytotec induction that led to a condition called amniotic fluid embolism (AFE). There is evidence that the number of women dying from AFE in the United States is increasing, and I have believed for some time that one reason the numbers are going up is that this diagnosis has become popular among doctors who have made an error that led to a woman's death and have chosen a diagnosis that may not be accurate but that they believe will help their case if the patient's family decides to sue.

In 1941, two physicians, Steiner and Lushbaugh, first identified eight cases of a syndrome they named "amniotic fluid embolism," in which amniotic fluid containing baby's skin cells, hair, and so on, leaks into the mother's bloodstream, blocks lung and heart functions, and, in 80 percent of cases, causes the woman's death.[5] Synthetic oxytocin (Pitocin) and other pharmacological agents now used to stimulate the uterus were not available for clinical use in 1941, but as these drugs gained popularity for inducing and augmenting labor in the 1960s and 1970s,[6] doctors observed an association between the use of uterine stimulants and AFE, and there was general consensus that inducing or augmenting labor with drugs increases the risk of AFE.[7]

Then in 1979, M. Morgan, a researcher, published a survey of the English literature on AFE that reported on 272 cases.[8] He wrote that although there is an alleged association of AFE with the use of uterine stimulants to accelerate labor, their use was mentioned in only 22 percent of cases. He concluded that in view of the very wide use of accelerated labor and the rarity of amniotic fluid embolism, there must be no direct association between the two.

For a number of reasons, Morgan's paper and conclusions were not scientifically valid.[9] The study reported merely anecdotal evidence based on cases found in a review of the literature (not an experimental trial or a case control study), his reasoning was scientifically flawed, he used an incorrect comparison group, and many of the cases he looked at were from the 1940s, before uterine stimulants were even used.

Then in 1990, Steven Clark, an obstetrician, reviewed the issue of a causal relationship between using drugs to stimulate the uterus and AFE.[10] There were no new data and no new cases in Clark's paper. He theorized about the pathogenesis of AFE and then relied on Morgan's paper, based on faulty scientific methodology, to emphatically claim that there is clearly no relationship between the use of oxytocin and the development of the AFE syndrome.

This statement started an assumption train that continues to the present day and has become the basis for the belief that AFE is something that "just happens"—a condition that doctors can neither cause nor prevent—in other words, the perfect defense in court. It was not until much later that we learned that at the time he published his paper, Clark was involved in a number of lawsuits involving AFE and had been brought in to testify that the doctors and hospitals were blameless because there is no relationship between uterine stimulant drugs and AFE.

In 1993, ACOG weighed in on the issue with a predictable opinion: "In the past, oxytocin was sometimes implicated in the genesis of amniotic fluid embolism syndrome. However, such a relationship has been refuted on both statistical and theoretical grounds."[11] Two papers were listed in support of this statement: Clark 1990 and Morgan 1979. ACOG called Morgan's paper "statistical grounds" and Clark's paper "theoretical grounds" and failed to recognize the fundamental scientific flaws in both papers. It is important to note that it was in the early 1990s that U.S. obstetricians began to use misoprostol (Cytotec) for induction of labor and induction rates were rapidly increasing.[12] Consequently, it was becoming more and more important to claim that uterine stimulant drugs were not associated with AFE.

In 1988, Clark established a national registry of AFE cases by inviting individuals to submit cases. Sixty-nine charts were submitted and forty-six met the criteria for inclusion. The registry accepted cases dating back to 1983. The cases were then analyzed and Clark and colleagues published a paper in 1995.[13] Again, however, several significant mistakes were made in the analysis, including an incorrect comparison group, rendering the study invalid.

In their 1995 paper, Clark and colleagues concluded by urging caution and saying that the authors fully recognize the potential biases of the registry, but they nevertheless reinforced Clark's previous finding, saying that their observations appear to refute the concept of a causative relationship between oxytocin and AFE on a clinical basis, supporting the statement of ACOG that such a relationship has been refuted on both statistical and theoretical grounds.

It is easier to understand how this inaccurate conclusion was arrived at when we consider that of the forty-six AFE cases collected and analyzed in his 1995 article, Clark, the senior author, had been retained by lawyers in 75 percent of them to testify that the condition was not preventable or treatable and that there was no relationship between AFE and induction of labor. Sadly, Clark has admitted destroying all the data used in the study—a most unusual and scientifically improper act, as it meant that the results could not be questioned or further analyzed.[14]

Following the 1995 paper by Clark and colleagues, the conclusion that there is no association between the use of uterine stimulant drugs and AFE began to find its way into obstetric textbooks. In the widely read and quoted twentieth edition of *Williams Obstetrics* published in 1997, of which Clark was one of the chief editors, in the section on AFE, there were seven references to papers that include Clark as an author.[15] The text stated categorically: "There is no causal association between oxytocin use and amniotic fluid embolism, and the frequency of oxytocin use is not increased in these women compared with the general obstetrical population."[16] The statement about the need for caution had disappeared.

In 1998, ACOG repeated its earlier position: "Oxytocin use has not been reported to be associated with this [AFE] complication."[17] This statement was supported by four references: Morgan 1979, Clark 1990, Clark et al. 1995, and Martin 1996. (There are no new cases in Martin's paper as it is only a short review.)[18] In 1999, ACOG made a strong statement regarding oxytocin use in labor and AFE in one of the organization's publications: "Although AFE was once thought to be associated with oxytocin-induced labor, there is no causal relationship between oxytocin use or antecedent hyperstimulation and AFE."[19] This statement was supported by two references, Morgan 1979 and Clark et al. 1995. Since it had been well established for years that uterine stimulant drugs often can lead to uterine hyperstimulation—too frequent contractions—it is interesting to note that antecedent hyperstimulation (too rapid contractions of the uterus during the labor before the onset of AFE) is now included in the denial. Since then, Clark's conclusion, based on faulty science and almost certainly designed to protect physicians from legal responsibility in maternal deaths, has continued to appear—expressed with ever-increasing certainty—in obstetric textbooks and ACOG publications, including *Williams Obstetrics,* 21st edition (2001); ACOG, *Prolog: Obstetrics,* 5th edition (2003); *Danforth's Obstetrics and Gynecology,* 9th edition (2003); and *Critical Care Obstetrics,* 4th edition (2004).

Since the 1990s, there have been sufficient case reports of AFE after Cytotec induction in the literature, and enough reports have been sent to both the U.S. Food and Drug Administration and Searle, the manufacturer of Cytotec, to justify including AFE as one of the risks of using Cytotec on pregnant women, both on the package insert and in the warning letter to all U.S. physicians discussed in chapter 4.[20] Nevertheless, AFE remains a popular diagnosis to use to protect a doctor or hospital from culpability when a woman dies in or near childbirth. I am familiar with more than one hundred cases of maternal mortality after labor induction with uterine stimulant drugs. In two cases (one in upstate New York and one at Yale–New Haven Hospital), the doctors who conducted the autopsy on the woman stated that AFE was the cause of death, and then, in both cases, gratuitously inserted into their autopsy reports a statement saying that in cases of AFE, no one can be blamed. Such statements are completely inappropriate in a pathologist's report, but they are hardly surprising, given the culture of tribal loyalty among doctors, obstetric silence or "omertà," and the fact that a doctor who says anything against another doctor in a courtroom—even in cases of serious malpractice—puts his career at risk (see chapter 2).

And now it looks as though the days are over when obstetricians, faced with a woman who has died during childbirth, are able to play the AFE "get out of jail free" card. First came my paper published in 2005 reviewing the existing scientific literature on AFE and demonstrating that it was false science that was used to try to deny any connection between uterine stimulants during labor and AFE.[21] Then in 2006, the first ever large population-based study of AFE cases, using a cohort of three million hospital births, showed nearly twice the risk of AFE (and three and a half times the risk of fatal AFE) when uterine stimulants were used to induce labor.[22]

In malpractice cases, for the most part, it is not difficult for defense lawyers to find sympathetic obstetricians to come to the aid of their clients and testify when there has been an adverse outcome and the doctor is accused of malpractice that "Dr. X chose the right course under the circumstances," or to testify, as Steven Clark has done so many times with AFE, that research shows a particular outcome was not preventable. But the lawyers who represent patients have a terrible time finding doctors willing to testify. In most cases, they are forced to bring in a physician from another state because local doctors are too afraid of retribution (which can take many forms, from loss of referrals from other doctors to removal from hospital staffs). I am sometimes contacted by lawyers asking if I would help them find a doctor in their area willing to testify.

A defensive mindset hurts the obstetrics system in the United States in many ways, but perhaps the strongest argument against it is simply that it doesn't work. Despite the fact that three-quarters of practicing physicians have effectively admitted to practicing defensively, there has been little slowdown in litigation as a result. This suggests that, at least to some extent, fear of litigation has become an excuse that allows doctors to continue to use interventions such as induction of labor and C-section that they prefer to use for other reasons. It also illustrates that doctors' fear of the "litigation crisis" has become a self-fulfilling prophecy.

When obstetricians, undoubtedly encouraged by the insurance industry, which stands to gain enormously by legislation to cap awards to families, talk about the litigation problem, they tend to blame hysterical women, greedy lawyers, and an unfair legal system. For the benefit of the media and politicians, they paint a picture of a legal system that is completely out of control. But research sponsored by the Institute of Medicine has shown this "crisis" to be a myth. One study conducted by two eminent professors looked at obstetrics and gynecology malpractice jury awards in forty-six counties in eleven states over five years. They found that the accepted wisdom blames the legal system for the problems faced by doctors. They state further that physicians and commentators have argued that there are too many lawsuits, too many jury awards for plaintiffs, and too many large awards in an unpredictable fashion. In contrast, their study found that few of these cases go before a jury, that plaintiffs do not usually win, and that there are identifiable patterns in what juries decide in the cases that come before them.[23]

The truth is that obstetricians bring litigation on themselves when they practice vigilante medicine such as Cytotec induction of labor and make little or no effort to develop an evidence-based practice. Clearly, if physicians waited to adopt new interventions until there was sufficient scientific evidence showing that the benefits outweigh the risks, it would result in fewer risks to the patients, reduce the chance of adverse outcomes, and reduce the chance that litigation will follow.

Another reason there is so much obstetric litigation is that most U.S. hospitals do not have an effective complaint process for women and families who have had a bad birth experience and want information on what went wrong. There is a movement in the United States toward transparency and accountability in health care services, but we still have a long way to go. Secrecy and self-protection are still the norm. When there has been a bad outcome at a birth, most attempts to get information from doctors and hospitals are stonewalled, sometimes in subtle ways.

Most hospitals have someone called a "patient liaison" whose job it is to meet with a family that has a grievance or suspects that a mistake was made. Liaisons are usually women (as one might expect) and tend to be highly paid, for they have a challenging job. A staff member of a department store complaint department can almost always satisfy a customer by quickly agreeing that, yes, the clerk was rude or incompetent, or, yes, the product was defective. All they have to do is apologize and reimburse the customer. But a hospital's liaison can never admit that a doctor or other staff member was incompetent or made a mistake. Instead they must "spin" the situation to put the hospital and doctors in the best possible light. It is a liaison's job to convince patients that there has been no malpractice. It is not her primary job to assist patients in getting all relevant information or resolving their issues. It is important to remember that no matter how sympathetically she listens, a patient liaison is a hospital employee and on the hospital's side. I have personally seen that liaisons will participate in a cover-up when necessary.

There are various laws that protect patients (discussed later in this chapter), but most patients don't fully understand the laws that protect them, and in my experience doctors and hospital "spin doctors" are in no hurry to educate them. It can be complicated because, although basic patient rights are insured by federal law, some rights, for example those regarding informed consent and disclosure of information, partly fall under state laws and vary from state to state. All hospitals that receive federal funding (about 80 percent of hospitals) must have a chief compliance officer and some form of "internal grievance process," but the details vary greatly from one hospital to another. Many patients aren't even aware that a complaint process exists and many hospitals are not eager to inform them. Those families that do file a complaint are likely to run into obstacles: hospital records that have been "lost" (the law says that a patient's medical records belong to the patient), fees required at every step in the process (e.g., for making copies of records), strange delays, and long, unintelligible legal forms. Hospitals work hard to attract maternity patients, and they work equally hard to keep any complaints hush-hush. Their goal is to appease the family while showing them in every way possible that they are ungrateful and irresponsible to complain.

Ironically, a very persistent, legally savvy patient can sometimes obtain information from a hospital without going to court. But for the average citizen who suspects that she has been wronged by an individual doctor or a powerful medical institution, going to court is the obvious answer. That is what our civil courts are for, after all. When a family can't get answers to their questions about their birth, it is perfectly reasonable for them to turn to the legal system that is there to protect them.

Another cause of obstetric litigation that we don't hear much about from doctors and hospitals is the betrayal and anger patients feel when their baby is damaged or dies. I believe these feelings are, at least in part, the result of false promises made by doctors and hospitals. Doctors and hospitals have a dilemma. They know perfectly well that childbirth does not always go smoothly, and may even result in the death of the woman or baby. But with maternity care in the private sector as a big money maker, doctors and hospitals must compete for patients. To survive, they must put their best foot forward, stressing their strengths and downplaying any negative aspects of the care they provide. There is a constant tension between the need for a successful marketing strategy and the need to behave ethically and professionally as medical providers.

In order to convince birthing women to give up the comfort and security of their homes and give birth in hospitals, doctors and hospitals find it necessary to feed pregnant women and their families promotional statements in pamphlets and in advertisements on radio and television that come extremely close to promising a perfectly safe birth and a perfect baby.

Come tour our lovely birthing rooms (but don't try to find out our obstetric track record, because we're not going to tell you). Often hospital maternity ads are not exactly lies, but neither are they responsible in the sense of providing balanced information on what may happen. That hospitals take this approach is an inevitable consequence of the marketplace for maternity services. The fact that patients believe the hype is probably due in part to their desire to believe and in part to the widespread view that with modern technology, a 100 percent safety record is actually feasible. But if you play God, you will be blamed for natural disasters. There is no country in the world where babies do not die or where women giving birth do not die. In the United States, more than one thousand women die every year around the time of birth, and around thirty-five thousand babies die every year around the time of birth—and sometimes it is due to a mistake in care.

Throughout history, women have accepted this harsh reality as part of the human condition, but attitudes have shifted in recent decades. Now we find obstetricians writing in the medical literature that childbirth has become very safe for both mothers and babies.[24] (This is the prevailing attitude despite the fact that the rate of women and babies dying is going up, so it is getting less safe, not more safe, to give birth in the United States.) Of course, average women don't read the medical literature, but statements like this reflect the obstetric attitude most doctors project to their customers— we are doing the best possible job and should never be challenged. As a result, parents have come to expect a perfectly safe birth. It is no surprise that when something does go wrong they feel deceived. But instead of understanding their role in generating false hopes, obstetricians turn right around and blame families for their expectations. In the very same article, the authors object to a couple's expectation of a perfect baby.[25]

Obstetricians, hospitals, and organizations such as ACOG invest an enormous amount of time and money in avoiding litigation and hampering the litigation process. Although they are quick to hold news conferences to tell the public about the awful litigation crisis—ACOG has issued eight news releases in the past two years on obstetric liability issues[26]—they make every effort to prevent the public from finding out about individual cases that might give women, families, and lawyers ideas about the mistakes being made during labor and birth.

When there is a bad outcome at a birth, the hospital internal "peer review" committee—consisting of fellow clinicians or peers in that hospital—will investigate, but these meetings are always private, and investigation results are not admissible in court. This confidentiality versus transparency issue is complex. On the one hand, if members of a peer review committee are not certain their findings will be confidential, they will not be open and honest and unafraid to be critical of their peers. This eliminates the possibility of learning from mistakes and improving practices and protocols at the hospital.

On the other hand, when investigations are kept private, transparency is lost. We lose the possibility that doctors who are not on the committee will learn from peer-reviewed cases as well as the ability to consider these cases in research. If a lawsuit ensues, valuable analysis—often the real truth of what occurred—cannot be revealed in court. And a family whose life has been profoundly affected is denied information. Certainly this level of confidentiality is not found in any other industry and is not fair to women and families.

The British have found a middle ground in the confidentiality/transparency issue in the form of a special investigation process for maternal mortality cases. When a woman dies around the time of birth, a group of experts (none of whom is on staff at the hospital in question) conduct a thorough investigation. When the investigation is completed, the investigators review their findings in a confidential meeting held at the hospital and attended by all staff involved in the case. This allows the staff to learn from the case and, if necessary, change their practices.

All names and other identifying details are then removed from the investigation data and the data is grouped with other maternal mortality data for the country. Every three years a government report is published that includes a thorough analysis of all cases. The report is available to everyone (practitioners, scientists, politicians, and the public). Medical researchers in countries that do not have this level of transparency in maternal mortality cases (such as the United States) use the data as well. For example, the data in chapter 3 on increased maternal mortality in elective C-section are from this British report. However, while the British maternal mortality system is certainly an improvement over what we currently have in the United States, it does not go much further in honoring the rights of families.

When they don't think they can win a case, lawyers for doctors, hospitals, and insurance companies settle cases out of court and include a gag order on families and their lawyers in the settlement that makes it a crime for them to discuss the case publicly. For this reason, it is very difficult for scientists, policy makers, and health care consumers to discover the extent of the litigation involving Cytotec induction. Obstetricians and hospitals don't want the public to know about these cases for fear that the news would encourage more Cytotec victims to sue and because it would damage the public image of obstetricians by increasing public awareness of the fact that they are using powerful drugs on women in labor that have not been approved by the FDA for this purpose. In a 2004 article, I reported on sixteen cases of induction with Cytotec with adverse outcomes and I have been asked to review several more cases since my article was published.[27] I am certain this is only the tip of the iceberg. Of the cases I'm familiar with, two were in Oregon, and both settled for well over a million dollars; one was in Washington State and it too settled for more than a million dollars; a case in New York State settled for more than a million dollars; and cases in Massachusetts, South Carolina, Texas, Florida, Connecticut, Maryland, and Pennsylvania all settled for very large sums. The only case I know of that settled for a large sum and did not include a gag order was the case in Idaho, and in that instance, the lawyers tried to get a gag order but the appalled judge would not allow it.

To my knowledge, to date every case of litigation involving Cytotec induction has been settled before coming to trial, with two exceptions, and those cases were partially settled but did go to trial. It's not hard to understand why. As discussed in chapter 4, when a doctor uses a drug that is not approved by the FDA or the drug company for induction, and their choice results in a damaged or dead woman or baby or both, any trial would likely draw media coverage and it would be hard for the doctor or hospital to win. Nevertheless, even with all the attempts to hide the tragic outcomes of vigilante practices with settlements and gag orders, the truth has a way of leaking out.

Lawyers with experience in obstetric litigation have told me that most cases are won by the defense because, in general, the public has a deep need to believe what doctors say, and because it is easy to find doctors willing to defend other doctors but very difficult to find doctors willing to testify against other doctors. Malpractice litigation is not a level playing field in other ways as well. The family in a case usually has limited means, whereas the defense (doctors and hospitals) have malpractice insurance, with very large resources at hand—nearly a David and Goliath situation. In most cases, the defense tries hard to delay going to trial. They can make it costly for the family by bringing in many doctors to testify for the defense (which results in a lot of expensive depositions), in the hope that the family will give up before the case can be heard by a jury. Cytotec litigation is an exception to the rule, as it is difficult to defend against the FDA and the pharmaceutical industry, and a family with a dead mother or a dead or brain-damaged baby is always an object of sympathy to a jury.

Another strategy used by obstetric organizations is to try to get the American public to feel sorry for the doctors who "can't afford" to pay their insurance premiums, despite the fact that on average, obstetricians take home in the neighborhood of $200,000 a year (after taxes and insurance expenses). President Bush has been sympathetic to their "plight" and urges giving doctors a break by capping awards to families for noneconomic damages at $250,000.[28] ACOG has taken it a step further and turned this into a game of semi-blackmail, suggesting that obstetricians won't keep delivering babies if something isn't done to help them. In an editorial in August 2002, ACOG complains about "the erosion of the ability to make a good living" and threatens that "without state and federal legislation, many rural areas will be without obstetricians because of difficulty getting professional liability insurance."[29] In a May 2002 news release, ACOG insisted, "Problems in the nation's medical liability system could severely jeopardize the availability of physicians to deliver babies in the U.S."[30] And again in a news release in July 2004, ACOG reported that a medical liability survey reaffirmed that more obstetrician/gynecologists are quitting obstetrics.[31] I can't help but believe that this kind of scare tactic is likely to backfire. In chapter 5, I discussed how doctors in Madera County, California, played the same game by refusing to attend births at the county hospital. Midwives were hired instead, at a significant salary savings, and the number of babies dying at birth fell dramatically.

When the topic of settlement caps comes up, I am inclined to remind people of the family in Idaho whose son was born with extreme brain damage due to an unnecessary Cytotec induction. All the medical specialists, including pediatric neurologists, who have seen this little boy agree that, now at five years of age, the child has severe cerebral palsy so he can't crawl, much less sit or walk; has severe mental retardation, so he can't talk and knows only family members; is unable to feed and swallow normally and must be fed with a tube; and is probably blind. The specialists also all agree that all these severe disabilities are due to what happened during labor and birth.

For more than four years, this family has provided around-the-clock nursing care for their son, a heroic effort that will probably need to continue for the next forty years. Every health care professional who has worked with this boy writes in the chart about the child's devoted and loving family. The cost of their son's medical care is staggering, but beyond the financial burden, the pain and suffering this family has endured, and will continue to endure for many years to come, is hard to imagine.

Contrast the money issues this family in Idaho has with the money issues of the two obstetricians who gave the mother her unnecessary Cytotec induction. There is nothing wrong with hard-working obstetricians earning a reasonable income. But it is unreasonable, even offensive, for obstetricians to try to increase their net income by lobbying for caps on the amount a jury can award a family in obstetric cases as a way to get their malpractice insurance premiums down. In the President's State of the Union Address in 2006, he called on Congress for the fourth year in a row to pass medical liability reform, and ACOG, commenting on this in a news release, calls such lawsuits "frivolous," a comment that could well be put into perspective by the family and their community in Idaho.[32] I do not believe that the American public wants obstetricians and insurance companies to become richer at the expense of families with damaged or dead women or babies.

In cases that do go to court, one of the most effective strategies used by doctors to limit damages for malpractice is called "community standard of practice." This is an extraordinary bit of reasoning that goes like this: Whatever a doctor is doing, if it is done by other doctors in that community, it can be called the "standard of practice" and should be considered proper regardless of bad outcomes. This is like saying that although the speed limit on the highway is sixty-five miles per hour, if a number of drivers are going eighty miles per hour, the acceptable speed on the highway is really eighty miles per hour. When this reasoning is argued in court, it means that to be relieved of responsibility, a doctor who has been sued for doing something terrible need only find a few doctors in his neighborhood or even from quite far away if in the same state who are willing to testify that they do it too. This reasoning is still common despite the fact that every obstetric textbook now teaches that evidence-based practice—that is, practice that is in accordance with what scientific evidence says is effective and safe—is the best standard of practice, and it is no longer acceptable to adopt as a standard of practice that which merely reflects what some doctors do.

As discussed in chapter 2, in the Idaho case that resulted in a severely brain-damaged baby, the obstetricians being sued were the only two obstetricians in a small-town joint practice, and they used this reasoning in their deposition. They were questioned concerning their management of the Cytotec induction, and it was established that they did not follow hospital protocol in their use of the drug. When Dr. X was asked whether he believed that it's okay for doctors not to follow hospital protocol, as he did not, he replied, "The judgment of the individual allows them to do that if they want to," and "The way that Dr. Y and I used [the drug] at the time is the standard of care." Dr. Y then added, "There is no national standard of care." When asked if he is familiar with the standard of care in his community, he replied, "I am familiar with what I do."

When asked, "Do you rely on FDA approval in any way in your selection of drugs to administer to patients?" Dr. X replied, "No," and added, "the use of a drug in pregnancy, whether the manufacturer endorses it or not, is my decision, based on clinical judgment." When he was asked if the selection and dose of drug is "his call and nobody else's," he replied, "It is." When asked if a hospital protocol is binding, Dr. X replied, "I don't think that it is. I think it has room for physicians to order more doses and choose routes and do what they feel comfortable doing." Dr. X also stated that he does not consider the textbook *Williams Obstetrics* to be authoritative. Dr. Y concurred, saying that he does not rely on obstetric textbooks.

When two obstetricians can say that they, and only they, establish their standards of practice, based on what they "feel comfortable" doing, and that they are free to ignore the FDA, hospital protocols, and obstetric textbooks, it is a dangerous form of vigilantism and medical anarchy. In a community such as theirs, where they are the only obstetricians in town and all the family physicians and nurses follow their lead, there is no way for a woman even to determine if she is receiving high-quality health care, let alone choose from among a range of birth options. Would you want to have a baby there?

The attitude taken by these two obstetricians is in keeping with a long tradition in the medical profession. When physicians are asked to account for their practices, and feel their backs against the wall, they pull out their ace, as Dr. X did in his deposition response: "It's a matter of clinical judgment." This is a kin to the concept of "community standard of care" and reduces the physician's culpability even further. Although the consensus wave of the future in medical practice is evidence-based practice, many doctors still believe that much of what they do for a patient is no more than a judgment call based on experience. This perspective allows them to insist that unless you were there at the time, and unless you have had as much clinical experience as they have, you can't question what they did. In other words, it is never appropriate to question a doctor's choices.

Some take it even further. In addition to having little or no training in science, most physicians in clinical practice also have little or no training in public health and epidemiology. Consequently, a surprising number of physicians have a hard time grasping the concept of evidence-based practice. They cannot understand how data gathered on a group of patients (C-section rates for a given hospital, for example) apply to an individual patient. Some of these physicians have published papers in clinical journals that object to applying recommended rates for C-section to individual hospitals and individual clinicians.[33] When defending their choices in a legal case, these doctors tend to take the out-of-date, reactionary position that it is necessary to consider all aspects of each individual case and, in the final analysis, use clinical judgment. This position, what anthropologists call "authoritative knowledge," has been very useful for obstetricians—not only as a litigation defense, but also as a weapon in their never-ending battle to protect their territory and as a way to reject what valid epidemiological evidence says they should be doing.

Another variation on the "only we can judge what we do" defense is to try to get the courts to require that only a board-qualified obstetrician can testify against a board-qualified obstetrician. Like most medical and surgical specialties, obstetricians have a "board" that consists of a small group of "senior" obstetricians (many on staff at medical schools and university hospitals). The board establishes a system of examinations, which an applicant can take to become "board-qualified." Although the system is supposed to provide quality assurance, it ironically has the opposite effect as well, in that it makes enforcing the obstetric omertà easier and the task of finding doctors willing to testify against an obstetrician much more difficult. Since the process of becoming "board-qualified" is not an "official" governmental one and is administered only by a nongovernmental organization of peers without any mechanism for oversight or regulation, it is inappropriate and dangerous for the courts to agree to this restriction. Nevertheless, this is now the law in some states.

On a national level, obstetric organizations such as ACOG have made no secret of the fact that many of their policies and recommendations are based not on a desire to promote practices that are good for patients, but on a desire to avoid or hamper litigation against their members. In chapter 2, I described in detail two recommendations in particular where ACOG has put protecting members from lawsuits above patients' needs. The first example is Committee Opinion number 207, published in September 1998, with the title "Liability Implications of Recording Procedures or Treatments," in which ACOG recommended against allowing a patient's family to create a birth video, saying that "recording solely for the purpose of patient memorabilia or marketing is not without liability, and each institution should weigh these competing concerns."

The second example is ACOG's Practice Bulletin number 5, published in July 1999, in which ACOG recommended against women attempting a vaginal birth after a previous cesarean (VBAC) except in a hospital with surgeons and anesthesiologists at the ready. The bulletin states, "That these adverse events during trial of labor have led to malpractice suits illustrates the need to reevaluate VBAC recommendations." These examples demonstrate ACOG's willingness to make or reevaluate its recommendations because of fear of litigation.

But there is another side to the litigation coin. ACOG recommendations also allow obstetricians to use litigation to their advantage, to frighten doctors and hospitals and control and maintain their monopoly. ACOG has such far-reaching influence in American obstetrics that an ACOG recommendation can be used as an attack (or defense) in court the same way an FDA approval can. This makes doctors and hospitals that go against ACOG recommendations more vulnerable to litigation.

The ACOG recommendation against VBAC is a good example of how this works. As I discussed in chapter 2, cases of uterine rupture among women who had previously had C-sections were going up (almost certainly due to an increase in pharmacological labor inductions). That was becoming a problem for ACOG members because under these conditions, the chances of a uterine rupture leading to the kind of bad outcome that precipitates a lawsuit are relatively high. Though ACOG could easily have addressed the issue by discouraging the use of pharmacological induction, it instead discouraged VBACs by recommending that women be permitted to attempt VBAC only in a hospital where an obstetrician and anesthesiologist are always present. In one fell swoop, this recommendation had a profound influence on obstetric policies at larger hospitals, where administrators were compelled to cut back on VBAC; made it legally risky for smaller hospitals, clinics, and birth centers to support VBAC at all; promoted unnecessary C-sections (creating more business for obstetricians); and limited birth options for millions of American women.

Another area of U.S. obstetrics where a fear of litigation has played an important role is in the investigation of maternal deaths. As discussed in chapters 2 and 3, we know that in the United States, at least half of maternal deaths are not reported anywhere.[34] We also know that nearly all of these women die in the hospital, not at home, and that with adequate medical attention, close to half of these women need not have died.[35] American women have a right to know that their chance of dying around the time of birth is increasing and why, and for many years, the CDC has pushed states to improve their maternal death audit processes. CDC staff members have worked with states to set up official maternal death surveillance groups.

While consulting on a case of maternal death due to Cytotec induction in South Carolina, I called the state health department to inquire about its process for investigating a case of maternal mortality. I was told that the state has four to six maternal deaths a year and it is not required by law that these cases be reported to the state. Furthermore, there is no place on a death certificate to indicate that it was maternal death (a death around the time of childbirth). That means that the state must pay someone to go through death certificates looking for maternal deaths, a difficult system with plenty of opportunity for mistakes. When a maternal death is found, the state health department reports it to the South Carolina State Medical Association, and the Medical Association is suppose to investigate. The physician responsible for the patient who died is to be called in for review in a closed session with only physicians attending.

The state medical association is a nongovernmental body with no legal authority, so all investigations are voluntary and have no power to actually change practices. Recognizing these weaknesses, the South Carolina State Health Department later started a maternal death surveillance group after urging by the CDC. Under the new system, when a maternal death was identified, the group sent two physicians and two nurses to the hospital where the death occurred as well as to the coroner. The team would abstract the records, remove all names, and report their findings to the maternal death surveillance group, which would then evaluate the case and make recommendations for changes in maternity care policy and practices. However, many obstetricians and hospitals feel threatened by any attempt to investigate maternal deaths, even in a process such as this where the names of doctors and patients are not made public and the goal is not to punish anyone but to understand what is causing these deaths, learn from the mistakes, and recommend improved practices. Not long after starting its work, the South Carolina maternal death surveillance group was discontinued. The official reason offered was "lack of funds." However, I was told in confidence that the surveillance group experienced resistance from doctors and hospitals from the beginning, in the form of "delays in turning over records, lost records, and failure to appear at meetings." Even today only a few states have a thorough audit of every maternal death, and only one state, Massachusetts, has a law, passed after intense lobbying by consumer groups for the measure and intense lobbying by medical groups against it, mandating that newspapers report maternal deaths.

In stark contrast with the extremely high rates of litigation against obstetricians, midwives, who attend around 10 percent of births in the United States, are rarely sued. Some of the reasons for this are discussed in chapter 5, including the deep personal relationship that develops between a midwife and a pregnant woman. When things go wrong, a midwife is there for the woman and her family, unlike most doctors and hospitals, who immediately construct a stone wall. Also, midwives are much less likely to promise a perfect baby, as the midwifery model accepts that sometimes women and babies die around the time of birth.

Midwives do carry malpractice insurance, but with lower coverage, as they don't have "deep pockets," and their premiums are also lower. In the rare case in which a midwife is sued, it is almost always after an out-of-hospital birth and after the family has been told by doctors that the reason for the death or impairment of the baby is the midwife and the out-of-hospital setting. In chapter 6, I described a case in Texas where a baby was born in an out-of-hospital birth center attended by midwives and the next day developed respiratory difficulty and needed to be hospitalized. Local doctors tried to use the case to change the regulation of birth centers in Texas. What was particularly interesting about this case is how, when the baby came to the hospital and the staff found out that it was an out-of-hospital birth, they assumed that the baby's difficulties were the result of bad management of the birth and told the parents that the baby had suffered from lack of oxygen during the birth. The hospital staff urged the family to sue the birth center and the midwives, and the family took their advice and sued. Investigation later found the cause of the baby's problems to be a genetic blood disorder, which had nothing to do with the birth or where the birth took place.

Also in chapter 6, I discussed the case of the baby with microcephaly born in an out-of-hospital birth center in which the doctors urged the family to sue the midwives and birth center, and in chapter 5, I discussed a case in which a home birth in Las Vegas was reported to the legal authorities as child abuse. Incredibly, doctors, who themselves hate litigation, are quick to report families to the authorities or urge families with a dead or damaged baby to sue the midwife or birth center.

Obstetricians, if they chose to, could learn a lot from midwives about how to practice maternity care in a way that does not encourage litigation.

This will not likely happen, however, for many reasons, one being that obstetricians are too upset by the litigation issue to be able to rationally assess their own role in it. They want the license to practice vigilante obstetrics and rightly see litigation as a threat to their being able to do whatever they jolly well want. This helps to explain the paradox of obstetricians protesting the litigation crisis while going right on with practices that inevitably lead to litigation.

So, while litigation may be a bad thing, as we have seen, it has become a necessary way to protect families. It provides a setting in which women and families can attempt to address concerns and hold doctors accountable in the one public forum that even doctors can't always evade.

Litigation has a second positive function as well: it is one of the few ways we have of putting the brakes on vigilante obstetric practices. In some cases, such as off-label use of drugs such as Cytotec, the normal mechanisms of drug regulation simply don't work, and our only avenues for promoting the proper use of drugs by doctors are public education and regulation by litigation. As I've said, there have been a number of cases of litigation following Cytotec inductions in the last decade, a fact that has not escaped the notice of ACOG and malpractice insurance companies. When the Searle Pharmaceutical Company sent a warning letter to all physicians regarding induction with this drug (see chapter 4), ACOG published an editorial in the *New England Journal of Medicine* saying that the letter *did* cause some doctors and hospitals to stop using Cytotec. ACOG went on to say that "ACOG received hundreds of inquiries from irate members who were concerned about the implications and the impact of the letter."[36] The fact that some doctors and hospitals were so scared that the Searle letter would leave them vulnerable to litigation that they stopped using Cytotec for induction illustrates the power of litigation to slow, if not stop, vigilante drug practices as well as its role as a symptom, alerting us to serious underlying problems in maternity care.

THE LEGAL RIGHTS OF WOMEN

In all the attention being given to the "litigation crisis" and the needs of doctors, hospitals, managed care organizations, and insurance companies, there is little or no discussion of the needs of the woman and how to protect her and her baby in this "crisis." And yet, until her needs are met, the crisis will not go away. The steps in the usual scenario that leads a woman or family to start litigation in obstetric cases are: (1) a bad outcome for the baby and/or the woman with evidence of significant emotional or physical harm; (2) a sense of betrayal on the part of the woman or family because the outcome is unexpected; and (3) the family's sense that they are being stonewalled when they try to find out what went wrong. The family turns to the court out of frustration as the only avenue available to them for finding out what actually happened. So outlawing litigation and capping settlement awards will not solve the crisis. Litigation will stop only when there is sufficient transparency and accountability in maternity care for a birthing woman and her family to know what happened to her and to her baby and why.

Ironically, it is because childbirth has been medicalized that pregnant and birthing women are turned into patients and are protected as patients through laws governing patients' rights. Although there is a great deal of attention in the media given to the legal protection of doctors and hospitals, there is so little attention given to the legal protections for pregnant and birthing women that most women know nothing about these protections, and many journalists, politicians, and even health care professionals also know very little. So the rest of this chapter will look at these protections, which are primarily about informed consent and a patient's right to refuse treatment.[37]

The concepts of informed consent and the right to refuse treatment are supported by constitutional law (the right to privacy and self-determination protected by the First and Fourteenth Amendments); federal law (the Emergency Medical Treatment and Active Labor Act and the Patient Self-Determination Act); international tort law (which U.S. courts sometimes cite); as well as state laws and state-mandated medical ethics. They are also covered in the ethical guidelines of the American Medical Association (AMA) and the American College of Obstetricians and Gynecologists (ACOG). These laws provide all patients, pregnant or not, with certain fundamental rights:

· The right to exercise self-determination and autonomy in making all medical decisions, including the decision to refuse treatment.

· The right to bodily integrity. Any form of nonconsensual touching or treatment that occurs in a medical setting constitutes battery.

· The right to be provided with the necessary information on which to base medical decisions, including a diagnosis; recommended treatments and alternatives; the risks, benefits, discomforts, and potential disabilities of proposed medical treatments; realistic expectation of outcomes; a second opinion; and any financial or research interests a physician may have in proposing certain treatments.

- The right to be informed of any potentially life-threatening consequences of a proposed treatment, even if the likelihood of experiencing such an outcome is rare.

- The right to make medical decisions free from coercion or undue influence from physicians.

- The right to have informed medical decisions witnessed, signed, and documented by the attending physician and another adult.

- The right to revoke consent to treatment at any time, either verbally or in writing.[38]

There are only a few situations that are recognized as exceptions to these rights, the first being when a patient is in an immediately life-threatening situation that requires treatment to save her life. Another is when the physician determines that revealing all facts would have a bad effect on the patient, but medical ethics hold that this "therapeutic privilege" is rarely, if ever, justified. Another is when a court orders a treatment, but it's important to note that courts have upheld the right of pregnant women to decline treatment even in situations where the lives of their fetuses are threatened. Finally, diagnostic tests that are required by law enforcement agencies, such as drawing blood to test intoxication levels in impaired drivers, are considered an exception.

The Patient Self-Determination Act also says that hospitals must inform patients of their rights when they are admitted.[39] Some states, such as New York, have expanded on federally protected patient rights, adding detailed points regarding maternity care as well as describing various grievance procedures available to women if a hospital fails to adhere to their rights.[40] Some individual hospitals have also created their own patient bills of rights, showing their intention to uphold the law by respecting patient autonomy.

The legal basis for medical informed consent and the right to refuse treatment came from the laws on battery. In a medical setting, battery is any touching or treatment of a patient that occurs without proper informed consent. This is extended to include medical treatments that are substantially different from the ones a patient consented to, or that are beyond the scope of the consent, as well as treatment administered by a physician other than the physician who obtained the patient's consent.

However, as the laws have evolved through actual cases, the courts have increasingly defined a lack of proper consent as negligence. For negligence to exist, the lack of proper consent or a failure to meet the standard of care must result in emotional or physical harm worthy of monetary compensation. It must be added that having to prove a failure to meet the standard of care is a slippery slope since, as discussed earlier in this chapter, the concept of standard of care is presently in transition as it becomes clear that defining standard of care as what other doctors in the community do rather than as evidence-based practice results in a "lowest common denominator" standard that severely weakens the patient's protection from questionable or dangerous practices.

The courts have been an important ally in protecting the right to informed consent for pregnant women, especially in recent years. Many people are under the impression that no physician has ever lost a malpractice suit for performing a cesarean. However, in 2005, in the case *Meador v. Stahler and Gheridian,* a jury awarded a $1.5 million settlement to a Massachusetts woman and her husband for her undergoing a medically unnecessary C-section that she had made clear she didn't want.[41] The woman had had a previous C-section and prior to going into labor had expressed her desire for a VBAC rather than an elective C-section. Her obstetrician agreed, but did not follow through on the agreement. The woman's attorney successfully claimed that, although her labor appeared to be progressing normally, her obstetrician misrepresented the risks of VBAC, ignored her expressed wishes for a vaginal birth, and compelled her to agree to a C-section in an emotionally coercive manner. The woman suffered physical complications from the C-section that left her largely bedridden and unable to work or meet family responsibilities for several years. Further, her loss of personal decision-making power concerning her body and the birth of her child caused her to suffer from post-traumatic stress disorder. A forensic psychiatrist testified that the lack of informed consent caused the disabling physical and emotional damages experienced by the woman and her family. The attorney also argued that the damages included a loss of "consortium" (sexual companionship) for the woman's husband, and that his loss of consortium was exacerbated by the physicians' failure to include him in the decision-making process, leaving him feeling powerless as well. The jury agreed with this argument as well, and nearly one-third of the total damages was awarded to the husband. Although this case doesn't have the same legal standing as an appellate court ruling, it does establish a useful precedent that can be used by other women whose lawsuits accuse an obstetrician of negligence due to failure to obtain proper consent.

There have been a number of cases in recent years in which physicians have gone to judges to obtain court orders when pregnant women refused to undergo C-sections.[42] In the majority of these cases, the courts sided with physicians and ordered the women to undergo C-sections against their will. However, the trend has now shifted in the other direction. Several appellate decisions (which hold the force of law) have upheld a pregnant woman's right to refuse a C-section, even in situations where her physician believes the life of the fetus is at risk. Apparently the courts now recognize how dangerous it is for medical professionals to make themselves the watchdog of the fetus. It is bad for society. It implies that the woman doesn't have the best interests of her baby at heart. It is dangerous to imply that the doctor cares more about the baby than the mother does. Also, there are religious issues involved, and it is inappropriate for doctors to try to impose their own or anyone else's religious beliefs on the woman and family, who may have different religious beliefs.

The most widely cited case in this area involves a woman named Angela Carder, a pregnant cancer patient who refused to consent to a C-section when she was twenty-five weeks pregnant, and said she wanted cancer treatments instead, which her doctors believed would kill her fetus.[43] Officials at George Washington University Hospital obtained a court order to force her to undergo the C-section, and both she and her baby died. Her estate appealed the court order and won. The Court of Appeals upheld a pregnant woman's right to make all medical decisions on behalf of herself and her fetus, arguing that to force invasive treatment on pregnant women would be putting the fetus's rights above the mother's rights. The court added that forcing invasive treatment on a pregnant woman would diminish the rights of born children whose parents could not, by law, be forced to undergo surgery or donate organs on their behalf. The court also ruled that the state's interest in the viability of the fetus and in preventing any potential harm the mother might cause to it by refusing treatment does not override her fundamental right to bodily integrity and informed consent or her right to refuse treatment.

In another case, the Illinois Supreme Court upheld a pregnant woman's right to refuse a blood transfusion.[44] Following these decisions and other related cases, ACOG issued ethical guidelines saying that physicians must respect the autonomy of pregnant patients and that using the courts to compel treatment is rarely, if ever, justified. These guidelines take a clear position on what has come to be called maternal-fetal conflict. They state, "Occasionally, a woman's autonomous decision will seem not to promote beneficence-based obligations to the fetus. In this situation, where there is insufficient time to obtain transfer of care, the obstetrician must respect the patient's autonomy, continue to care for the pregnant woman, and not intervene against the patient's wishes, regardless of the consequences."[45] The guidelines go on to remind physicians that, even in the case of a court order, physical force is never justified.

ACOG's ethical guidelines and ACOG's Committee Opinion paper on informed refusal take an even stronger position on cases where refusing treatment poses no substantial risk to the fetus, saying that patient autonomy in making medical decisions must be respected at all times, that physicians must obtain informed consent for any medical or surgical treatments, and that a patient's decision to forgo treatment based on cultural or religious beliefs and personal preference or comfort must be honored.[46]

Although failing to meet ACOG's, or any other medical organization's, ethical guidelines is not a crime, these guidelines have been useful in some malpractice cases, and violations have been used as grounds for revoking a physician's license to practice or have led to other disciplinary action in some states and hospitals.

Another area where ethical guidelines have been important is patient abandonment. In chapter 2, I mentioned a case in Oakland, California, with an adverse outcome after the woman in labor was given Cytotec for induction of labor. Incredibly, the laboring woman had repeatedly refused the Cytotec because she wanted a natural birth until the obstetrician threatened to discharge her "against medical advice" unless she agreed to have her labor induced with Cytotec. Tragically, not knowing her rights, she gave in to the doctor's demand to use Cytotec for an unwanted induction and as a result she and her baby died.

Many people, unfortunately including many physicians, are under the impression that in instances such as this, where they disagree with their physicians about a course of treatment, their doctors have the right to simply discontinue care. But this is mistaken. Ethical guidelines and federal law (the Emergency Medical Treatment and Active Labor Act, EMTALA) say that a doctor may terminate care only after reasonable notice and after providing for necessary interim or emergency care. Physicians who fail to meet these guidelines can be charged with patient abandonment, which is grounds for malpractice and can result in loss of license. As a general rule, physicians who wish to discontinue care in a nonemergency situation must notify the patient in writing, give thirty days' notice, and offer a general referral to other obstetricians in the area. And if ongoing care is needed at the time the physician wishes to terminate care (certainly the case with pregnancy and especially during labor), then the physician is obligated to make sure the patient has successfully transferred to another doctor.

An example of widespread failure to honor the rights of pregnant and birthing women is hospitals mandating that pregnant women with prior uterine surgery must undergo cesarean sections in subsequent pregnancies. As discussed earlier, there has been a trend among hospitals to require that a woman who has had a C-section must have C-sections in future pregnancies. This is in direct violation of the laws that protect patient rights, including a pregnant woman's right to refuse treatment. The same legal principles apply to doctors who neglect to inform patients that elective repeat C-sections also involve risks and that VBAC is a medically sound alternative. This means that women who have had repeat C-sections only because of hospital policies banning VBAC can sue for negligence if they or their babies experience any complication they weren't informed of prior to the surgery, particularly if they weren't informed that VBAC was an alternative.

It's important for women who want to have VBAC to know that the Carder case has had a very chilling effect on the willingness of doctors or hospitals to use the courts to force women to undergo C-sections. Many doctors and hospitals continue to coerce women to consent to a C-section by threatening them with a court order, but they and their attorneys are well aware that if they go through with it, and the mother decides to sue, they're looking at a long and expensive legal battle that they will lose in the end. In most cases, a woman who is threatened in this way will be successful if she informs the staff that she knows it's an empty threat, that the law is on her side, and that she plans to appeal the ruling all the way to the Supreme Court if need be. State and federal laws make it clear that hospital policies mandating C-section violate the legal rights of pregnant women and constitute violations of professional ethical standards as well.[47]

There are a number of things women can do during pregnancy to make sure that their rights are not violated. One strategy is to customize a hospital's boilerplate consent form. Most patients don't know that they are not required by law to sign the hospital's consent form and that they have the right to change it to reflect their wishes regarding specific treatments. Many physicians tell patients that their hospitals' consent forms do not protect them from lawsuits, but this is not the whole story. If your wish to refuse treatment is documented, under U.S. law it's very difficult, if not impossible, for a hospital or doctor to be held liable for not doing the procedure. On the other hand, if a patient's wish to refuse a C-section is documented and the patient is given one anyway, the doctor and hospital are subject to criminal battery charges, regardless of whether the woman or baby were harmed by the C-section.

A pregnant woman who finds that her hospital is not willing to comply with her wishes for her labor and birth can also file a complaint with the chief compliance officer of the hospital. All hospitals that receive federal funding (approximately 80 percent of hospitals) must adhere to a set of rules called the Center for Medicare and Medicaid Service's (CMS's) conditions of participation (CoP). These rules require hospitals to honor patient rights as defined by the Patient Self-Determination Act, the Consumer Bill of Rights and Responsibilities, EMTALA, and the large number of actual cases that uphold a patient's right to refuse treatment, to be fully informed of the risks, benefits, and alternatives of any proposed treatment, and to participate in all treatment decisions.

Hospitals that fail to adhere to the CoP are subject to heavy fines and risk losing their right to qualify for Medicare and Medicaid funding. In addition, the CoP require that hospitals institute an internal grievance process and give patients the information they need to know about how to file a complaint and where to appeal in the case of an unfavorable ruling.

Once a woman is in labor, she can often get doctors to comply with her wishes by telling them that she is aware of her rights under EMTALA. EMTALA was originally enacted to prevent "patient dumping"—hospitals refusing to admit a woman in labor for whatever reason, often because it appears that she will not be able to pay for maternity services. Before EMTALA, some hospitals would station guards in the hospital parking lots to intercept women in labor and turn them away. Now hospitals are required to admit women in active labor, explain the risks, benefits, and alternatives of all proposed treatments, and honor their treatment wishes, including their right to refuse treatment, regardless of their ability to pay.

Under the act, no patient who requires emergency care, which is defined to include laboring women, can be transferred to another hospital until after they've been "stabilized." In the case of a woman in labor, stabilization is defined as the delivery of both the baby and the placenta. EMTALA begins to apply when a patient comes within 250 feet of the hospital building. So EMTALA can get the woman in labor into the hospital and, once inside, if her wishes are not honored, the CoP can make sure they are. There's no question that it can be difficult to sue a doctor for malpractice and that most states do not adequately discipline physicians who commit malpractice, but it can still be worthwhile to sue an obstetrician, especially one who fails to obtain proper consent or who coerces a patient into consenting to a medically unnecessary procedure, such as C-section, that results in physical or emotional harm. Any form of physical force to perform a medical procedure without a patient's consent constitutes grounds for battery (a criminal action) as well as for malpractice (a civil action). Lawsuits can cost a doctor or hospital a great deal of time and money, and until more women pursue this route, physicians will continue to see C-section as a no-fault course of treatment.

Short of filing a lawsuit, filing a complaint with a state medical board can be a very effective means of changing the birth climate in a given state. Though few complaints actually cause physicians to lose their licenses, they can lead to other disciplinary actions, such as the loss of hospital privileges or the loss of professional credentials. In addition, many states have searchable databases of complaints, malpractice suits, and disciplinary actions against physicians, so a complaint is public information and may deter patients, which can have financial repercussions for the physician. At the very least, filing a complaint with the medical board, the hospital, and the insurance company establishes a record (letters of complaint usually remain on file permanently), so that if other patients complain about the same physician, the organizations will see a condemning trend.

Flying under the radar in the issue of obstetric litigation is the insurance industry, which has its eye on the health of its bottom line, not of women and babies. There does not appear to be any transparency, much less accountability, in the establishment of malpractice insurance premiums. Even ACOG's suggestions for reforming the "litigation crisis" start off with a call for consideration "of insurance market reforms, to answer the question: why are premiums so volatile for doctors?" The insurance industry, including those who provide malpractice insurance, certainly appears to have a healthy bottom line. They are an important but nearly invisible element in the obstetric litigation crisis and their role urgently needs investigation and transparency.[48]

In the face of all the legislation reviewed here protecting pregnant and birthing women, ACOG's threat to abandon women in labor because obstetricians have high insurance fees rings hollow. Clearly, the government recognizes that childbirth is of central importance to the health and future of society, and politicians will not abide any serious threat to it. It is sad that so much of the litigation crisis dialogue is so adversarial. Pitting pregnant and birthing women against those doctors and hospitals who abuse their rights is, one hopes, only a temporary but necessary strategy in giving birth decision-making rights back to women and families.

EIGHT VISION OF A BETTER WAY TO BE BORN

I navigate by the stars. I may not reach them soon but they guide me in the right direction.
NORWEGIAN SAILOR'S PROVERB

In this chapter I offer my vision for a better way to be born in the USA. I consider it a guide to keep us heading in the right direction, a goal to work toward. In chapter 9, I will offer some practical ideas for getting from where we are to where we need to be.

My vision of a healthy maternity care system for our country is built on two sets of principles. The first set of principles guides the work of the Coalition for Improvement in Maternity Services (CIMS).[1] These are included in chapter 1 but are worth repeating:

- Normalcy: treat birth as a natural, healthy process.

- Empowerment: provide the birthing woman and her family with supportive, sensitive, and respectful care.

- Autonomy: enable women to make decisions based on accurate information and provide access to the full range of options for care.

- First, do no harm: avoid the routine use of tests, procedures, drugs, and restrictions.

- Responsibility: give evidence-based care used solely for the needs and in the interests of mothers and infants.

The second set of principles were unanimously approved by more than two thousand participants at the International Conference on Humanization of Birth held in Fortaleza, Brazil, in the year 2000:

- Humanized birth means putting the woman giving birth in the center and in control so that she, not the doctors or anyone else, makes all the decisions about what will happen.

- Humanized birth means understanding that the focus of maternity services is community-based (out of hospital) primary care, not hospital-based tertiary (specialist) care.

- Humanized birth means midwives, nurses, and doctors all working together in harmony as equals.

- Humanized birth means maternity services that are based on good scientific evidence, including evidence-based use of technology and drugs.[2]

A NATIONAL HEALTH CARE SYSTEM

It is clear that many of our serious maternity care problems would be immediately and profoundly improved by establishing a national health care system. This is a fundamental difference between the maternity care provided in the United States and the care provided in those countries that have lower mortality rates for mothers and babies than we do—every one of those countries has unobstructed access to care for *all* pregnant women. In the United States, there have been efforts to extend insurance coverage to pregnant women, but these efforts have not prevented the number of uninsured pregnant women from increasing.[3]

In the United States, the maternal mortality rate of Hispanic women is twice as high as that of Caucasian women. Among African American women, the maternal mortality rate is four times as high as that of Caucasian women. Each year, African American babies die at twice the rate of Caucasian babies.[4] This is not a matter of race. It is a reflection of our inadequate care for women and families living in poverty.

Today fewer and fewer American women and families who are in need of maternity care have health insurance. Employment-based health insurance, the only serious source of coverage other than Medicare or Medicaid, is in decline. The number of American workers covered by employee-based health insurance has recently fallen by 4.9 million people, and we can expect this trend to continue. Many American companies have reduced medical benefits or are planning to reduce benefits in coming years, and it is becoming more common for large companies such as Wal-Mart to hire employees who do not work enough hours to be entitled to medical insurance.[5] This trend may be coming to an end now that Maryland has passed a law requiring Wal-Mart to increase its spending on health insurance, and other states may follow. But even if this is the case, it will be a long, drawnout patching process.

A national health care system would not only mean medical services for all pregnant women and babies, it would also allow us to monitor maternity care practices far more effectively. It is extremely hard to assure highquality services for an entire country when we know very little about what is actually going on. Only two out of fifty states currently require hospitals to disclose their C-section rates to the public, and even in those states there is a lot of noncompliance with the law. We have very little solid information on the use and outcomes of procedures and drugs, such as Cytotec for inducing labor, that have not been adequately tested for safety. Without a national health care system, physicians and hospitals have no tradition of reporting, whether it be reportable infectious diseases such as tuberculosis and AIDS, adverse drug reactions, medical mistakes, or even usual practices such as cesarean section, making the monitoring of health care nearly hopeless. Maternal mortality cases are grossly underreported (some say that fewer than half are reported).[6] The FDA believes that less than 10 percent of cases where there has been an adverse reaction to a drug are reported.[7] Despite the fact that we have laws requiring doctors and hospitals to turn over records to patients and their families upon request, there are so many obstacles to getting case information that families feel that their only option is to file a lawsuit. With a national health care system in place, monitoring becomes part of quality control and can be easily facilitated by withholding reimbursement for noncompliance, a mechanism that has been used successfully in other national health care systems.

A national health care system would also greatly improve quality control of physician practice in the United States. Currently, every state has a medical board that grants doctors licenses to practice. When a malpractice complaint is made to the state medical board, it must investigate, and if it deems appropriate, the board has the power to take a doctor's license away. However, in reality, state medical boards rarely take any action of consequence. I am a licensed physician in California, and for decades I have received an annual summary of the malpractice cases the California State Medical Board has investigated and what action has been taken. Almost all the cases involve drug or alcohol abuse by the physician. There are very few instances in which a specific case of malpractice is actually investigated. This is not surprising, as the board consists of fellow physicians, and as noted in chapter 2, asking physicians to control other physicians is fraught with difficulty due to tribal loyalties. This system provides very little protection for the American public. Even when a state board does rule against a physician, he or she can simply move to another state and practice there. Clearly, a national program of quality control, as part of a national health care system, would be much more effective—with rulings against physicians held in a national database (and made accessible to the public), more thorough investigations, and more neutral investigators.

Those who advocate keeping our present system, which is clearly unfair and sometimes even cruel to many families having babies, often argue that we are getting better care than we would with a national system. But there is a wealth of evidence that, although we pay far more than other countries for our health care, we are not getting better care.

The first evidence comes from the Organization for Economic Cooperation and Development (OECD). The OECD gathers survey data to compare the health systems of its thirty member countries (including the United States), which are all industrialized. One OECD survey concludes, "U.S. health spending towers over that of other countries with much older populations. Prominent among the reasons are a highly complex and fragmented payment system that entails high administrative costs."[8] Another OECD survey concludes, "The data show that the United States spends more on health care than any other country. However, *on most measures of health services use, the United States is below the OECD medium.* These facts suggest that the difference in spending is caused mostly by higher prices for health care goods and services in the United States."[9] In other words, the OECD has found that the United States gets less in the way of health care than other industrial countries do but pays a lot more because of the high prices charged for the care.

For further evidence that the United States does not have better health care than other countries, we need only look to the fact that we have higher mortality rates for women and children and shorter life expectancies than other countries.[10] Anecdotally, I can say that for several decades I have made repeated, extended visits to every other industrialized country—

including every OECD country—and have never found health care inferior to what we have in the United States.

There is also an unsupported belief among many American policy makers and politicians that private insurance is more cost-effective and efficient—that is, it allows us to get the best health care possible for the best cost and with a minimum use of time and resources. This idea is entirely false. The United States spends more than twice as much per person on health care as Britain does and almost twice as much per person as Germany and Canada do.[11] There are many reasons for this, including health care providers, hospitals, and health maintenance organizations looking to maximize profits; health insurers wanting to maximize profits; higher administrative costs because our system is more bureaucratic; and higher costs for drugs and medical supplies because our system is fragmented and providers do not have the leverage to bargain successfully with drug companies and other suppliers.

A decade ago, Taiwan shifted from a U.S.-style health care system to a Canadian-style single-payer health care system, and in six years, the percentage of Taiwanese people covered by health insurance rose from 60 percent to 97 percent. Furthermore, the expanded coverage cost no more than the previous coverage because of savings in bureaucratic costs.[12]

The fact that health services in the United States, which combine private and public-sector funding, cost more and are less efficient than health services in other countries illustrates a principle that has been proven again and again in many countries around the world. Human services—including health, education, and social welfare—must be in the public sector. They are labor-intensive, expensive, and require highly skilled people. It is not possible to make them broadly accessible, high-quality, and, at the same time, financially profitable.

In addition, to be effective in the long term, human services must be prevention-oriented, and that requires a willingness to wait years to see results. We must spend time and money today, when the desired results—improved health combined with a reduced need for medical care, leading to long-term cost savings—will take years to show. This approach is fundamentally incompatible with the need to focus on the bottom line at the end of every fiscal year.

Commenting on a series of *New York Times* articles on the rising tide of diabetes, Paul Krugman points out: "The U.S. system of paying for health care doesn't let medical professionals do the right thing. There's hardly any money for prevention. . . . '[I]nsurance companies will often refuse to pay

$150 for a diabetic to see a podiatrist who can help prevent foot ailments associated with the disease . . . [but] nearly all of them cover amputations, which typically cost more than $30,000.' . . . The point is that we can't deal with the diabetes epidemic in part because insurance companies don't pay for preventive medicine or disease management, focusing only on acute illness and extreme remedies."[13]

Ironically, maternity care includes prenatal care, which is preventive care, but although publicly funded prenatal care is typically high-quality care, private prenatal care is often characterized by visits that are too short because of cost considerations. As I mentioned in chapter 5, studies have shown that midwifery prenatal visits are much longer than obstetrician prenatal visits, but many midwives have complained to me that if they are working in the private sector in private obstetrician groups or HMOs, they are under constant pressure to keep prenatal visits short.

Nearly all education and social welfare services in the United States are already in the public sector, and, truth be told, health services are not really "private" currently, as they are heavily financed, directly and indirectly, by public funds. Many programs in private hospitals receive public funding. And medical schools, nursing schools, and postgraduate specialty training programs, such as obstetrics, are all government-subsidized, though their graduates will go on to work in the private sector. Essentially what we have today are doctors and hospitals that want the public to fund their programs and their training, but still want to be free to provide services (or not) in whatever way they want, with little or no regulation, transparency, or accountability.

GIVING BIRTH OUT OF THE "SICK HOUSE"

Normal, low-risk birth should never have been moved to the "sick house." (*Krankenhaus,* the German word for *hospital,* translates to sick house in English.) Hospitals are highly symbolic of the medical model of birth— twenty-first-century cathedrals with priests in white robes. A hospital is usually one of the biggest buildings in town, the halls are quiet, and outsiders are awed when they enter and feel reverence for those walking by dressed in white. The doctors are mostly male and the underlings (nurses and others) are mostly female, which creates an ambience antithetical to providing a woman-centered birth. We will achieve real woman-centered childbirth only when we get birth out of these institutions. In my vision of a better way of birth, pregnant women with no serious medical complications—80 to 90 percent of pregnant women—would be able to choose between giving birth in an out-of-hospital birth center or at home. For these low-risk women, giving birth in a hospital would not be an option because it represents a considerable unnecessary drain on the economy and, more important, because it presents serious risks to both the woman and the baby.

As the rates of invasive obstetric interventions increase (the rate of C-section, for example, is approaching one in three births in the United States), so does the need to keep those women who are having low-risk pregnancies safe by keeping them out of the hospital. There are precedents for no longer offering a medical procedure for low-risk birth. Several previously widely practiced medical procedures are no longer available because of their proven risks. For example, you can't get a doctor to perform blood-letting or to take an X-ray during a patient's pregnancy. I also believe that it should not be an option for affluent low-risk women to pay for their own care in a private hospital, because that drains the economy as well, since public funds are used to train doctors, nurses, and other health care workers and to build the hospital.

It is basic logic that if you want to be as safe as possible while driving your car, avoid using the freeway during rush hour. Stay out of harm's way. Sadly, there are severe limitations on what a woman can do to stay out of harm's way—that is, to avoid unnecessary invasive obstetric interventions—while giving birth in a hospital setting. In a hospital, a woman simply does not have enough power to change the way things are done. A woman attempting to change the way her obstetrician and hospital manages her labor and childbirth would be like a woman attempting to change the driving habits of all the drivers on her local freeway. As illustrated by the Massachusetts court case discussed in chapter 7, in which a woman who wanted to give birth vaginally after a previous C-section was coerced into an elective C-section, even when a woman has her doctor's promise that certain interventions will not be done, there is no guarantee that the doctor will remain true to his word.[14]

Another reason hospitals are not safe for low-risk births is that there are more dangerous infectious agents—bacteria and viruses—in hospitals than in any other community setting. There is a good chance that anyone who spends time in the hospital will acquire an infection. The CDC estimates that one in every twenty people hospitalized will develop a hospital-acquired infection (HAI), leading to ninety thousand deaths every year in the United States from HAI.[15] The risk of contracting an HAI increases when invasive procedures such as epidural anesthesia and C-section are performed.[16] In fact, 20 percent of women having C-sections have postoperative fever, the most common cause being an HAI.[17]

Hospitals are well aware of the risk of infection and try hard to minimize it, but it is a never-ending struggle, as dangerous new infectious agents are introduced in every hospital every day by sick patients. Furthermore, infections picked up in the hospital tend to be caused by germs that are resistant to most antibiotics, including the most powerful recently developed antibiotics. The most common HAI is methicillin-resistant *Staphylococcus aureus* (MRSA), which is resistant to nearly every antibiotic we have.[18] You don't want one of these. The bottom line is, if a woman doesn't want her baby to pick up a serious infection during or after birth, she should not give birth in a hospital.

Beyond these safety considerations, there are important social and philosophical reasons for moving birth out of hospitals. Childbirth is not a medical issue; it is a social issue that may or may not have medical consequences. Day care for children, spousal abuse, and care of the elderly are all social issues that may or may not have medical consequences. If maternity care were included with other social and family services, it would mean an entirely different approach. I would then expect to see family-centered maternity care. This might include home visits; attention paid to prevention issues, such as nutrition; screening tests provided selectively (not routinely), with fully informed choice; counseling as needed; and good continuity of care before, during, and after pregnancy and birth, with emphasis placed on the woman and her family knowing the care provider. Maternity care will become fully integrated into social and family services only when it has escaped the hospital.

Childbirth is a very personal, emotional phenomenon, analogous to sexual intercourse. Most people would balk at an expert coming in to tell them how to make love. In fact, if you want to make lovemaking impossible, have a stranger walk in. Childbirth is like sex in that it is much more than a physical act and it requires privacy and intimacy. Childbirth is not just about a head coming out, just as sex is not just about a head going in. Sexual intercourse has medical risks as well (one of the partners contracting AIDS or gonorrhea, for example), but that doesn't justify having a doctor in the room. There is a basic physiological fact that strongly favors childbirth outside a hospital: women have hormones (endorphins, oxytocins) that do not function normally in a strange environment or if there is a stranger present. In order for a woman to have a personal, private birth experience, it is essential to get her out of an institution that by its very nature is impersonal and not private—the hospital.

The key issue in the question of where to give birth, however, is who is in control. Physicians, hospitals, electronic fetal monitors, and drugs do not have babies—only the mother of the child can do that. To give birth, a woman must open up her body, wide. This profound social and biological act requires everything a woman has and is. All maternity services should reflect this fundamental fact and should be designed to assist and support the woman. Most of the present care system for birthing women in the United States is designed not to assist the mother but rather to control her.

Doctors control women with fear. They have succeeded in convincing the great majority of American women that they cannot safely give birth outside the hospital; that nearly half of them have uteruses that are non-starters and need to have labor induced or augmented with powerful drugs; that up to two-thirds of them cannot tolerate labor pain and must be made numb from the waist down with an epidural block so they cannot feel the birth of their babies; that one-third of them cannot push out their babies but must have it pulled out with forceps or a vacuum or cut out by C-section. When we try to make women believe that they can't give birth without the help of men, machines, and hospitals, we take away their confidence and their belief in their own bodies—and with their confidence gone, any feelings of power and autonomy also disappear. Women in the United States have become victims of a medical vision of female reproduction, and that needs to change. The most effective way to avoid this medicalization of birth is to stay away from where it goes on—the hospital.

A family must be allowed to own the birth of their child and to create the birth experience they want and need. The only way families can do that is if women are in control of their own bodies. The doctor is not the important person at a birth. It is the woman's childbirth. It is her life. It is her family. It is her baby. As a physician with decades of experience, I can assure you that at any birth, the level of concern and value is very different for the woman and family than it is for the doctor. For the doctor, it is one out of hundreds of births. For the family, it is one of very few, or the only one. When a woman is seventy years old, she will almost certainly remember every detail of giving birth, whereas the doctor who was there will have forgotten it a week later. We've gone astray in this regard. To honor the family and preserve the sanctity of birth, we must get birth out of an institution that is designed and managed for the care of the sick.

We live in a diverse society that includes people of many religions and cultures, and childbirth has always been associated with religious and cultural traditions. In fact, religious and cultural issues are so integral to maternity care for some families that the issue of separation of church and state arises. In chapter 6, I told a story of an orthodox Jewish family who insisted on their right to a home birth attended by a midwife, and when their birth later became a legal case, they refused to answer questions about the birth of their child before a grand jury—a representative of the state—for religious reasons. In an out-of-hospital birth, a family can orchestrate their special childbirth needs either in their own home or in a neighborhood birth center where there are people to assist who share their beliefs. In the United States, families have the right to practice their religion. They have the right to have Santa Claus at their birth if they want to. And there is no way a hospital can begin to provide for the special childbirth needs of all religions and cultures.

In addition to providing assistance with low-risk, out-of-hospital births, neighborhood women's centers, staffed primarily by midwives, would also provide a wide array of primary care services for women, including social services such as individual counseling, support groups, and services for abused women. They would also provide preventive health services such as family planning, cancer screening, prenatal care, postnatal care, breastfeeding support, and so on.

This is not a new idea. Groups of women in the neighborhood who gather to support and serve one another have existed in one form or another for thousands of years, but they are scarce today in the United States. These gatherings have traditionally been informal networks of female relatives and friends, surrounding the local midwife. For much of history, they have flown under the male radar, so they have not been formally documented in what has been a male-dominated authoritarian society. It is highly likely that Hanna Porn, the midwife in Massachusetts who was persecuted at the beginning of the twentieth century (see chapter 5), attracted such a group of women. But over time, midwives were driven out of American communities and it became unusual for members of extended families to live near one another. Neighborhood women's gatherings began to fade away as well, although they still exist in some parts of the country.

In Europe and other parts of the world where midwives have not been driven out, these groups thrive. I have personally spent time with out-of-hospital midwives in London, Amsterdam, Copenhagen, Sydney, Kyoto, St. Petersburg (Russia), and elsewhere, and have seen the groups that surround them. Sometimes the members of the group are a familiar sight at the midwife's home, and sometimes they are not, but they come out of the woodwork when needed. In the 1990s, a midwife in a small town in the south of France was attacked by the local obstetrician, who had a vendetta against her and was trying to get her license to practice revoked. He used the excuse that she attended planned home births, even though home birth was not illegal. A group of local women quickly organized, circulated a petition, and presented it to the city council. They also contacted me, and others who support the midwifery profession, and requested letters of support.

I've seen the same support appear when a midwife in the United States is caught up in a witch-hunt. Groups of local women come to the rescue. When a Mennonite midwife in Ohio was in trouble with the law for not testifying in a grand jury investigation (she refused to break her code of confidentiality), an outpouring of support came from women all over the Midwest.[19]

A home birth midwife in London, Mary Ann Scruggs, came up with the idea of forming self-help groups of pregnant clients who would give one another prenatal care, with a midwife as a teacher and consultant to the group. The midwife would teach them to take one another's blood pressure, test one another's urine, measure the growth of one another's uterus, and so on. When a question came up regarding pregnancy and birth, one member of the group would research the question and report back, and the midwife would guide the discussion. I thought it a brilliant idea—a way to bring a self-help group approach to the informal neighborhood women's groups already in place. Mary Ann and I tried to get funding to do an experimental trial of this method of prenatal care. We were not successful, but I still believe it has great potential. My vision of neighborhood women's centers would build on these existing informal women's networks. Mary Ann and I were attempting to reinvent the wheel. In chapter 6, we saw that birth houses—neighborhood women's centers—have existed in Japan for centuries, and in chapter 5, we saw that Inuit midwives in the Arctic regions of Canada serve as the village "wise women."

There are a number of fine examples of maternity care systems that successfully provide for out-of-hospital births for low-risk women, showing that it can be done. Perhaps the best known is the system in the Netherlands. As I explained in chapter 6, the Netherlands has a long tradition of planned home birth. As recently as thirty years ago, half of all births in that country were planned home births. Though the percentage fell to about one-third of all births in the 1980s, it has been climbing again in the last ten years. The Netherlands does not have significantly higher perinatal and maternal mortality rates than other Western European countries do, and it has lower perinatal and maternal mortality rates than the United States does.

How do the Dutch do it? For one thing, they have a national health care system that provides maternity services to all families with no barriers to care, such as income qualifications to meet. A woman in the Netherlands having a low-risk pregnancy can choose to give birth at home or in the hospital, but there are significant incentives for choosing home birth. If a woman gives birth at home, a home helper (paid by the government) will come for two weeks to help take care of the house and any other children, so the mother can focus on caring for her newborn. (This service is not available after a hospital birth.) A woman giving birth at home is likely to know her midwife because the same midwife will have provided at least some of her prenatal care, whereas if a woman gives birth in the hospital, she will be attended by the midwife on duty, whom she will not have met before. Since hospital midwives usually work eight-hour shifts, a woman giving birth in the hospital will probably have her attendant replaced by another stranger during her labor. With a home birth, the midwife typically comes when labor starts and stays until she has checked the mother and baby after the birth. She then comes to the home once a day for several days to check the mother and baby again and answer questions. These incentives are certainly applicable to a vision of out-of-hospital birth in the United States. Americans could learn a lot by close observation of the Dutch home birth system.

Denmark also guarantees a choice of place of birth to all Danish families. Like every other highly industrialized country except the United States, Denmark also has a national health care system. In Denmark, midwives attend all low-risk births either in the hospital or in the family's home. When midwives in Denmark graduate from midwifery school, they take an oath to attend any birth, anywhere, anytime. If a pregnant women has decided to give birth at home, when her labor starts she calls the local hospital and asks for a midwife to be sent to her home. By law, the hospital must comply with this request. If a complication develops during the birth and it becomes necessary to transfer the woman to a hospital, this transfer is handled smoothly and easily, as the midwife is already well known in the hospital. The home birth rate varies within Denmark (it is around 10 percent of all births in some districts), and Denmark's mortality rates for birthing women and newborn babies are among the lowest in the world, far lower than those in the United States. The United States could learn a lot from studying the communication between midwives attending out-of-hospital births and hospital staff in Denmark.

An excellent example of how changing the place of birth changes obstetric practice comes, ironically, from Brazil, a country known for its astronomical C-section rates (as high as 80 percent in some regions). The federal government in Brazil is aware of the country's C-section crisis and has been trying to improve the situation even in the face of lobbying efforts from those in the medical profession who want to maintain the status quo. Wisely recognizing that it would be extremely difficult to change hospital obstetric practices under the circumstances, at the beginning of the twenty-first century the government endorsed a plan to build a network of out-of-hospital birth centers and has agreed to help fund it.

The move to out-of-hospital birth in Brazil is supported by Brazilian women, who are getting increasingly angry at how they are treated in hospital maternity care. A group of women scientists in Brazil conducted a study that looks at violence against women committed by health care workers in health care facilities including childbearing services in hospitals.[20] They analyzed all research reports and surveys of patients from the previous decade that revealed how women were managed and treated by heath care workers in hospitals, and identified four forms of abuse of women by doctors and nurses in Brazilian hospitals: neglect, verbal abuse, physical abuse, and sexual abuse. The authors note: "These forms of violence recur, are often deliberate, are a serious violation of human rights, and are related to poor quality and effectiveness of health-care services. This abuse is a means of controlling patients that is learnt during training and reinforced in health facilities. Abuse occurs mainly in situations in which the legitimacy of health services is questionable or can be the result of prejudice against certain population groups."[21] The paper goes on to suggest ways to prevent abuse. It is an important contribution to our understanding of hospital maternity services, and in my opinion, it should be read by every obstetrician, midwife, and obstetric nurse in every country. This paper also makes it abundantly clear that moving childbirth out of the hospital will bring about dramatic improvement in maternity care.

Even within the United States, there are models for providing high-quality out-of-hospital maternity services. One example can be found in Taos, New Mexico, where a group of maternity providers has succeeded in giving women a real choice of place to give birth. Two obstetricians—a husband and wife—and several midwives work together in a group practice.

The group offers pregnant women a choice of giving birth at home, in an alternative birth center, or in a hospital, as well as a choice of birth attendant—midwife or obstetrician—for each location. Because this group is the only obstetric practice in town, it has been able to gather good statistics on its practice. The data show a steady increase in the number of pregnant women choosing to give birth in an out-of-hospital setting.[22]

Another outstanding example of providing out-of-hospital birth in the United States is found in rural Tennessee. For more than thirty years, The Farm, a small community outside Summertown, Tennessee, has offered planned home birth attended by a group of midwives. Of the 2,200 babies born at The Farm between 1970 and 1990, 96 percent of the births were attended only by midwives. Since there were no complications, there was no need for a doctor to be involved. The Farm's excellent track record for home births has been the subject of a scientific analysis that looks at the intervention rates and birth outcomes.[23]

The Farm serves as a model for home birth and has also become a source of inspiration to midwives, doctors, nurses, doulas, and others interested in humanizing childbirth. Ina May Gaskin, the leader of The Farm's midwives, has been a pioneer of the home birth movement in the United States as well as globally. Her 2003 book, *Ina May's Guide to Childbirth,* is a classic that I believe should be read by all in this field because Ina May Gaskin is the most important person in maternity care in North America, bar none. Hundreds of maternity care providers (myself included) have visited The Farm to observe the work done there. Ina May also helped organize the Midwives Association of North America, an organization that has been the driving force in the renaissance of direct-entry midwifery in the United States.

MIDWIVES TO ATTEND LOW-RISK BIRTHS

In my vision of a better way to provide maternity care in the United States, midwives would have primary responsibility for women with low-risk pregnancies, while obstetricians would have primary responsibility for pregnant women with serious medical complications. This has always been the system in other highly industrialized countries, and women cherish their midwives and do not see obstetricians as preferable for normal birth. In 2005, the Crown Princess of Denmark gave birth assisted by her midwife. Having obstetricians—surgical specialists—provide primary care for pregnant women has been shown to be one of the reasons for bad maternity care outcomes. To quote a recent *Health Affairs Journal* article: "Increasing the supply of specialists will not improve the United States' position in population health relative to other industrialized countries, and it is likely to lead to greater disparities in health status and outcomes. Adverse effects from inappropriate or unnecessary specialist use may be responsible for the absence of relationship between specialist supply and mortality."[24]

The majority of maternity services would be community-based—located in neighborhoods, not in medical facilities—and the 10 to 20 percent of women with high-risk pregnancies would be cared for in the hospital. If the United States had a national health care system, American obstetricians would no longer be able to maintain their monopoly and negotiate with a wide group of insurance companies, government agencies, and managed care organizations to maintain a good profit. Without this financial incentive, I believe obstetricians' motivation for continuing to manage more than three million low-risk pregnant and birthing women a year would quickly vanish. My decades of personal experience with American obstetricians convinces me that most of them are bored with routine prenatal care and with trying to manage low-risk hospital birth from a distance, and they are tired of the inconvenience. If this practice were no longer highly profitable, I believe that most obstetricians would be more than happy to leave the management of low-risk pregnancies and birth to midwives. In the meantime, it is inevitable that doctors in the United States will let economic issues interfere with their practice decisions.

It will take time for American obstetricians to gain sufficient experience with midwives to develop deep respect for their professional skill and expertise. Removing the economic barriers between obstetricians and midwives would accelerate the process and move the two groups toward the true collaboration we see in countries where they are not competing for patients. It is also clear that in other highly industrialized countries where obstetricians are not struggling to maintain their monopoly over maternity services for economic gain, their tribal qualities, including omertà (see chapter 2), are less apparent, allowing a more collegial relationship with their coworkers.

Under the new distribution of labor I've described, it is essential that midwives and doctors work together in harmony, as equals, each recognizing the unique professional contributions of the other. With this equality and mutual understanding would come clarity in the relationship—and an end to the idea that doctors must supervise midwives and are responsible for midwifery practice.

In truth, this strategy of trying to supervise midwives and take responsibility for their practice has already backfired. As I discussed in chapter 5, in areas of the United States where obstetricians have insisted that midwives work under their supervision and have succeeded in getting legislation to mandate this, they are required by law to assume some responsibility for what midwives do. Where obstetricians have tried to convince legislators that midwives are not as safe as obstetricians or that home birth is dangerous, insurance companies have bought into the falsehood as well and have raised premiums for backup obstetricians.[25] In countries around the world that have more effective maternity care than the United States does, obstetricians do not supervise midwives, nor are they responsible for what midwives do.

It is also important that all those who provide services to pregnant and birthing women understand that, although midwives and physicians are both highly trained professional "experts," maternity care is a service and the work of both midwives and doctors is to serve the women in their care. This is a key concept in a modern maternity care system, as it redefines the role of "patient," understanding that the woman giving birth is not a passive sick person but someone who is experiencing a profound life-cycle event. When we view midwives and doctors as in a service role, it supports the view that the pregnant woman is in the central position—as the one being served.

Some physicians have always understood that their role is to be of service to their patients. Many doctors, however, see the field of medicine not as a service but as a profession. In an editorial, the deputy editor of *Obstetrics and Gynecology,* the journal published by ACOG, wrote: "Keep medicine a profession instead of a service."[26] By saying "instead of," ACOG is implying that it is not possible to be a service provider if you are a professional, creating a false dichotomy, as there is general consensus in the United States that medical doctors are service providers. But by calling themselves "professionals"—elite experts providing professional consultation—rather than service providers, obstetricians are giving themselves elevated status, certainly above that of a patient. In U.S. medical schools, medical students model themselves after their professors and learn to view themselves as members of an elite group. There is a lot of emphasis placed on how important doctors are and little discussion of how important patients are, and no one talks about medicine being a service. In particular, it is my experience that many obstetricians/gynecologists chose their specialty without fully recognizing that while they will be playing the role of highly skilled surgeon some of the time, at other times their role will be to serve—assist and support—a woman and her family as they go through a major life event. So for some doctors, what I'm describing represents a fundamental paradigm shift, which when made cannot help but affect not only their attitudes but their practice. An obstetrician who practices with a strong anti-regulation ethic, for example—taking an attitude of "I can do anything I want"—will find that this ethic breaks down when he views himself as performing a service, because when one is performing a service, one has an inherent obligation to the people one serves.

We can look to other countries for models of how midwives can be the primary care provider in low-risk births. In Scandinavia, a woman's family doctor (not an obstetrician) confirms her pregnancy and rules out any serious medical problems. From then on, the woman receives maternity care from local midwives, and in most cases, will not be seen by a doctor again during the pregnancy. The midwife handles all prenatal visits, and when the woman goes into labor, she chooses either a hospital or a home birth. If she chooses a hospital birth, the midwife attends her in the hospital, admits her, assists her during the labor, assists her at birth, assists after the birth, and discharges her from the hospital without the woman ever having seen a doctor.

In some areas of Western Europe and Scandinavia, a low-risk pregnant woman can choose a small group of midwives who share a practice. The woman will usually get to know all of the midwives during prenatal visits over the course of her pregnancy, and when she goes into labor, one of them will come to the home or hospital and assist for the entire time, even if the labor is thirty-six hours long. This allows the woman to receive one-on-one continuous care with a known midwife—so this scientifically proven ideal scenario is not pie in the sky, but quite feasible. All those countries in Western Europe and Scandinavia where midwives handle prenatal and birth care for low-risk women exclusively have lower mortality rates for birthing women and their babies than the United States does.

In Japan, the network of midwife birth houses provided a significant cadre of independent midwives in the first half of the twentieth century. But after World War II, during the American occupation, the Americans not only insisted that birth houses be closed but insisted that all midwives must train first as nurses and must work under the supervision of obstetricians. Until then, Japan had not medicalized birth but handled it as a normal part of the life cycle and as a normal part of Japanese family life. The country had a large, strong, independent midwifery profession. The U.S.-

imposed restrictions resulted in the tragic loss of this cultural tradition, but independent midwifery did not die. As it was not against the law, a few obstinate, independent midwives maintained their birth houses. As soon as the Americans left, a resurgence of birth houses in Japan began, and more and more midwives are leaving hospital practice to work as community midwives in birth houses. This Japanese experience confirms what we have seen in the United States, that in the end, attempts to eradicate midwifery are not successful. In every society, there will always be midwives working to maintain women's freedom to control their own reproductive lives, and there will always be women who will avail themselves of midwifery services.

In July 2001, while in Tokyo, I met with fourteen leading obstetricians from the Japanese Society of Obstetricians and Gynecologists (all men). We discussed current obstetric practices in Japan, and they voiced their opposition to birth houses. When I asked why they opposed birth houses, they replied that they are dangerous. I then asked if they had scientific evidence that birth houses are dangerous, and they admitted that they did not. The resurgence of birth houses in Japan continues, despite this obstetric disapproval. There are many lessons to learn from Japan. Two that are particularly relevant: It is difficult for an occupying army to impose changes to something as basic to a country's culture as childbirth, and even in a society as patriarchal as Japan, women still play a central role in their own reproductive lives and are somehow intuitive enough to ignore unjustified warnings from high-ranking men.

In New Zealand, the maternity system is similar to Scandinavia's, but a woman having a low-risk pregnancy can choose either a midwife or a family physician to provide her prenatal and birth care, and whichever provider she chooses receives the same flat fee for all the woman's maternity care, covered under the country's national health service.

Canada is a particularly relevant model for the United States for using midwives for primary maternity care for low-risk women. Until recently, Canada was the only country in the world besides the United States to banish midwifery, making it possible for doctors to take over the care of low-risk pregnant and birthing women. But then something extraordinary happened. In the 1980s, a midwife in Toronto transported a woman having a home birth to the hospital, where the baby died. The obstetricians in the hospital notified the police, and shortly after, an inquest was called to investigate the midwife because midwifery was illegal. As in the United States, midwives had gone underground decades earlier, due to persecution by a coalition of doctors, nurses, and politicians. But, of course, some women still wanted to have home births, and there were always underground midwives to attend them.

The lawyer defending the midwife in Toronto had great difficulty finding a Canadian physician willing to testify at the inquest, and I was invited to come and testify.[27] The inquest had a jury of twelve, and I spent about six hours on the stand. My goal was to educate these twelve Canadians about midwifery, a profession they knew nothing about. At the end of the inquest, the jury recommended to the government that it investigate the possibility of legalizing midwifery—the opposite of what the obstetricians who reported the midwife to the authorities had intended. This case was the beginning of a long struggle to reestablish midwifery in Canada. This struggle was not always easy. At one point, a top physician/official in a medical organization in Quebec Province stated that if Quebec legalized midwifery, it might as well legalize prostitution too. Today, twenty years after the coroner's inquest in Toronto, midwifery is legal in every province of Canada and there are midwifery schools gradually training enough midwives to attend all low-risk pregnant and birthing women in Canada.

As part of this process, the editor of the *Journal of the Society of Obstetricians and Gynecologists of Canada* contacted me and told me that he, like most Canadian-born obstetricians, knew nothing about midwifery until he was lucky enough to be exposed to the profession while doing postgraduate training in the United Kingdom, where midwives are the designated professionals assisting all woman having low-risk births, as they are in other parts of Europe. He wanted to help educate Canadian obstetricians about midwifery and asked if I would write an article for the organization's journal reviewing all aspects of midwifery, including the scientific evidence for midwifery practice. I agreed and wrote the article, which was published in his *Journal.*[28]

Canada's experience in reestablishing direct-entry midwives as primary care providers for low-risk women has lessons for the United States. Even in countries such as the United States and Canada, where the present generation of doctors has no experience with midwifery, nor does the public, it is still possible to introduce midwifery, although it takes time. If a few obstetricians understand the importance of midwives, it is important to use them to promote changing attitudes. In time, educating the public and politicians leads to legislation, which essentially forces doctors to adapt to the change, and over time gradually come to accept it.

As described earlier, there are also areas of the United States where midwives provide primary care to low-risk pregnant and birthing woman, specifically Taos, New Mexico, and The Farm in rural Tennessee. There are also hundreds of independent direct-entry midwives and nurse-midwives across the United States assisting women in planned home births. And an even larger cadre of nurse-midwives in the United States are bringing midwifery care to a significant group of women having hospital birth. So inroads have been made.

It is interesting that some of the important innovations in maternity care in the United States have occurred in the country's more remote areas. Midwifery made a comeback in the United States when no one else wanted to attend births in Appalachia. A group of nurses trained to become nurse-midwives and created a new profession.[29] In chapter 5, I discussed a case where the value of midwifery was proven in Madera, California, in a natural experiment that compared midwife-attended birth with doctor-attended birth in a rural community hospital.

Some of the most progressive legislation and practice of midwifery in the United States continues to go on in rural, less populated settings such as New Mexico and Oregon. In these two states, not only are direct-entry midwives licensed, there are state midwifery boards separate from the state nursing boards, and the midwifery boards are made up of direct-entry midwives who investigate complaints. So in these states, midwifery practice is regulated by true peers. I was invited to observe a meeting of the New Mexico State Midwifery Board. As I left, there was no doubt in my mind that the midwives on the board were committed to strengthening midwifery in their state.

In sharp contrast, I have attended meetings at the state nursing boards in Washington State and South Dakota. These boards are responsible for regulating midwives as well as nurses, but both boards are made up entirely of nurses. In these board meetings, the members were openly hostile to direct-entry midwifery and repeatedly expressed the opinion that only nurse-midwives should be allowed to practice.

In more rural states, there may occasionally be a local doctor who manages to get a local district attorney to bring groundless charges against a local midwife (as happened in a small town in Oregon in 2005), but generally, the public and the authorities are quite positive about their midwives. This suggests that midwifery can flourish in the United States in areas where there is less pressure from organized obstetrics to limit midwifery practice because practice in those areas is less attractive to doctors. Perhaps a key to shifting to midwifery for low-risk births is to establish laws or other disincentives that make that practice less appealing to doctors.

Throughout the United States currently, there are group practices that include obstetricians and nurse-midwives, and some of these groups allow a woman having a low-risk birth to choose a midwife rather than a doctor as her primary birth attendant, if she prefers. In some of these groups there is tension because the midwives find it difficult to practice full midwifery with obstetricians looking over their shoulders, but these tensions can often be worked out with a great deal of learning on both sides. These groups represent another precedent, a proven track record for having midwives provide pregnancy and birth care for low-risk women in the United States. Although these mixed groups are not by any means an ideal model, they are certainly a step in the right direction on the way to having all low-risk women assisted by midwives. Gradually the mix in these groups can evolve to increase the number of midwives and reduce the number of obstetricians, so that midwives handle all low-risk pregnancies and births and obstetricians handle only high-risk pregnancies and births.

Some believe that women should always have the right to choose to have an obstetrician "attend" their childbirth, and I would expect those opinions to continue for awhile in a future in which midwives are the primary care providers for women having low-risk pregnancies. In response to these people, I believe we must look to the precedents that already exist for limiting patient choice to safe and appropriate alternatives.

If I have a brain tumor and want my general practitioner to do the brain surgery, it will not happen. Even if the general practitioner agrees to do it, there is no hospital that would allow it because of the high risk involved. There are many regulations and protocols in place in hospitals and states that govern what the various health care providers can do and how and when they can do it. The entire prescription drug system is also predicated on controlling which drugs a patient can purchase—without patient choice. So for reasons of safety, there are limits on what a patient can choose. If a practice is out of the scope of training and experience for a practitioner, as attending low-risk birth is for obstetricians (and will become more so over time), hospitals should not allow the practitioner to do the practice. When we consider the case of obstetricians handling low-risk birth, it is not only that they do not have the proper training and experience, it is not possible for them to give one-on-one *continuous* assistance throughout a woman's entire labor and birth. If it is not possible for them to provide what we know to be the safest service, they should not be allowed to provide the service. In the future, neurosurgeons will do brain surgery and midwives will attend low-risk births.

SHARED RESPONSIBILITY FOR HIGH-RISK MATERNITY CARE

Obstetricians are absolutely essential in the overall system of care during pregnancy and childbirth. They are the experts in high-risk maternity care and should have primary responsibility for managing serious medical complications. However, midwives are the experts in normal birth and high-risk women still have many of the normal needs associated with all pregnancy and birth. For this reason, the team assisting a woman with a high-risk pregnancy should include a midwife.

Incorporating obstetric and midwifery expertise in an egalitarian team effort will be a key challenge in the maternity care of the future. How can midwives and obstetricians communicate effectively when they have such different models for birth and such different experience and skills? Who decides when a low-risk birth becomes high-risk?

One answer to the question of who decides is illustrated by my daughter's childbirth in a large hospital in Copenhagen, Denmark. She was having her first baby and received all her prenatal care from midwives. At 6 A.M. on her due date, she began having contractions, so she went to the hospital. Because her labor was not yet active, a midwife at the hospital ruptured her bag of waters and sent her home. At noon she returned in active labor and was admitted by the midwife, who then attended her labor. Her cervix dilated slowly but steadily, until there was just a lip left.

By this time it was late evening, and the baby had not descended any further. Using a stethoscope, the midwife listened to the fetal heart and detected evidence of mild fetal distress, so for the first time during the labor my daughter was hooked up to an electronic fetal monitor. The monitor corroborated the signs of mild fetal distress, so the midwife gave my daughter oxygen to breathe and called in the midwife supervisor and the obstetrician on duty in the hospital. The obstetrician and supervising midwife confirmed the remaining lip on the cervix and the mild fetal distress and the two midwives and the doctor discussed what to do. It had been fifteen to twenty minutes since the mild fetal distress was first found, and although all agreed that action was necessary, there was not a feeling of emergency. The supervising midwife said, "Before we turn to surgical solutions, give me a couple of minutes. I think I can get this baby out."

The more experienced midwife took command, essentially giving orders to the other midwife, the obstetrician, and the recently arrived pediatrician, all of whom were now assisting her. She did a vaginal examination and found the baby's umbilical cord wrapped around its neck. In no more than two minutes, she managed to release the cord and push the remaining lip from around the baby's head. Then she put my daughter in a more vertical position, which made my daughter push even more. A couple of minutes later, just after midnight, my granddaughter was born. The pediatrician found her to be in good condition.

This birth story illustrates a midwife managing a low-risk birth, a low-risk labor becoming high-risk, the midwife calling for the obstetrician because of the complication, an egalitarian consultation between midwife and obstetrician, the value of a highly experienced midwife when a complication develops, and the value of trying a nonsurgical approach first. I have told my daughter that there is no doubt in my mind that if she had been in a U.S. hospital, she would have had a C-section—something she didn't want. My daughter's case also illustrates the mutual respect that evolves when obstetricians and midwives work together, as they always have in Denmark.

Communication between the midwife and the obstetrician is also essential when a woman has chosen to give birth out of hospital. When there is a question about the progress of labor or fetal distress, the midwife can contact the hospital and have an egalitarian discussion with the obstetrician over the phone. This communication is an important element in out-of-hospital birth, both because it brings another type of expertise into the case and because it facilitates transport to the hospital if that becomes necessary. When providers outside and inside the hospital know one another and are comfortable working together, if a case is transported, lots of time can be saved and any necessary personnel and equipment can be lined up quickly.

Because the Netherlands has a national health service (which eliminates economic competition between midwives and doctors) and also has a high percentage of home births, that country also illustrates a high level of respect between doctors and midwives, and the communication between them is, generally, excellent.

Finally, we must not forget that when obstetricians participate in managing a high-risk birth, the principles of informed choice, empowerment, and autonomy are just as valid as in a low-risk birth. In high-risk cases, it is just as important that ownership of the birth remain with the woman and her family. Doctors are human, and birthing women, whether their births are low-risk or high-risk, are human. To err is human. A woman must have the right to have any errors committed during her childbirth be her own and not someone else's.

INCREASED MONITORING, TRANSPARENCY, AND ACCOUNTABILITY

In the midwifery model of care, a midwife develops a close relationship with the pregnant woman over many months and ordinarily discusses whatever is going on in their prenatal visits. With these close relationships, midwifery care is, by nature, much more transparent than obstetric care and midwives are more accountable to the women they serve in such a close, interpersonal way. Providing low-risk maternity care in an out-of-hospital setting also facilitates transparency and accountability, as the woman and her family are better able to see and understand what is going on in these smaller settings. Another benefit: when the pregnant woman and her family are responsible for making the choices, the provider is much less likely to feel that there may be something to hide, so transparency and accountability come naturally and less monitoring is needed.

Although I believe that low-risk births should not be managed in hospitals and that midwives, not obstetricians, should be providing the primary care in these cases, I acknowledge that this will not be a reality for some time to come. In the interim, we must look at improving hospital birth.

There are essentially two kinds of transparency and accountability—to the patient and to the public. In maternity care, transparency and accountability to the patient must mean that the woman and her family are active participants in the birth of their child. The more woman-centered maternity care is achieved in hospitals, the more transparency and accountability to the family we will see. And the more transparency and accountability we insist on, the more woman-centered maternity care we will see. Over time, we can expect to see the present tendency of hospitals to stonewall families after an adverse birth outcome disappear—and with it will go much of the litigation against doctors and hospitals, a most civilized solution to the present so-called obstetric malpractice litigation crisis.

It is also natural and important for a woman to want to know more generally what is going on in the hospital where she is considering giving birth. Knowing what her birth options would be in a given hospital—choice of birthing positions, whether she could choose to eat and drink during labor, her freedom to choose a VBAC, rates of C-section in that hospital, and so on—is the only way a woman can make an informed choice. If a pregnant woman can choose between two hospitals and there is no transparency, how will she find out that in one there is a 30 percent chance that she will have a C-section and in the other there is a 15 percent chance?

Working against women in this area is the fact that it may be against the interests of the hospital to disclose information on their birth practices, as they are trying hard to "sell" their services to pregnant women. Hospital administrators are always looking for ways to cut costs and lure patients. (This is why inducing labor with Cytotec is a windfall for hospitals. Cytotec costs less than other drugs and allows a doctor to tell a woman that if she gives birth in his hospital, she can have her baby when she wants to.) A hospital is an institution and will always behave as any institution, and that includes protecting its institutional secrets.

The second type of transparency and accountability is to the public, which includes reporting to local and state health agencies and providing political bodies and the media with information when they request it. It is essential that all hospitals and individual heath providers, including obstetricians, be open to providing information on their obstetric practices—including rates of C-section, epidural anesthesia for normal birth, and pharmacological induction of labor—as well as on their birth outcomes, including rates of maternal mortality, neonatal mortality, uterine rupture, and adverse drug reactions.

Today U.S. hospital maternity services are not transparent to the public, and until this changes it will be impossible to enforce regulations, correct deviations in standards of care, and promote responsibility. For example, we saw in chapter 1 that even though New York State has a law requiring hospitals to report to the public on their maternity practices such as rates of C-section, many hospitals do not comply and, as there is no health care system in place, there is no good way to enforce the law.

Many people believe that physicians in the United States are resistant to the idea of national health care because they would make less money, but I think that an equally strong reason is the fear physicians feel around disclosing what they're doing and being held accountable for it. A national system would certainly mean more monitoring and regulation and would infringe on doctors' freedom to do whatever they want with no judge in sight.

In our current semiprivatized health care system, hospitals and doctors have understandable needs—to reduce costs, increase profits, avoid litigation, improve efficiency, maintain staff satisfaction—and these needs sometimes conflict with the needs of patients and their families. It is fashionable for a hospital to have a poster on the wall in its lobby titled "Patient's Rights" that affirms informed consent. But a woman who comes to that hospital to give birth will be asked to sign a standardized informed consent form that contains no information for her benefit and gives blanket permission for the hospital's doctors to do whatever they decide is necessary. This is an example of how current hospital needs discourage transparency and accountability—both to patients and to the public—and interfere with the changes that must be made to increase monitoring and quality assurance.

Monitoring and regulation are more aspects of health care where the United States can look to other countries for clues. The United Kingdom, the Netherlands, and Denmark are all countries that illustrate the way a national health care system serves as a framework into which regulation and monitoring can be incorporated. With a national system in place, backed up by legislation, with government regulations to define practices, and with standardized payment mechanisms for providers, it is far easier to regulate and carefully monitor practices, as well as to ensure proper informed consent for patients.

Any vision of how to regulate and monitor maternity services in the United States must begin with establishing some form of national health service, as this will inevitably lead to better transparency, better accountability, better regulation of health care practices, and better enforcement of these regulations. The United States needs a national health care system in which there is as much regulation, monitoring, transparency, and accountability as is found in other Western industrialized countries, without any loss of democracy in government at all levels, open competition in free markets, and individual freedoms.

When this is in place at the federal level, there will be agencies to regulate medical practices including maternity care, similar to the FDA, but with more power to enforce. These agencies will report to the U.S. Congress certainly, but they will also bring relevant information on medical practices to the public. And care must be taken not to allow such federal agencies to come under the inappropriate influence of doctors and hospitals. This transparency will lead to accountability because the information will include the names and locations of providers and health care institutions. We have done well in regulating and monitoring a can of fruit in the United States, and we can now say that we have a respectable level of transparency and accountability in food safety. We must do as well or better for the birth services we provide for woman and families.

ENHANCED MATERNITY CARE EDUCATION

In my vision for a better way to provide maternity services in the United States, federal and state governments would continue to fund the education of maternity care providers. The federal government currently provides considerable funds for the postgraduate training of obstetric residents in hospitals.[30] However, rather than funding going to train ever more obstetric residents in hospitals, most of it should go to train midwives to provide primary maternity care in out-of-hospital settings. In this area as well, there would be transparency, in that the government would report to the public regarding whose education was being funded and would provide justification for these decisions.

The United States trains more obstetricians every year.[31] Why? Who decides how many obstetricians will be trained? ACOG has provided the federal government with estimates of how many new obstetricians are needed, and these reports are used to inform funding decisions. It's hardly surprising that ACOG insists that the United States needs more obstetricians—every medical specialty insists that the world needs more specialists in their area. With obstetricians in the role of hospital-based specialists that provide care for high-risk pregnant and birthing women, however, we will need far fewer obstetricians. With midwives becoming the primary provider for low-risk pregnant and birthing women, we will need many more midwives.

According to the American College of Nurse Midwives and Midwives Alliance of North America, the United States has around 41,000 obstetricians and 5,000 midwives. That's eight obstetricians for every midwife. Great Britain has 35,000 midwives and 1,000 obstetricians, thirty-five midwives for every obstetrician (according to the British Royal College of Midwives and the British Royal College of Obstetricians and Gynecologists). Looking at it another way, the United States has one obstetrician for every hundred births, while Great Britain has one obstetrician for every thousand births. Having one obstetrician for every hundred births is beyond excessive—it's ridiculous, and it's one of the reasons the United States spends nearly twice as much per birth as Great Britain. Having one midwife for every 800 births in the United States is also ridiculous.

The education of maternity care providers must be based on good evidence of what is needed rather than on lobbying by doctors. I also believe that the public has a right to participate in deciding whose education will be funded, given that public funds are being used, and I would want to see any large funding allocations reviewed in televised hearings in a public setting and approved only after a thorough discussion among the public and their representatives.

The curriculum for training obstetricians must also be revised. Although obstetricians will be focusing on cases with serious complications, it is still important for obstetricians to know what normal looks like in order to distinguish between normal and pathological. In my vision, as part of their training, obstetricians would have to observe midwives attending at least ten normal births in out-of-hospital settings. This will go a long way in opening their eyes to what normal birth is—something women do, not something that happens to them—and will give them another way to see and attend birth, as well as some much-needed respect both for midwives and for women.

Midwives will also train first-year obstetric residents in the management of common complications that can be handled without resorting to surgical interventions—for example, turning breech babies late in pregnancy, managing VBAC, managing vaginal breech birth, managing shoulder dystocia, and managing other less common fetal birth positions such as posterior lie. This will also create frequent opportunities for information exchange between obstetricians in training and midwives. There is at least some precedent for this. Ina May Gaskin, the direct-entry, home birth midwife and author mentioned earlier, developed a special maneuver for managing shoulder dystocia (when a baby's shoulder gets stuck after the head is already out). This breakthrough maneuver has been published in the obstetric literature.[32] Gaskin has also trained obstetric residents in this maneuver in a number of hospitals in the United States, and the "Gaskin maneuver" is now widely practiced by obstetricians.

In Scandinavia, Great Britain, and many other industrialized countries, first-year obstetrical residents are routinely trained by midwives, which not only passes on midwifery knowledge to young doctors but helps them to see the essential role midwifery plays in maternity care and encourages communication and respect between the two groups. There is a precedent for providing obstetricians in training with experience in planned out-of-hospital birth as well. In some training programs in the Philippines, obstetricians can't be certified until they've attended at least ten planned out-of-hospital births.[33]

PUBLIC EDUCATION ABOUT MATERNITY CARE

One reason women have been so willing to give up their autonomy when it comes to childbirth is that they are afraid, and much of this fear is the result of ignorance. In modern American society, where most people live only with nuclear family members, there are rarely opportunities for young girls to actually witness childbirth and ask questions. What we have instead are a lot of childbirth books that tell women to trust doctors and turn their care over to them because birth is a medical event and demands highly trained experts.

An educated public would grease the wheels of change in a number of ways, one being that it would make women better consumers when they considered birth options. Education would also make women feel more confident taking ownership of their own experience. When women begin to understand that maternity care is a women's issue, change really takes off.

Beginning early in elementary school, children would be taught the wonders of human reproduction, and this education would continue into high school. Midwives would be invited to schools to talk about conception, pregnancy, and childbirth. Girls and boys would see films on childbirth and go on field trips to the neighborhood women's center. Adolescent girls would have an opportunity to observe actual childbirth, just as they have throughout history until recently, when childbirth was moved to the hospital and girls were forbidden to join their mothers.

Midwives working in local women's centers would play a large role in educating children in local schools, and also in educating women. The center would facilitate self-help and support groups for pregnant women in which women can offer one another prenatal and postnatal care under the guidance of the midwife while learning about their bodies, pregnancy, childbirth, breast-feeding, early childhood care, and family planning. (See the discussion earlier in this chapter on self-help prenatal groups.)

The media also play an important role in educating the public. As the average birth experience changes in the United States, I would expect to see the media, especially television, depict childbirth as a normal part of family life, with scenes of childbirth as it occurs in women's centers, with midwives attending and with no medical trappings. I would also expect to see more books about pregnancy and childbirth that emphasize the social, cultural, and physiological aspects of normal birth and its place in the life cycle, and that show that women can take responsibility for what happens to them during pregnancy and birth.

The United States has a serious problem with unwanted teenage pregnancies. Denmark and the Netherlands share the honor of having the lowest rates of unwanted teenage pregnancy in the world. What is their magic? They both do an excellent job of educating young people about human reproduction and sexuality, starting in the first grade. By the time their citizens are twelve years old, they know how to prevent unwanted pregnancy. In many additional places in the world, public education about pregnancy and childbirth is in place and there is no shame about the body, no shame about sexuality, no shame about birth. Shame leads to ignorance, which leads to more shame—and ignorance and shame also lead to unwanted pregnancies and higher rates of maternal and infant mortality. The solution to this vicious ignorance/shame cycle is education. Just say no to ignorance and shame.

NINE HOW TO GET WHERE WE NEED TO BE

Never doubt that a small group of thoughtful, committed people can change the world. Indeed, it is the only thing that ever has.
MARGARET MEAD

We Americans are consumed with the need to believe that we are number one. But here's a wrenching fact: forty-one countries have better infant mortality rates than the United States does. In 2002, our infant mortality rate went up, not down, and if the United States had an infant mortality rate as good as Cuba's, we would save an additional 2,212 American babies a year.[1] And mothers? Women are 70 percent more likely to die in childbirth in America than in Europe, and the rate of women dying in childbirth in America has been going up every year for more than twenty years.[2]

But things are changing in maternity care in the United States, and in this chapter I will look at how things are changing and how we can work to promote the vision of maternity care I described in chapter 8.

HOW OTHERS ARE MAKING PROGRESS

Just as those who never make mistakes can never learn from them, so too those who must always be number one can never learn from others. So to begin, it helps to view changes in maternity care from a global and historical perspective, paying particular attention to how services tend to improve or evolve. In the chart "Global Evolution of Birthing Practices," I've focused on the autonomy of birthing women and midwives because I see that as the

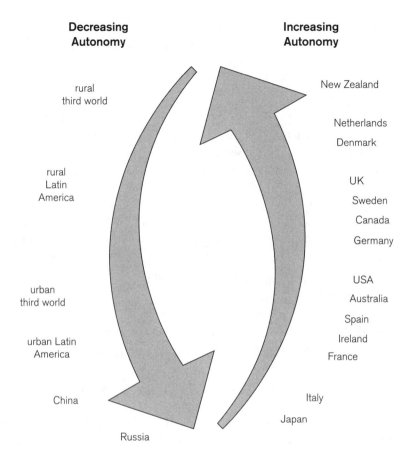

rural
third world

New Zealand

Netherlands
Denmark

rural
Latin
America

UK

Sweden

Canada

Germany

USA

urban
third world

Australia

Spain

urban Latin
America

Ireland

France

China

Italy

Japan

Russia

Global evolution of birthing practices.

key variable for determining where a country or region is in the evolutionary process. In countries at the top of the chart, women and midwives have
a high degree of autonomy; in countries at the bottom, they have little or
no autonomy. The chart illustrates where countries lie at this time. I've put
them in these positions based on the knowledge of their maternity care systems I've gleaned from personal visits as well as from published reports,
World Health Organization reports in particular. Of course the placement
is a bit arbitrary—the evolution of maternity care is by no means static and
one might argue that the Netherlands should be higher on the chart than
New Zealand, for example—but the overall pattern is certainly valid.

Until around three hundred years ago, all countries in the world were at the top of the circle, with almost all birthing women having control over their own childbirth. Midwives were autonomous care providers who assisted women during childbirth. Essentially, the woman and midwife worked together without outside interference because of the nearly universal cultural taboo against men getting involved in women's reproductive activities. Just as in the past menstruating women had been isolated, birthing women were isolated with no men allowed nearby.

With the gradual introduction of men and "barber-surgeons" (precursors of today's medical surgeons) into maternity care, both birthing women and midwives gradually lost their autonomy in childbirth, and as childbirth became less woman-centered, countries slowly moved down the left side of the circle. Today, many developing countries are in this early part of the maternity care evolutionary cycle. Their urban areas are "modernizing" maternity care by bringing in obstetricians and hospitals, while the women in rural areas still use indigenous midwives.

Eventually, a country reaches the bottom of the circle, where the global goal of "development" has penetrated and the government and the population are eager to be "modern." China, Russia, and much of Latin America serve as examples here. Birthing women in these countries are no longer allowed to decide what happens during their pregnancy and birth, and midwives are nothing more than slaves to doctors.

I have worked in Russia for many months and have seen the conditions with my own eyes. All births take place in hospitals, with the woman giving birth placed on a cold, hard table with her feet up in stirrups, surrounded by doctors, with midwives running around doing doctors' bidding. A woman is assigned to a maternity hospital and has absolutely no choice about anything to do with her pregnancy and birth. No family members, husband included, are ever permitted into the maternity hospital, where the woman remains for ten to fourteen days after birth. It is not unusual to see husbands standing outside in the hospital yard waving to their wives, who are leaning out windows several stories up and waving back.

Then something happens in the countries at the bottom of the chart. It varies from country to country, but whatever it is, when things get really bad and women's reproductive freedom is abused severely enough, some precipitating factor or series of events finally brings women's attention to the power doctors hold over their reproductive lives. This leads to women's disillusionment, anger, and resentment and a call to action. This reaction may go more quickly in developed countries, where there is at least some degree of freedom and women's rights in place, but it can also be the start of these rights and freedoms.

Although midwives in countries at the bottom of the chart tend to be divided into those who accept the status quo and those who want to change it, this precipitating factor angers the midwives as well. They join with the angry women (often forming coalitions that also include scientists, journalists, some politicians, and some doctors and nurses) to start the long, difficult process of regaining their women's autonomy in childbirth and reproduction, moving the country up the right side of the circle.

Looking at how this played out in particular countries can provide important lessons for us in how to go about getting the United States to where it needs to be. In chapter 8, I described how this happened in Canada, where the arrest of a home birth midwife in Toronto led to a coroner's inquest, which led ultimately to the government legalizing midwifery.

Germany is another good example of the struggle to regain autonomy. In the 1980s, the national organization of German obstetricians went to the federal government and demanded that all out-of-hospital births be forbidden by law. Suddenly, German midwives woke up, German women's organizations woke up; they formed coalitions and worked together to plan an opposition strategy. They collected ammunition in the form of scientific data and policy documents from other countries and from WHO and descended on their legislators and the media. It was a battle, but in the end they were successful. Out-of-hospital birth was not outlawed in Germany, and there is now a strong, wide-awake lobby of German women and midwives who stand ready to oppose any further attempts on the part of German obstetricians to take away birth options.

As a result of this struggle, a large number of German midwives have since left hospitals to become community midwives attending births at home and at out-of-hospital birth centers. Today, approximately one-quarter of the midwives in Germany are working primarily outside of hospitals, and the number of out-of-hospital alternative birth centers (ABCs) has increased from one in 1990 to more than seventy in 2003.[3] This happened despite fierce resistance from the German obstetric establishment, which repeatedly told women that out-of-hospital birth would put their babies in jeopardy. Germany demonstrates that it is possible to change a maternity care system without the blessing of obstetricians, an important lesson for the United States. It seems there is at least one thing more powerful than the medical establishment: women, when they are angry and get organized.

Around the same time, there was a similar angry reaction among women in New Zealand. A professor of obstetrics at a university hospital conducted an experimental, randomized trial to try to further confirm if a particular screening test for cervical cancer worked: the Pap test, named after the doctor who first described it, Dr. Papanicoleau.[4] The study looked at women who had positive Pap tests. The group with positive screening tests was divided in half: one half received follow-up and treatment for cancer, and the other half received no treatment. Over time, an increasing number of women in the group that received no treatment died from cervical cancer—but the experiment continued. Then a journalist got wind of the situation and wrote about the study. Women in New Zealand were outraged. The country's entire obstetric profession lost credibility.

Around the same time, midwives in New Zealand were trying to improve the country's maternity care and to resist the extreme medicalization of birth going on in other countries, such as the United States. When New Zealand women became disillusioned with obstetricians, many turned to midwives to assist their births, and New Zealand legislators began paying more attention to what midwives and women wanted. They created a new system of maternity care, and now every woman having a low-risk pregnancy in New Zealand can choose her own midwife or family physician for prenatal and birth care (leaving the obstetricians to care for women with high-risk pregnancies), and she can choose where to give birth as well. As I mentioned in chapter 8, all maternity care is covered by the national health service in New Zealand, and all providers, whether doctors or midwives, receive the same flat fee for providing pregnancy care and attending births of low-risk women. New Zealand now has rates of unnecessary obstetric interventions that are among the lowest in the world, with a national C-section rate close to 10 percent. And it has lower perinatal and maternal mortality rates than the United States does.[5]

In Brazil, a different precipitating factor recently triggered a reaction among women: the country's extreme C-section rate. Brazil has one of the highest national average C-section rates in the world, and in some private Brazilian hospitals the rate is above 90 percent.[6] For a time, Brazilian doctors were able to convince women and health officials that they were only doing what women wanted. Their reasoning: in Brazil's macho society, a man wants his woman to have "a honeymoon vagina," and we doctors are helping women achieve this by saving them from vaginal births. But then, in 1985 and 2000, two large international maternity care conferences were held in Brazil, and the media surrounding these conferences helped educate

Brazilian women about the dangers of extreme medicalization of birth and the need to humanize birth care.

As a full-time World Health Organization staff officer, I helped organize the World Health Organization Consensus Conference on Appropriate Technology for Birth, held in Fortaleza, Brazil, in 1985. The conference reviewed scientific evidence on technologies used during childbirth and went on to make a series of recommendations, including that the rate of C-section should never be more than 10 to 15 percent of all births.[7] These WHO recommendations have become the global standard for the appropriate use of birth technology and were of particular relevance to Brazilians, not only because the conference was held in their country, but because their own rates are so extreme.

Then in 2000, a follow-up conference in Fortaleza covered a broader topic: how to humanize all aspects of childbirth. I was involved in planning this conference as well. We hoped to attract as many as a thousand participants from all over Latin America and from other countries. To our surprise and delight, there were more than two thousand participants, including many from Brazil—a broad range of women's organizations, social scientists, midwives, nurses, obstetricians, perinatal scientists, politicians, and journalists. There was good coverage of the conference in the media. The enthusiasm level was very high; one could feel change in the air. There was no doubt that these people were committed to changing birth practices, and a resolution was passed urging countries to demedicalize and humanize childbirth.[8]

In the years following these two conferences, there was a lot of anger among women in Brazil over their maternity care, and coalitions were formed to work for a better system.[9] These groups have worked closely with the national government in Brazil to establish a network of out-of-hospital birth centers (partially government-funded) and to change the country's policy for reimbursing public hospitals for C-sections—hospitals with excessive C-section rates are not reimbursed by the government for these unnecessary surgical procedures.

A group of Brazilian scientists, stimulated by the movement in Brazil to humanize birth, conducted a research study to determine whether women in Brazil truly prefer C-section to vaginal birth. Interviewers spoke with a large sampling of women, during pregnancy and again after childbirth, and concluded that Brazilian women do not want or choose C-section, but instead have it imposed on them by their obstetricians.[10]

Though precipitating events vary in countries where a shift in maternity care has taken place, it's possible to see common themes and draw some conclusions. I believe there are lessons those of us who want to bring about change in the United States can learn from this evolutionary process.

First, it appears that the medicalization of maternity care and the loss of women's and midwives' autonomy must become extreme for a reaction to set in. It is only when women's reproductive freedom is being severely abused in one way or another that women and midwives get sufficiently angry to take action. There is no doubt that at present in the United States, certain aspects of maternity care are getting worse—as evidenced by the frequent witch-hunts for midwives; false information given to women about the risks of labor induction; rising induction rates; rising C-section rates; hospitals refusing to do VBAC; and the widespread against-label use of a powerful and dangerous drug to induce labor unnecessarily. Now we must work to get information on these worsening aspects of maternity care out to the public—and especially to women's organizations and women's magazines, books, and television programs—to stimulate action.

Another feature of this circle of evolution of birthing practices is the interrelationship between the autonomy of women and the autonomy of midwives. Simply put, if women in a country do not have the power to make their own birth decisions, there will be no autonomy for midwives, and if midwives do not have the authority to practice independently, the autonomy of women is much more difficult to achieve. Women understand that their feelings of strength and freedom are closely tied to having control of their bodies, including control of their reproduction and childbirth. And midwives know that they will never have autonomy without the full support of the women in society. This is why the quality of maternity care in any country is closely tied to the level of autonomy of women and midwives and why I used autonomy as the critical factor when placing countries on the circle of evolution of maternity care in the chart earlier in this chapter.

As women and midwives struggle up the right side of the circle of evolution of birthing practices and regain autonomy, maternity care simultaneously becomes more women-centered, more humanized, and more evidence-based. Western European countries serve as an excellent example of the relationship between autonomy for women and midwives and healthful birthing practices. In Western Europe, there is a gradient in the equality and independence of women in general from north to south, with women in northern countries such as Denmark having a lot of rights and independence and women in southern countries such as Italy having far less. There is a similar north–south gradient in the authority and independence of midwives in these countries, and the quality of maternity care follows. For example, C-section rates are 10 to 15 percent in Scandinavia, in the 20 to 30 percent range in central Europe, and 35 percent in Italy. (See www.who.int/reproductive-health.)

To Americans who are used to thinking that their country is number one in the world, the position of the United States in the circle of evolution of birthing practices often comes as a surprise. Although women in the United States have made enormous strides in their place in society, when it comes to maternity services, American women have made too little progress. The women's movement in the United States has focused on the workplace, economic equality, and certain health issues such as cervical and breast cancer, eating disorders, and abortion rights. These issues are certainly important, but there is no question that the women's movement in America has neglected issues of maternity care.

As a result, today in the United States, women are still willing to put themselves in a doctor's hands and say, "Take care of me." They are all too willing to believe an obstetrician who tells them that they have the freedom to choose C-section, without demanding full disclosure of the serious risks of C-section for themselves and their babies. In general, pregnant and birthing women in the United States have limited valid information, limited true choices based on full disclosure of risks, rising rates of unnecessary and risky interventions such as pharmacological induction of labor and elective C-section, unfavorable and rising rates of mortality for pregnant and birthing women and their babies, and a serious lack of transparency, accountability, monitoring, and regulation of obstetric practices—hence America's ranking on the circle of evolution. One of the main reasons that obstetrics in the United States is out of control is because obstetricians do not have the restraining influence of a larger, strong midwifery profession and larger, strong women's groups focused on maternity issues as do obstetricians in other industrialized countries.

HOW THE UNITED STATES CAN MAKE PROGRESS

There are a number of things that can be done to eliminate the subtle violence against women and families presently taking place in American maternity care. The ten strategies discussed here include practical steps for mobilizing the necessary forces in the struggle to emancipate women, midwives, and maternity care from the monopolistic control of organized obstetrics (and some obstetricians), so we can move up the circle of evolution to better birth practices.

I. EDUCATE THE PUBLIC

It is crucial to the movement for humanizing birth that the American public understand childbirth, midwifery, and the present abuses in our maternity care system. Thanks to soap operas and sitcoms, most of the American public currently thinks birth is a surgical procedure carried out not by a woman but by a doctor (the hero). It is important for the producers who create these programs to understand that they are not just telling a story, they're modeling a "reality" that can have long-term consequences for viewers. They are in a position of considerable power, and they must do all they can to make the model a responsible one. Participants in the movement to humanize birth can write to the media and help educate them to what birth really is and what it needs to be. This is undoubtedly a long process but an important one. Sometimes it is possible to find an individual—actor, producer, writer—who is sympathetic to these issues and willing to help to influence others. Recently a well-known actor, Tom Cruise, spoke out against taking postpartum depression seriously, insisting that it is psychiatric nonsense—and of course his comments made all the news outlets. But then a well-known actress, Brooke Shields, who had suffered from such depression and wrote the book *Down Came the Rain: My Journey through Postpartum Depression,* also spoke out, insisting that it is a real problem and deserves attention.[11] The result of this back and forth in the media is much more public awareness of the problem.

Even a news journalist who is putting together a serious medical story (TV, radio, newspaper, magazine, or online) and wants to present all sides of the issue faces a dilemma. If the journalist goes to just any doctor, he or she will almost certainly get the medical establishment party line. If there is another legitimate side to the issue but this alternative opinion is not looked on with favor by the medical powers that be, it is likely that the journalist will never get access to the alternative point of view because no physician will be willing to discuss it on the record. I've heard this story time and time again, most recently when a woman and her baby both died after a Cytotec induction in California, and a TV journalist could not find one doctor in the area willing to talk on camera about the risks of induction with this drug.[12]

In educating the public, it is important that the information given be accurate. In chapter 4, we saw that a leading obstetrician who should know better claimed on a TV news program that in 2002 Cytotec was approved for induction of labor at term by the FDA, and that he was unwilling to stand corrected on the air even when told that the FDA had just told the TV producer that Cytotec was not approved by the FDA for this use. It is appalling that the public should be given such false information.

Any group that wants to maintain a monopoly and is worth its salt knows that controlling the media must be a key part of its strategy. Organized obstetrics in the United States puts enormous energy into what is often called "public relations." The American College of Obstetricians and Gynecologists (ACOG) issues frequent news releases carefully worded to lend credibility to its point of view and even stages news conferences—in chapter 7, we saw that ACOG issued eight news releases in two years on the subject of the "litigation crisis." I was once invited to do an interview about Cytotec induction for a major television network program, *Dateline NBC*. When the show's producer asked ACOG to have a representative interviewed on the same program, ACOG asked the producer if I was going to be interviewed as well, in order to get my interview dropped (ACOG was not successful).[13] Authoritarian rulers want only their own point of view available to the public. Is that what we should expect from those providing care to our women and babies?

Other major TV news programs have covered the Cytotec induction catastrophe. In addition to the already mentioned *Dateline NBC* segment on November 4, 2001, and the CBS San Francisco news segment on May 6, 2004, the *CBS Evening News* had a segment on Cytotec on June 20, 2005, and the Canadian Broadcasting Corporation (CBC) had a segment on its national news magazine *The National* in October 2002. It is encouraging that, without exception, every one of these TV programs has presented the point of view that the reporters and producers are shocked and appalled that doctors would use such a powerful drug without FDA approval and wreak such havoc on so many families. The TV segments show the label on the bottle the Cytotec pill comes in with a circle around the silhouette of a pregnant woman with a diagonal line through it, and they show families with severely brain-damaged babies and families with no mother after Cytotec induction.

Occasionally, thanks to a journalist's commitment to balanced reporting on other issues in addition to induction of labor with Cytotec, another view of childbirth sneaks in. Because a journalist for *U.S. News and World Report* had met me and we had discussed birth issues, she decided to do an article on C-section that was excellent and balanced.[14] After a birth activist contacted a journalist at the *San Francisco Chronicle* and told her that the FDA had just moved to warn patients of Cytotec's serious risks when used for labor induction, an excellent article appeared in that paper the next day.[15]

Local television and print media are often more likely to be open to another point of view on childbirth. When a family in Las Vegas was being hassled because they chose a home birth, when a woman died at the time of birth following Cytotec induction in a small town in upstate New York, and when obstetricians in Des Moines tried to shut down an ABC, local journalists and their editors got riled up and jumped in with excellent editorials and good investigative reporting on issues such as freedom of choice in childbirth, respecting family sanctity in childbirth, and the safety of births at birth centers and at home.

Another source for education of the public in the American way of birth are those newspapers, magazines, and Internet magazines focusing on controversial issues. The first real "break" in news regarding the dangers of Cytotec induction came from an article in the activist magazine *Mother Jones*.[16]

Mothering is an excellent magazine containing many carefully researched articles on childbirth, for example, one titled "Induced and Seduced: The Dangers of Cytotec."[17] *Midwifery Today*, a monthly journal for midwives, has many excellent articles on the state of affairs in American midwifery, which are well written and easy to understand. *Salon* (salon.com) also has good articles on obstetric issues, sometimes written by midwives. But watch out for some of the magazines found in doctors' offices, many of which are full of sycophantic drivel about how wonderful doctors will save the woman and her baby. It is sad to see these articles, because once in a while doctors are really necessary during pregnancy and birth and do save lives. It is a disservice to obstetricians to have their role glorified and romanticized in slick magazines.

It is also fair to hope that books written for popular consumption would be an excellent source of education on childbirth, but there is a real problem here as well. I once went to a large bookstore in Washington, D.C., and surveyed all the books on the pregnancy and childbirth shelf. There were twenty-eight titles, and twenty-three of them I would put solidly in the category of obstetric party-line dogma, the kind that insults the intelligence of women and urges, "Do what the doctor says, dearie."

There is a simple test women can use to determine whether or not a book or magazine article is worth reading. I call it the trust test. If the book or article says, "ask your doctor," "trust your doctor," or "listen to your doctor," it has failed the trust test and should probably go back on the shelf. If it says, "trust yourself," "trust your body," or "trust the scientific evidence," then it is probably worth reading. The quotation at the beginning of chapter 3, in which the author of a popular book titled *The Girlfriends' Guide to Pregnancy* urges the reader to choose C-section for convenience and cheat her insurance company, is typical of this surfeit of insulting and misleading books.

Fortunately, books for women who want the correct facts about pregnancy and childbirth do exist. I can recommend anything by Ina May Gaskin, Henci Goer, Sheila Kitzinger, Robbie Davis-Floyd, Elizabeth Davis, and Barbara Katz Rothman.

Multidisciplinary conferences are another important means of educating the public about the need for change in maternity care. A conference can reach a wide variety of groups from health care providers to politicians to the media, like the conference in the year 2000 in Brazil described earlier. Women's groups and consumer groups can get together in a coalition, either locally or on a larger scale, and invite key people in the field of maternity care to help them choose topics and speakers for a conference. If necessary, they can bring in people who have organized conferences in the past to help. One thing those with experience in maternity care conferences will always stress is that it is important to include the media from the beginning.

As discussed in chapter 8, I also believe it is important to begin teaching children about birth at a young age to kick-start a change in attitudes toward pregnancy and childbirth. Interested parents and teachers can recruit school nurses to be expert consultants and help in the preparation of teaching plans, as well as working with midwives and others in the community.

2. REVISE EDUCATION FOR MATERNITY CARE PROVIDERS

As I discussed in chapter 8, we currently have far more obstetricians than we need in the United States, and far too few midwives. Because public funds are used for training maternity care professionals in the United States—nearly every training program for obstetric residents is heavily subsidized by the federal government, although there is far less subsidizing of midwifery training—that means that, in theory, the public can work through their government representatives to influence such funding decisions.

But how are these who-will-be-trained decisions made? I decided to find out and, after several hours of telephone calls, I finally managed to get through the federal bureaucracy to determine that somewhere in the federal Department of Health and Human Services there are people who approve the funding of training of health professionals, including heavily subsidizing hospitals that train obstetric residents. It was clear that I would not be able to get further without spending many, many more hours on the telephone. Ultimately, those I spoke with were unwilling to tell me who makes the decisions about such funding, except to say that ACOG advises them. I was told that although such information is in theory available to the public, no one ever asks for it. I can say that they were certainly not eager to provide the little information I received, despite the fact that I used the magic words, "This is *Doctor* Wagner calling."

In addition to federal funding, whenever obstetricians train in state or local government facilities, including state university hospitals and county hospitals, state or local government is subsidizing obstetric training.

The public needs to be made aware of this government subsidizing of obstetric training with far more transparency and accountability than now exists. Individuals and organizations committed to the humanization of birth need to be persistent in pursuing this information and then getting it out to the public. The public has a right to participate in deciding whose education will be publicly funded.

Obstetricians want the public to believe that they are leaving obstetrics in droves because of the litigation crisis. Well, thank God! Bring in the midwives and start public funding of midwifery training instead.

The training of midwives, both nurse-midwives and direct-entry midwives, is slowly growing in the United States. That we now have regulations in the federal Department of Education for the training of direct-entry midwives was the result of a big effort sustained over many years by a coalition of midwives groups. Now midwifery organizations and advocacy groups need to study how many midwives will be needed when all low-risk pregnancies and births are attended by midwives, and set targets for training them. Here the Canadian experience is relevant again. Midwifery organizations need to collaborate on recommendations for expanding and subsidizing midwifery training and become advisors to the same government departments that ACOG works with.

3. REGULATION BY LITIGATION: PRESERVE THE RIGHT TO LITIGATE

Litigation may not be the most elegant way to bring about change in American maternity care, but right now it serves three important functions. First, it helps put the brakes on excessive obstetric practices. In a way, trial lawyers actually have functioned like the sharks they are so often compared to. If an obstetrician sticks his hand outside the limits of good evidence-based practice, thereby increasing the risks of adverse outcomes for the woman and baby he's supposed to care for, a legal shark will swim by and bite it off, as it were, by suing for lots of money—a strong incentive for evidence-based practice. But politicians have been killing off the sharks. Wave after wave of "tort reforms" are making obstetricians increasingly sue-proof by putting caps on how much the patients can sue for, and are creating obstacles to litigation, for example, requiring that a local judge determine whether or not a proposed case of malpractice litigation is "legitimate."

The second function litigation serves is to guarantee individuals and families an arena where they can seek justice if they feel that they have been abused by powerful forces in the medical world. The right to seek justice is fundamental to the American democratic ethic and is enshrined in the U.S. Constitution. Doctors are not gods operating outside the law; they must be accountable to their patients. If doctors become sue-proof, patients will lose their rights and any chance at justice.

The third function litigation serves is to drive obstetricians out of the business of attending women having normal, low-risk births. In a high-risk childbirth situation, the woman and her family understand that there may be adverse outcomes, they are more likely to be given information because interventions are more likely to be necessary, and family members are less likely to feel disillusioned by what has taken place. In a low-risk hospital birth, there is a greater chance that unnecessary interventions will be used, leading to unnecessary adverse outcomes, and the obstetrician is less likely to have established a close relationship with the woman and family and less likely to provide information.[18]

If the United States trains midwives as fast as possible and stops training so many obstetricians, existing obstetricians can safely stop providing care for low-risk births and focus their practice on gynecology and serious medical complications of pregnancy and birth. The net result will be a much-improved maternity care system. The more lawsuits obstetricians must face, the faster this day will come.

If litigation is evil, as obstetricians would have us believe, I believe that it is a very necessary evil, as it is a source of protection for women and babies. We must do what we can to fight any attempt to take this protection away. When legislation is proposed for tort reform to make doctors sue-proof, concerned citizens interested in optimal maternity care must work against it by contacting their legislators and the media. Lawyers and their organizations can help by making clear to the public that litigation has a legitimate role in maternity care.

4. TAKE POLITICAL ACTION FOR HUMANIZED BIRTH

Birth also has political dimensions (especially regarding who has decision-making power), and political action plays a role in each of the steps covered in this chapter for getting to where we need to be. Too often, politics is seen as "dirty." But in today's world of maternity services, it is the reality. It is inevitable that obstetricians will resist change, as they presently have power, money, and, for the most part, no one to answer to. So it is essential that supporters of the movement to humanize birth be politically active. Politicians and government agencies that make crucial decisions about maternity care and the training of providers of maternity care must be thoroughly educated on the issues. ACOG is very active politically, as we have seen from the organization's letters to politicians, journal articles, and news releases, and advocates of humanized birth can make sure that policy makers and politicians are aware that the point of view put forth by organized obstetrics is not the only point of view. They can demand that policy decisions be based on scientific evidence—and even bring specific studies to policy makers' attention when necessary. Advocates can make politicians and policy makers aware of the scare tactics used by the more reactionary elements in the medical establishment. Finally, advocates of humanized birth can prepare themselves to address erroneous statements made to the media and others—such as those often made about the safety of midwives and out-of-hospital birth—and the standard "What if something goes wrong?" argument. (For responses, see chapter 6.) And on occasion, advocates need to organize political events or outings. It can make a big difference for an organized group to attend a hearing on pending legislation on tort reform or licensing midwives, or to hold public rallies that bring the issue and the legislation to the attention of the public and the media.

Legislators can be most helpful as well. Often if a single legislator takes on an issue close to her or his heart, amazing legislative action follows. One important strategy is to locate such legislators and work closely with them. At the request of local advocates of humanized birth, I have met with such legislators in Vermont, South Dakota, California, and elsewhere, and I admire what they have accomplished. On the other hand, one legislator in Ohio, a nurse by trade, has successfully blocked progressive legislation on midwifery year after year. A reliable source told me that the night before legislation on midwifery was voted on in the state legislature in Wyoming, a group of doctors called those legislators who were their patients and told them all manner of nonsense about the dangers of midwives and out-of-hospital birth. Sadly, the midwifery bill was voted down. This is called "playing hardball."

One strategy often used by obstetricians whose goal is to influence legislators is to attempt to overwhelm them with technical language. Organizations and physicians who do this are implying that only doctors can understand the intricacies of maternity care. I've found that these groups and individuals are often the same ones who take the approach, "Trust me, I'm a doctor." As I mentioned in chapter 2, the best way for politicians and policy makers to respond to this approach is with a simple request for scientific data. It can also be illuminating for legislators to ask someone who is making scary statements about out-of-hospital birth how many out-of-hospital births he or she has attended.

Not all of the political struggle to humanize birth goes on at the state level. I was part of a group from a nonprofit called the Tatia French Foundation (named after a woman who died—her baby died also—after being given Cytotec for labor induction) that visited a legislator at the House of Representatives in Washington. The purpose of the meeting was to draft legislation to better control off-label drug use and to have more transparency on drug risks, especially risks for pregnant and birthing women. I have attended meetings at the FDA where consumers testified to the need for better transparency and controls over off-label use of drugs.

There are many issues in the effort to humanize birth, and nearly all require political action. The most important overarching issue, though, is to find a way to guarantee free access to maternity care for all pregnant and birthing women in the United States. Other critical issues include legalization for direct-entry midwives; freedom of midwives to practice full midwifery, collaborating with obstetricians but without their supervision; freedom of women and families to have control over what happens at the birth of their children; freedom of women and families to litigate after an adverse obstetric event; better transparency, accountability, and regulation of maternity care; and midwives' right to an even playing field when competing with obstetricians in finding women and families to serve. Only a couple of key issues can be addressed here.

For the most part, the key political struggle to license direct-entry midwives—and thereby provide women who choose planned out-of-hospital birth with a legally sanctioned person to assist at their childbirths—has been fought successfully state by state. Occasionally, a major bill is put to a vote in a state legislature, but often the key battles for the autonomy for midwives—and women—go on in state midwifery boards, state nursing boards, and state medical boards (often called medical quality assurance boards). These may sound like staid, boring government entities, but they can have far-reaching influence on women's lives—for good or ill—and are also where witch-hunts against midwives usually play out.

I have appeared before such boards or provided written opinions in about half the states, because in a case brought before such a board, the defendant has the right to bring "experts" to testify on her or his behalf. I testified before several nursing boards that were trying to nail nurse-midwives who left hospital positions and began practicing home birth midwifery, and before others that were trying to prevent non-nurse, direct-entry midwives from creeping into their domain, even though in most cases direct-entry midwifery was not illegal in that state.

Not one of these nursing boards included even one midwife of any stripe, and most board members hadn't a clue about midwifery, much less about out-of-hospital birth. They were righteous in their indignation and clung to their dogma and their "protection" by obstetricians.

Most of these board hearings are open to the public, and large groups of women and families served by these midwives came to the hearings to show their support for their midwives and for midwifery in general. The lawyers for the midwives were for the most part serving pro bono. And there were usually journalists present who brought the case to the attention of the public, usually in support of the midwife—another case of midwives, doctors, women and families, lawyers, and journalists all working together.

At these board meetings, I am frequently asked why I strongly support midwives. I reply that I am not an advocate of midwifery; as a scientist, I am an advocate of evidence-based maternity care—or the care that has been proven to reduce adverse outcomes to a true minimum—and since all the scientific evidence proves that midwives are the safest attendants for low-risk birth, of course I advocate midwifery for all low-risk births.

From these experiences and others, it has become clear to me that in most cases, the struggle is fundamentally a turf battle between nurses and midwives or between doctors and midwives, and the bottom line—a woman's right to have a home birth with a trained birth attendant—gets little attention, unless someone makes a point of expressing the woman's perspective.

Another political battle is fought in the land of insurance companies. ABCs need insurance, but some insurance companies decline to do business with them or charge higher premiums to physicians who provide backup services to ABCs. As a result, ABCs are being squeezed from both directions. It has also been difficult for midwives attending home births to get malpractice insurance. Why does this happen? As we've seen, the scientific evidence refutes any suggestion that births at ABCs or at home attended by midwives are a bad risk. So it is likely that insurance companies are relying on medical consultants who are simply preaching the obstetricians' party line. Some midwives have worked creatively to obtain insurance with some success. And where ABCs and home birth midwives are being denied insurance because their competitors are advisors to the insurance companies, it is an issue that may eventually have to be addressed in civil court as restraint of fair trade.

Obstetricians can be quite creative in finding reasons to maintain the status quo in maternity care or to make only doctor-friendly changes. I've sat in legislative hearings in a number of states, including Virginia and California, and listened to doctors, nurses, and lobbyists for medical and obstetric organizations say some unbelievable nonsense about childbirth—such as that any woman who chooses a home birth is selfish and doesn't care about her baby or she wouldn't make a choice that may kill her baby.

On the other hand, I sat in a legislative hearing in Vermont once and listened as doctors, midwives, and women's groups testified to the value of midwives and the need for direct-entry midwifery legislation in their state. (They got it.) I also attended a rally under the dome in the capitol building in Indianapolis and heard hundreds of women and families demand direct-entry midwifery legislation in their state. (They didn't get it.)

Sometimes one committed individual can make a difference in the struggle up the evolutionary circle. Meet Maddy Oden. Her daughter and the daughter's newborn baby both died during childbirth after her daughter was given Cytotec to induce labor, even though she had repeatedly told her doctor she did not want her labor induced and had been given no information about Cytotec. Maddy channeled her terrible grief into constructive action and started the Tatia French Foundation (named for her daughter) to work for better maternity care. The foundation has sponsored large public conferences on birth issues, has lobbied Congress and the FDA in Washington, D.C., and Sacramento, and has informed a broad range of journalists about birth issues. Political action taken by a broad range of groups and individuals is a necessary component in the struggle to improve maternity care in the United States.

There is another group of health care providers, who, like midwives, have had to fight for their place in the sun in health care. Chiropractors fought for decades to be licensed and to be acknowledged by health care organizations and medical professionals as legitimate members of the health care team. Over time, they have won many battles in many states, despite the efforts of many medical organizations and some individuals to keep them out. Midwives could learn a few things from these politically successful chiropractors, such as perseverance (it was a long, difficult struggle for them), how to use support and testimonials from a broad range of satisfied patients, and the value of placing emphasis on open competition on a level playing field without any restraint of trade.

The political process can seem painfully slow at times, but progress is being made. As time passes, more and more states pass legislation to license certified professional (non-nurse, direct-entry) midwives, and thereby guarantee the families in these states free choice of birth options with qualified assistance for all options. These successes have a momentum of their own. When I testify in hearings, I can now point out all the states that have passed this legislation and say that it's reasonable to assume that the legislators in these states are intelligent, have listened carefully to all opinions, and have made their decision to approve the legislation with the safety of the families in their states firmly in mind.

This political progress would not have been possible without the active participation of midwifery organizations and consumer organizations, which can be quite savvy in their approach. It's fun to see the look on the faces of legislators when they come into a hearing room full of breast-feeding women and kids running around. This serves to remind legislators in a visceral way that the issue before them is all about women and babies, not just about doctors getting a bigger piece of the pie. Some legislators clearly love it and others clearly hate it but are smart enough not to object. It's called democracy.

5. STRENGTHEN MONITORING AND REGULATION OF OBSTETRIC PRACTICES

One reason for the vigilante obstetric practices I've discussed in this book is that the monitoring and regulation in our maternity care system are inadequate. Obstetricians are free to behave as if they're in the Wild West and there's no sheriff or judge in town. This creates obstetric lawlessness, and patients who have become victims have figured out that the only way to get the sheriff and judge to come to town is to litigate.

How inadequate are the systems for monitoring and regulating maternity care practices in the United States? Think of a can of soup. In the United States, every ingredient that goes into a can of soup must, by law, be printed on the label—full disclosure required. In most hospitals in the

United States—places where women give birth and life-and-death decisions are made—no disclosure is required. Only two out of fifty states have laws requiring hospitals to disclose information on their maternity services. These laws are the result of a long fight by women's groups against fierce resistance from medical groups, and even in these states, the fight continues because compliance with the law is poor. Many doctors are also strongly opposed to disclosing what they're doing. Could it be that they've got something to hide?

States currently regulate maternity care after the fact in a reactionary manner. When somebody reports that something terrible has happened, they look into the situation. There is almost no effort made to monitor maternity practices in order to prevent harmful practices or to bring harmful practices to light. In Washington State, obstetricians in a private hospital were performing C-sections on 60 percent of their pregnant patients, but neither the hospital nor the state took any action and there have been no consequences for these overzealous surgeons. Consequently, these dangerous levels of mostly unnecessary and always risky major abdominal surgeries—C-sections—continue.

Many people who work in public health believe passionately in the value of prevention, but if that's true, why aren't state health departments monitoring maternity practices and going after "outliers," the fancy name for people working at the extremes of practice? The answer is simple: public health officials are too often afraid of organized medicine and practicing doctors.[19] One way to address this dilemma is to get the public health establishment, which is, in general, progressive and courageous, to be more proactive with its members. Every couple of years at the annual meeting of the American Public Health Association (APHA), excellent statements and recommendations are made (for example, the APHA has made strong recommendations for the right to home birth and the need for midwifery), but then everyone goes back home with no follow-up. It is easier to be brave far from home. If the APHA had its own monitoring system to determine whether its members were complying with a key maternity care recommendation, maybe local public health officials would begin to find the courage to do the right thing.

In addition to monitoring hospitals, public health agencies need to monitor individual practitioners. Every state has a process in place to investigate and punish practitioners if a complaint is made and the person is "found guilty," but, as I discussed in chapter 2, tribal loyalties prevent doctors from reporting doctors, except under extreme conditions, so these state medical quality assurance systems are weak at best. As suggested in chapter 8, establishing a national health care system would go a long way to solving this. If monitoring and regulation start at the federal level—far from the scene of the accident—tribal loyalty is less of an issue.

Since it's clear that government agencies are not doing the job, consumer groups have come in and tried to monitor individual practitioners. For example, one situation of concern to consumer groups is the fact that a physician can lose his license because of bad practices and simply move to a new state and open a new office. Naturally, people in the new practice area might like to know this about the new doc in town, but states do not make the names of doctors who have been disciplined by their medical boards available to the public. To correct this situation, the Health Research Group in Washington, D.C., publishes a book that lists the name of any doctor who has been disciplined by a medical board in any state.[20] Anyone can order this book and look up a doctor to see if he or she has been disciplined in the past. This is an important step in the right direction.

Hospitals are required to keep reports of "adverse events," which usually are reported to the state. That means that state health departments are a mother lode of information on medical practices. A group called the Center for Medical Consumers in New York is one of the first groups I know of to mine this lode.[21] They've collected data showing the volume of surgery performed by individual physicians in New York State, listed by the physician's name, as well as the death rate from coronary bypass surgery for each doctor listed by name. This is a good start.

Increased monitoring and regulation by federal and state agencies of maternity care practices, including drug use, is an important long-term solution to vigilante obstetrics. Until we have maternity care sheriffs and judges in our local communities who are not afraid of hospitals and doctors and are willing to name names, we will not truly have accountability in medicine and protection for women and families.

6. FORM COALITIONS

Imagine for one minute what would happen if the thirty thousand labor and delivery (L&D) nurses in the United States decided that they would no longer take care of birthing women, take grief from omnipotent doctors and hospital administrators, and get none of the credit. If L&D nurses called a work stoppage for even one day, and there was no one to monitor the ten thousand women who give birth each day in the United States, the entire hospital maternity care system would collapse, along with the obstetrics profession.

Such labor action (double entendre intended) will not happen, of course, because L&D nurses are committed to serving birthing women, but the idea illustrates the power L&D nurses have to force change if they really want to and have the courage. Groups have a lot more power than individuals, generally speaking. Groups of health professionals can work in their own community to promote improvements in pregnancy and birth care. They can go beyond pushing for a pretty new "birth suite" in the local hospital to lobbying hospital administrators to spend less money on high-tech equipment of dubious value and more money on increasing the number of midwives on staff.

In many cities and states and on a national scale, diverse midwifery groups, women's groups, and consumer groups that share a concern for improving maternity care have found one another and formed coalitions. These coalitions are often successful because the issues in maternity care transcend the usual group boundaries. Groups that hold right-wing family values join with groups that hold feminist values, groups working for religious freedom join with groups working for individual freedoms, and so on. Compromise is essential. I remember attending a conference where a maternity care coalition was forming (the Coalition for Improving Maternity Services) and listening to an anti-circumcision advocate who was being opposed by a Jewish physician. Eventually agreement was reached in the form of a recommendation against *nonreligious* circumcision.

If groups generally have more power than individuals, then groups of groups (coalitions) have even more power. In my experience, coalitions form when women feel that their basic rights are being threatened. Women's rights groups in the United States have been relatively quiet on maternity issues until recently, when the media reported on a case of attempting to force a C-section in Pennsylvania and a case in Utah in which a woman who refused a C-section was accused of murder.[22]

Midwifery groups in the United States, while performing vital functions during recent years, have also spent too much energy fighting one another. An effective strategy is for midwives' groups to form coalitions, not only among different midwifery groups but also with women's groups and consumer groups. In chapter 1, I described some coalitions that include midwifery groups as well as other grassroots organizations that are working with midwifery groups to improve maternity care through strengthening midwifery. With the renaissance of midwifery in America and the energy they get by collaborating in coalitions, midwives are becoming more assertive and coming to realize that they must fight for what they do in the service of women.

Consumer action is an important part of the American way of life. It's the primary reason we now have informative labels on soup cans. Consumer groups in maternity care are working for better labeling of hospitals and obstetricians. These groups usually start at a grassroots level, when a woman or a small group of women has a negative birth experience. Then slowly the group grows. For example, a woman whose uterus ruptured after Cytotec induction organized a group using the Internet that now includes more than three hundred women who have suffered ruptured uteruses during birth.[23] The Internet is a powerful tool for grassroots efforts.

ICAN is the acronym for the International Cesarean Awareness Network, a consumer group working to reduce unnecessary C-sections in the United States.[24] ICAN activities include protesting at a meeting of ACOG where the glories of choosing C-section were being promoted and organizing petitions against the ACOG recommendation that VBAC be done only in hospitals where a surgeon and anesthesiologist are present round the clock.

The following story illustrates what a consumer group such as ICAN can do, as well as how unbalanced and biased medical journalism can be. On June 4, 2002, the *Wall Street Journal* published an article with the headline "Growing Number of Physicians Warn of Serious Risks from Vaginal Deliveries."[25] The article states that a number of "high-profile doctors" (*high-profile* doesn't necessarily indicate competence or credibility, of course) are challenging the conventional wisdom that vaginal childbirth is the best way to have a baby. (It's hard to be more anti-nature than that.) The article goes on to say, "At the very least, [these "high-profile" doctors] say obstetricians need to give their patients more information about the risks of vaginal delivery just as they would a C-section or any other medical procedure."

The *Wall Street Journal* article claims that one-third of women have suffered injuries while giving birth—urinary or fecal incontinence, pelvic pain, sagging pelvic organs, sexual dysfunction—and quotes a professor of obstetrics, gynecology, and urology who calls vaginal birth "the silent epidemic of motherhood." It goes on to blame the increase in injuries to women giving birth on the public health effort to reduce the nation's C-section rate. The article implies that public health scientists are to blame for the increasing incidence of birth-related injuries to women, not doctors.

Jill MacCorkle of ICAN wrote a letter to the editor criticizing this article, and thank God the *Wall Street Journal* printed it:

> Welcome to the world of obstetrics, a Mad Hatter's Tea Party where the harm caused by doctors intervening in birth is blamed on Mother Nature and the proposed solution is even more drastic intervention.
>
> The birth injuries described are not inherent to the process of birth. Decades of research have shown that it is interference in the natural process that causes the vast majority of long-term complications such as incontinence, uterine and vaginal prolapse, and sexual dysfunction. More than 80 percent of first-time mothers in the U.S. have an episiotomy, an outdated and discredited procedure that causes nearly all of the deep perineal tears and rectal injuries that it is suppose to prevent. Episiotomies are virtually guaranteed for assisted deliveries involving forceps or vacuum, both of which also cause short and long-term harm to a woman's body.
>
> Having thus created the damage, doctors are now attempting to cover up the problems through more unnecessary trauma in the form of elective cesarean section. While this offers the illusion of informed choice, it is merely trading one set of complications for another.
>
> More cesareans will mean higher rates of maternal mortality and an increase in complications such as uterine rupture, placental abnormalities, and hysterectomy. The only viable solution is to reduce the medical mismanagement so prevalent in birth today. By doing so, we can both lower the cesarean rate and ensure that most women will emerge from childbirth without long-term damage to their reproductive organs.[26]

I couldn't have said it any better. Though it is great news that this brilliant, scientifically sound summary of the situation got published, it is a shame that far fewer readers saw it than saw the original article. The obstetric myths about surgical birth continue and the vigilantes ride on, sometimes in cahoots with unbalanced or biased journalism.

Another consumer organization working to improve care for women giving birth is Citizens for Midwifery. They have an excellent Web site featuring thoughtful explanations of what midwives do, the evidence for midwifery practice, and how women can support expanding midwifery in America.[27]

There are also several large organizations of childbirth educators (people who teach prenatal classes) in the United States representing more than one hundred thousand members.[28] Although I believe that it is safe to assume that all of the thousands of childbirth educators want the best for birthing women, I still feel that it's useful to apply the "trust test" to this group and separate those who tell women to "trust the doctor" from those who tell women to trust themselves and their own bodies and to carefully evaluate what the doctor says.

Childbirth educators in the second category are often in a dilemma similar to what L&D nurses experience. Their allegiance is split between the women they teach, on the one hand, and doctors and hospital administrators, on the other. Those who offer classes in a hospital and were hired by hospital staff have to be careful what they say or they risk being fired. If they're fired, they lose their chance to help pregnant women. So if a childbirth educator is teaching a hospital prenatal course, and in one of the sessions an anesthesiologist talks about the glories of epidural for normal labor pain without once mentioning the serious risks of the procedure because he doesn't want to "scare the ladies," the educator must make a serious choice on whether to confront him or otherwise present alternative views so the women in the class can learn the whole truth.

I lectured once in Medford, Oregon, and a local childbirth educator described this very dilemma. She was hired by a big hospital and was experiencing a lot of frustration that she could not tell the pregnant women in her classes all she knows. We corresponded, and she hung in there as long as she could, but finally she had to leave the hospital and give prenatal classes "out-of-hospital." In the end, it is a personal decision. Some educators find a way to compromise sufficiently to keep their hospital jobs and help the women who are there. Other educators find they do better if they offer "out-of-hospital" childbirth education, where they feel free to tell the whole truth. In general, I have found childbirth educators to be committed women who do their work for pennies because they care.

Even the childbirth educators whose classes are not controlled by doctors and hospitals struggle to find a middle ground, because they know that their students will probably give birth in hospitals, where there is little possibility for them to have a real say in what happens. However, I've found that most childbirth educators are well aware of the obstetric monopoly and its negative effects. It is good news for women that there are thousands of childbirth educators out there who will teach them to trust themselves and their own bodies and insist on the kind of birth they and their families want, not what their doctors want.

Childbirth education organizations have also set standards for their classes and for pregnancy and birth services and have been active in organizing communities and lobbying for improvements in maternity care. For example, these groups were instrumental in forming the Coalition for

Improvement in Maternity Services (CIMS), which has become a leading force in the movement to humanize birth.[29] Maternity care in the United States would be a lot further down the birth evolution circle if it weren't for all the women who give so much of themselves out of a deep commitment to their sisters: midwives, L&D nurses, doulas, childbirth educators, and community activists.

In 1918, a small group of middle-class women in New York City who were concerned with the inadequate care available for pregnant and birthing immigrant women started the Maternity Center Association (MCA).[30] They developed programs for prenatal care and prenatal education classes. In 1920, they produced a handbook for maternity services that described standards of care, many of which would be wonderful to have today—for example, one-on-one nursing care during labor and birth. In 1931, the MCA started the first formal training program for nurse-midwives in the United States, and in 1975, the association opened the first out-of-hospital ABC in the United States. The MCA has historically had a threefold mission: to provide services, to demonstrate the value of innovations, and to advocate for the spread of key innovations.

In 1999, the MCA changed direction, moving from a focus on the edges of maternity care—home birth and birth in out-of-hospital ABCs—to making mainstream birth (that is, hospital birth) more accountable. It adopted a new plan, called "Maternity Wise," built on evidence-based maternity care practices.[31] The MCA's new modus operandi is to do research leading to education and advocacy. The group does research to measure present practices, and then locates relevant evidence and identifies gaps between evidence and present practices. It takes action based on its findings. One MCA program, for example, focused on the nature and management of labor and labor pain, which led to a series of systematic reviews published in a leading American obstetric journal.[32]

Between 2000 and 2002, the MCA conducted a national survey of maternity practices. Instead of gathering data from doctors and hospitals, the surveyors interviewed women who had recently given birth about what had happened during their childbirths. This was an important break-through in research into obstetric practices. Women certainly remember what happened to them during one of the most important events in their lives, and they are not afraid to tell the truth. They have no need to put the best spin on the practice. This *Listening to Mothers* survey then used these women's voices to measure gaps between the practices used on them and the scientific evidence. The survey also took a step toward correcting the serious lack of transparency and accountability of maternity care in the United States.

The MCA has used the results of its survey to advocate for change. For example, in July 2004, the MCA released a report titled *What Every Pregnant Woman Needs to Know about Cesarean Section*.[33] This excellent report gives the data from the survey, gives the scientific evidence, and then makes recommendations. (In January 2006, MCA changed its name to Childbirth Connection, but its goals and activities are unchanged.)

In chapter 3, we saw how in Brazil the C-section rate soared in the 1980s and 1990s and many Brazilian obstetricians insisted that this was what Brazilian women wanted. Then in 2001, a paper was published of a large, prospective survey of Brazilian women proving that they did not want cesareans.[34] Now in the early 2000s in the United States, many obstetricians have been claiming that the steady rise in cesarean rates is largely due to women's requests for C-sections. Then in March 2006, Childbirth Connection (formerly MCA) released the results of another *Listening to Mothers* survey of birthing women in which women were asked whether they would choose cesarean birth without medical necessity.[35] The survey found that one of the 1,300 respondents (.08 percent) who might have chosen an initial or "primary" cesarean without medical indication did so. And 10 percent of the respondents had felt pressure from a health care provider to have a C-section. American doctors, like their Brazilian brethren, have been blaming women for what in reality the doctors want.

A much more recent grassroots organization in the maternity care field is the White Ribbon Alliance for Safe Motherhood.[36] The group has taken as its symbol a white ribbon dedicated to the memory of women who have died during pregnancy or childbirth. The group focus is maternal mortality and it is active in more than seventy countries around the world.

In the United States, the White Ribbon Alliance for Safe Motherhood has a national working group that brings together community organizations, such as midwifery and public health organizations, that share a concern about the fact that the U.S. maternal mortality rate has not been reduced in more than two decades. The group also brings attention to racial disparities in maternal outcomes and in women's access to maternity care in the United States. A major event for the White Ribbon Alliance in the United States is its yearly campaign for Mother's Day, when people are urged to wear white ribbons to raise awareness of the threat to safe motherhood in the United States, as evidenced by the increasing number of maternal deaths.

In countries around the world, coalitions have played a key role in bringing about change in maternity care. CIMS has become an important force for change and is recognized by the United Nations. CIMS has developed the Mother Friendly Hospital Initiative, consisting of ten steps to a mother-friendly hospital. These ten steps, available on the Internet,[37] are worth reading by every woman in the United States who is pregnant or may some day be pregnant or may some day be the mother or friend of a pregnant woman. They paint a clear picture of what is needed to stop the abuse of women and babies in maternity care in the United States. The ten steps, when accomplished, transform an obstetrician-controlled hospital environment into a place where women and families control childbirth.

Hospitals can apply to the group for designation as "Mother Friendly." CIMS will then send a team to do an on-site review to see if the hospital qualifies. Any hospital employee or anyone who is a patient in a hospital can bring the program to the attention of hospital management and suggest that the hospital apply. Applying for "Mother Friendly" designation and committing to meeting the qualifications are also one way hospital administrators can join the movement to improve maternity care.

The Mother Friendly Hospital Initiative is modeled after the World Health Organization–UNICEF Baby Friendly Hospital Initiative, which outlines ten steps to promote breast-feeding. Indeed, step ten in the Mother Friendly Hospital Initiative links the two initiatives, stating that a hospital designated as Mother Friendly "strives to achieve the WHO–UNICEF Ten Steps of the Baby Friendly Hospital Initiative." More than eighteen thousand hospitals around the world have been designated as Baby Friendly by UNICEF. So far, forty-eight U.S. hospitals have been designated as Baby Friendly, and more are added each year.[38] There is now an effort to combine these two initiatives, so that in the future a U.S. hospital can be designated as Mother/Baby Friendly.

In the United States, grassroots consumer groups for maternity care are growing every year although they may not yet be as powerful as ACOG and the medical establishment. But throughout history we have seen that, in democratic societies, these groups play a pivotal role in eventually bringing about change at all levels. As discussed earlier, they have played an important role in bringing about improvements in maternity care in Germany, New Zealand, and Brazil. Small community groups and Internet groups can consider joining larger coalitions such as CIMS. Individuals can also join coalitions such as CIMS—I am an individual member—and it is not necessary to be a health care worker.

For years, the citizens of Virginia have been trying to get legislation passed
to license certified professional midwives (CPMs or direct-entry midwives)
to attend planned out-of-hospital births in their state. In 1999, draft legislation was being considered and a hearing was held by the Joint Commission
on Health Care of the state legislature. In July 1999, a doctor from the
Virginia Department of Health testified before this Commission. His testimony shows one way public health agencies can fail in their primary mission—to protect the people. Instead they can be quite eager to protect doctors by not telling the people that the emperor (doctor) has no clothes, that
is, that doctors are behaving in a way that is detrimental to people's health.[39]

In 1999, the Department of Health in Virginia had no data on the outcome of planned home births in the state. All it had was information on all
out-of-hospital births, and these couldn't be separated into planned versus
unplanned. As I discussed in chapter 6, without data on *planned* home
births specifically, it is scientifically impossible to draw conclusions about
the risks of planned home births and the risks of having home birth midwives attend births. A "high-profile" doctor from the Virginia Department
of Health presented the department's data, saying nothing about the serious problems with the data he presented. He also never mentioned the fact
that the lack of data on planned home birth was due in part to the lack of
legislation to license direct-entry midwives in Virginia. The lack of legislation has driven home birth midwives underground and, since they are not
licensed, they are not allowed to report a birth, making it impossible to separate out-of-hospital births into planned and unplanned.

This doctor from the Department of Health did, however, take the time
to present a number of graphs and tables, all of which looked terribly
scientific but were essentially meaningless, given the faulty data. For example, in these tables, CPMs are included in a category called "other attendants
of out-of-hospital birth," which also includes taxi drivers, policemen, and so
on, so that midwives attending planned home births are not separated from
people who assist a birth simply because the woman didn't make it to the
hospital in time.

Another part of the presentation by the doctor from the Department of
Health was designed to show how very dangerous birth can be, and
included a list of medical emergencies. The list included meconium (fecal
waste on the baby) and breech, neither of which is an emergency, and no

attempt was made to document whether or not midwives in out-of-hospital settings can deal with these situations. The review of the literature on home birth was also totally inadequate and severely biased.

The representative of the Department of Public Health in Virginia drew four conclusions at the end of his presentation. The first one was that "present regulations do not safeguard the health and safety of pregnant women and their infants." It's ironic that the speaker apparently did not realize that this is a strong argument in favor of legislation to license CPMs. The second conclusion, "Consumers may not be well informed about midwives," is nothing but speculation as the Department of Public Health has no data on what Virginia consumers know or don't know about midwives. The third conclusion, "Home birth may present a significant risk due to emergencies," is a typical attempt to scare politicians, and, as explained earlier, was not based on hard data that separated planned from unplanned home births. In fact, as discussed in chapter 6, scientific literature shows that planned home birth is a safe option, but, as I've said, this doctor had no data on planned home birth in Virginia.

The fourth and final conclusion, "Midwives may not be equipped to handle emergencies," is laughable. There was no evidence that this public health doctor had conducted research on planned home birth or on the capabilities of home birth midwives, or evidence that he had read all the relevant studies and understood them. And it is most unlikely that he had ever personally attended a planned home birth. So it was quite clear that he didn't have the foggiest notion what home birth midwives are equipped to handle.

As I mentioned earlier, I was a director of maternal and child health in the California State Department of Public Health. In this capacity and subsequently, I have, sadly, seen many examples of public health officials who are more focused on job security than on ensuring the health of the public. Other examples in this book include the director of public health in Connecticut who went after what he called "lay midwives" and compared home birth with home brain surgery. In chapter 6, I mentioned that the Illinois State Health Department has joined with obstetricians in insisting that all ABCs must meet all the public health regulations of a hospital—a strategy that is clearly not meant to protect people but rather to keep ABCs out of Illinois.

Want another example? A family in the U.S. military service wanted a home birth and applied to their commanding officer for permission to use a certified professional midwife, licensed in the state where they were stationed, and for this midwife to be reimbursed by the military. A Mickey Mouse passing of the buck ensued until their request reached a top-ranking military health official in Washington, D.C., who in turned asked the chief of obstetrics at Walter Reed Army Hospital for an opinion. And, no surprise, this obstetrician was opposed to home birth, so the family's request was denied. This story illustrates another common public health bureaucratic ploy: never take responsibility, but instead protect yourself by passing responsibility to someone else who will do what you want to do.

For those trying to improve our dangerous American way of birth, public health agencies are often part of the problem, not part of the solution. But this can and will change. The American Public Health Association has passed resolutions in favor of midwifery, has presented important papers on planned home birth at its annual meetings, and has published important papers on midwifery and on home birth in its *Journal*. Of course, this is all at a national level, where it's less likely that jobs are on the line, but it is still encouraging.

Most public health officials at the state and local level have the right training, have their brains in gear, and have their hearts in the right place. But perhaps they need a bit of strengthening of their backbones. I've found that as long as taking a particular action won't make medical practitioners mad, public health officials may say or do the right thing, but when there is a conflict between the needs of the people and the needs of doctors, they will usually choose to protect their careers by supporting doctors. Still, when the movement for humanized birth gains sufficient momentum in the United States, I believe public health professionals will be more than glad to join the movement. As the public and maternity care advocates become more aware of the potential role public health officials can play in improving maternity care, I hope they will push harder at all levels to keep them honest—and expose them to the media when necessary.

8. FOLLOW THE MONEY

There are precious few situations in life where the cheaper alternative is also the better alternative—and maternity care is one. If we eradicate the unjustified obstetric monopoly in the United States, with its extreme medicalization of birth, and replace it with humanized maternity care, we can vastly improve the care of women and babies, lower death rates for both women and babies, and *save vast sums of money* at the same time.

A few facts:[40]

· Percentage of gross national product spent on health care
  1966: 6 percent
  1992: 12 percent[41]

- Percentage by which U.S. health care expenditures exceed those of
  Canada: 40 percent
  Germany: 90 percent
  Japan: 100 percent

- The twenty-two countries with lower infant mortality rates than
  the United States: Japan, Sweden, Finland, Switzerland, Canada,
  Singapore, Hong Kong, Netherlands, France, Ireland, Germany,
  Denmark, Norway, Scotland, Australia, Northern Ireland, Spain,
  England and Wales, Belgium, Austria, Italy[42]

- Percentage of countries with lower infant mortality rates than the
  United States that provide universal prenatal care: 100 percent

- Percentage of U.S. women who receive little or no prenatal care: 25
  percent

- Chances that a woman with little or no prenatal care will give birth to
  a low-birth-weight baby (less than 5.5 pounds) or premature baby (less
  than thirty-seven weeks of gestation): 1 in 2

- Factor most closely associated with infant death: low birth weight

- Percentage of infant deaths linked to low birth weight: 60 percent

- Average cost of long-term health care (through age thirty-five) for a
  low-birth-weight baby: $50,558

- Average cost of long-term health care (through age thirty-five) for a
  baby of average birth weight: $20,003

- Cost of newborn intensive care for one infant: $20,000 to $100,000

- Cost of prenatal care for thirty women: $20,000 to $100,000

- Percentage of births attended principally by midwives (certified nurse-
  midwives and certified professional midwives):
  United States: 10 percent
  European nations: 75 percent

- Percentage of countries with lower infant mortality rates than the
  United States in which midwives are principal birth attendants:
  100 percent

- Average cost of a midwife-attended birth in the United States: $1,200

- Average cost of a physician-attended vaginal birth in the United States: $4,200

- Health care cost savings obtainable by using midwifery care for 75 percent of pregnancies in the United States: $8.5 billion per year

- Cost per year of using routine electronic fetal monitoring during every childbirth: $750 million

- Number of well-constructed scientific studies in which routine electronic fetal monitoring during every birth has been proven more effective than the use of a simple stethoscope to monitor the fetal heart: zero

- Health care cost savings obtainable by eliminating the routine use of electronic fetal monitoring in every birth: $675 million per year

- U.S. C-section rate:
  1965: 5 percent
  2005: 30.2 percent[43]

- Cesarean section rate targeted by the World Health Organization (WHO) and the U.S. Department of Health and Human Services (HHS): 12 percent

- The eighteen industrialized nations and states with lower C-section rates than the United States: Czech Republic, Japan, Hungary, Netherlands, England and Wales, New Zealand, Switzerland, Norway, Spain, Sweden, Greece, Portugal, Italy, Denmark, Scotland, Bavaria, Australia, Canada

- Percentage of women in the United States with C-sections who undergo repeat C-sections today: 91 percent

- Ratio of women dying from C-section to women dying from vaginal birth: 4 to 1

- Average cost of a C-section birth: $7,826

- Health care cost savings obtainable by bringing the U.S. C-section rate into compliance with recommendations from WHO and the federal Department of Health and Human Services: $1.5 billion a year

Everyone bad-mouths HMOs and managed care, but if it's true that large health organizations care more about the bottom line than anything else, that is both bad news and good news. If they are looking for ways to save a buck without putting their clients in danger, making changes in maternity care is an obvious course. As more HMOs catch on to this, we will see more and more of them change their practices to align with the facts listed here. Doctors are forever criticizing HMOs for saving money at the expense of good medical practice; here's an area where HMOs can fight back with hard data that prove just how much money obstetricians are wasting through attending normal, low-risk births and using unnecessary and harmful interventions and practices.

Federal and state governments also need to find ways to save money, and they can save a lot of it by changing how they fund the training of birth attendants. Midwives usually make one-quarter of what obstetricians make, and their training takes two or three years instead of four years for medical school plus one year for internship plus three or four years for specialty training equals eight or nine years to train an obstetrician/gynecologist. If governments support the training of midwives rather than obstetricians, large savings are inevitable. Authorizing the reimbursement of midwives rather than obstetricians for providing care to welfare recipients is another example of a way to save lots of money while improving patient care.

Money can also be used to encourage changes in inappropriate obstetric practices. In Brazil, the government has changed how hospitals are reimbursed in an effort to lower C-section rates: if a hospital's C-section rate is more than 35 percent, that hospital will receive no government money for C-sections. Within two years, there was a dramatic fall in the C-section rates in these hospitals.[44]

9. USE SCIENCE TO IMPROVE MATERNITY CARE

Scientific evidence is a powerful tool for promoting changes in maternity care that will move us closer to the vision presented in chapter 8. Here are several examples already discussed in this book:

- Evidence shows that when the C-section rate goes over 15 percent, the maternal mortality rate increases.[45]

- Evidence shows that midwives are safer than doctors to attend low-risk births.[46]

- Evidence shows that planned home birth for women with low-risk pregnancies is as safe as hospital birth.[47]

The phrase *evidence-based practice* is a buzzword of sorts in obstetrics now. Those who want to see more humanized birth care practiced in the United States can use the evidence I've presented in this book to demonstrate to obstetricians, politicians, journalists, and others the gap between what science says our obstetric practices should be and what the actual practices are, as revealed in surveys such as the MCA's *Listening to Mothers* survey.

This leads to another point: It is essential that groups that are fighting for humanized birth work closely with scientists and others who are capable of separating bad data from good data and who understand how scientific evidence is applied to actual practices.

When the Pang and colleagues paper on home birth in Washington State was published in August 2002, I was impressed with how many midwives and others in humanized birth groups who contacted me understood precisely why the methodology in the paper was faulty, making the findings invalid.[48] Midwives have made enormous progress in their ability not only to conduct good research but also to interpret research results. *MIDIRS* is an outstanding midwifery journal that teaches midwives how to look at data, critically evaluates research from around the world, summarizes it, and pulls it together.[49] Many other midwifery journals publish good research, as well, often research conducted by midwives, many of whom have had training in science. There is no question that the caliber of scientific papers in journals such as *MIDIRS* is higher than that found in obstetric journals. I believe that this is largely owing to the need to promote doctor-friendly interventions in medical and obstetric journals, a bias that is not found in midwifery journals. And there is an urgent need to improve the caliber of the obstetric literature.

I believe the next important step in maternity care science is involving more consumers in the research—not just as research subjects, but as contributors.[50] The National Perinatal Epidemiology Unit at Oxford University works closely with community groups in the planning and evaluation of their research, and the U.S. National Institutes of Health include consumers on their expert committees. In the United States, nongovernmental organizations focusing on a particular disease or disability use scientists and doctors to provide them with technical assistance so they can correctly define the problem and collect and analyze the data, and then the people in the organization can use the results as they see fit to improve their own health and health care. By the same token, groups focusing on maternity care can get technical assistance in defining the issues of greatest interest to them and in locating the best evidence on those issues. Then they can use the results to guide their activities and political actions.

The research on planned home birth attended by CPMs in the United States and Canada discussed in chapter 6 is an excellent example of the kind of research we need to see more of in the future. The leaders of the study spent only a small amount of money (infinitesimal compared to the cost of medical research), which they raised from interested parties, and they recruited established, competent researchers. The researchers worked closely with the midwives on planning and while conducting the research, but maintained scientific distance from them during the data analysis and report writing phases.

In general, there is an urgent need to generate new scientific data on obstetric interventions. One avenue for new research is to look at how obstetric interventions during pregnancy and birth may correlate with the occurrence of disorders such as autism, attention deficit disorder, and other learning disabilities. This research could be done relatively easily using a retrospective, matched control methodology. This involves identifying individuals with the problem (which is easy to do if there is an organization of those with the problem), and matching them by age, gender, and other factors to a group that is not suffering from the problem. Then look back to see if those with the problem received a statistically significantly higher amount of the intervention in question than the group without the problem. A lot of research is not much more than organized common sense.

Another type of obstetric research that is in very short supply: no one has done long-term follow-up studies on interventions such as ultrasound scanning during pregnancy, epidural block for normal labor pain, or induction of labor with powerful drugs to see whether there are later consequences. As I mentioned in chapter 3, I once met an obstetrician in Florida who bragged that he had performed more than five thousand Cytotec inductions and had never had a problem, but when I asked if he had ever followed up to see if any of these five thousand women and children had long-term aftereffects, he admitted that he had not. Any medical scientist will tell you that it is not scientifically responsible to assume that invasive interventions with known serious risks carry no significant long-term effects. But no one is studying these issues, despite the fact that obstetrics has a long history of using interventions such as X-rays and drugs and later discovering that they have harmful long-term effects.

We also need new data on what works. Scattered around the United States are health care providers who are attempting to improve maternity care. Often these are not formal "experiments" but just maternity care providers trying to do it better by collecting data to measure the effects of various practices. If they keep careful records of their practices, the data can be analyzed and may demonstrate important findings. The work of the midwives at The Farm in Tennessee and the work of the maternity group in Taos, New Mexico, are two excellent examples of this.

We must never forget that while organized obstetrics may be working to maintain the status quo in maternity care, there are many thousands of obstetricians, midwives, nurses, doulas, childbirth educators, and consumers out there who are committed to improving maternity care.

10. WORK TOWARD CHANGING CHILDBIRTH ONE BIRTH AT A TIME

A most important strategy for improving childbirth is for birthing women to take individual action to manage their own pregnancies and childbirth. What can a pregnant woman do? How can she get the maternity care best suited to her and her family, with an appropriate use of technology, while, at the same time, influencing the direction of maternity care by voting with her feet?[51] She can take the following steps.

A pregnant woman can *choose the primary maternity care provider right for her,* talking to the midwives and doctors available to her, getting data on their practices, and reminding them that giving birth is one of the most important events in her life and her family's life and she will go to whatever lengths necessary to have it done right.

A pregnant woman can *choose the place to give birth that is right for her.* I hope that this will eventually be a choice between her home or a neighborhood women's center, but presently the choice is between her home, an ABC, or the hospital. She should not allow anyone to scare her into a choice not truly her own.

A pregnant woman can choose the kind of birth she wants by reviewing all the options and then *creating a birth plan* that she shows her doctor or her midwife, and making sure it is part of her prenatal and birth chart.

A pregnant woman can *use scientific evidence* when choosing whether or not to have a certain technology used on her, since to be appropriate, the benefit and the safety of a technology must be judged by those on whom it is used and not by what doctors call "community standards."

A pregnant woman can *insure that her wishes are carried out* by having a support person with her during her childbirth, ready and able to advocate strongly for her interests, in keeping with her written birth plan.

A pregnant woman can *document her childbirth* by having a family member use a small handheld video camera.

A pregnant woman can *find out what happened* if her birth had difficulties or there was a bad outcome, because she has the right to information about one of the most important events in her life—the birth of her baby.

As more women and families make choices about their own childbirth, and as all who want to improve maternity care in the United States do what they can to act on the evidence in this book, the scientifically unjustified obstetric monopoly will gradually crumble and there will be a level playing field for midwives and obstetricians. In time, the level of collaboration and professional respect between midwives and obstetricians will improve, and we will see a free and open market of maternity services for families in the United States.

NOTES

ONE. MATERNITY CARE IN CRISIS

1. The FDA has stated explicitly that Cytotec is not approved for labor induction. See FDA Drug Information Sheet, "Misoprostol (Marketed as Cytotec)," May 2005, posted at www.Druginfo@cder.fda.gov.

2. See M. Plaut, M. Schwartz, and S. Lubarsky, "Uterine Rupture Associated with the Use of Misoprostol in the Gravid Patient with a Previous Cesarean Section," *American Journal of Obstetrics and Gynecology* 180, no. 6 (1999): 1535–40; and H. Blanchette, S. Nayak, and S. Erasmus, "Comparison of the Safety and Efficacy of Intravaginal Misoprostol with Those of Dinoprostone for Cervical Ripening and Induction of Labor in a Community Hospital," *American Journal of Obstetrics and Gynecology* 180, no. 6 (1999): 1543–50.

3. For an excellent overall review of the data on risks of pharmacological induction of labor, including studies showing that uterine stimulant drugs increase labor pain, see H. Goer, *The Thinking Woman's Guide to a Better Birth* (New York: Penguin Putnam, 1999).

4. For information on who "attends" birth in highly industrialized Western countries outside the United States, see World Health Organization, *Having a Baby in Europe* (Copenhagen: World Health Organization, 1985). This publication is a detailed description of national maternity care systems in European countries. There has been no significant change in these systems since it was published. Midwives continue to attend most births in these countries.

5. For information on who "attends" birth in the United States, see *A National Survey of Obstetric Practices,* published October 24, 2002, by the Maternity Center Association of New York City (now named Childbirth Connection). Also, data on the number of U.S. births attended by midwives and doctors can be found on the Web site of the National Center for Health Statistics, www.cdc.gov/nchs.

6. S. Daniels and L. Andrews, "The Shadow of the Law: Jury Decisions in Obstetrics and Gynecology Cases," in *Medical Professional Liability and the Delivery of Obstetrical Care,* ed. V. P. Rostow and R. J. Bulger (Washington, D.C.: National Academy Press, 1989), 2:161–91. However, U.S. record-keeping practices prevent a definitive statistic on who "attends" births in the United States—that is, who is actually present during the labor and delivery. Birth certificate data is considered the official government data on who "attends" a birth, but if an obstetrician is responsible for the overall management of the women's care during the labor and birth, the obstetrician's name will appear on the birth certificate even if that obstetrician is present for only a few minutes or not at all. Further evidence that obstetricians are absent during their patients' labor can easily be gathered by a visit to any labor and delivery ward in any U.S. hospital at any time, day or night.

7. J. B. Gould, C. Qin, and G. Chavez, "Time of Birth and the Risk of Neonatal Death," *Obstetrics and Gynecology* 106 (2005): 352–58.

8. Daniels and Andrews, "Shadow of the Law."

9. For more information on labor and delivery nurses, including their roles, responsibilities, and distribution, visit the Web sites of the Association of Nurse Advocates for Childbirth (www.anacs.org) and the Association of Women's Health, Obstetric and Neonatal Nurses (www.awhonn.org).

10. The effectiveness of continuous one-on-one support by the same caregiver for women during labor and birth has been demonstrated by systematic reviews of randomized controlled trials; see M. Enkin et al., "Social and Professional Support in Childbirth," in *A Guide to Effective Care in Pregnancy and Childbirth,* 3rd ed. (New York: Oxford University Press, 2000), pp. 247–54. This textbook also includes "Fragmentation of Care during Childbirth," in a table of practices that should be abandoned (table 5, on p. 500). In addition, a randomized controlled experimental trial showed that women having the same caregiver throughout labor and birth had fewer drugs for pain, less Pitocin for augmentation of labor, shorter labors, and fewer babies showing distress at birth. S. Flynn, "Continuity of Care during Pregnancy and Birth: Effects on Outcome," *Journal of Family Practice* 5 (1985): 375–80.

11. The American College of Obstetricians and Gynecologists (ACOG), after review of the evidence, states that for low-risk births, intermittent auscultation of the fetal heart with a stethoscope is as reliable as electronic fetal heart monitoring and ACOG does not recommend routine electronic fetal

heart monitoring of all women in labor. See www.acog.org. An excellent review of the evidence regarding routine electronic fetal heart monitoring of all labor and birth is found in Goer, *Thinking Woman's Guide,* pp. 85–98.

12. For a discussion of the risks of using Pitocin for labor induction, see Enkin et al., *Guide to Effective Care in Pregnancy and Childbirth,* p. 388. For an excellent review of the risks of labor induction, see Goer, *Thinking Woman's Guide,* pp. 49–74.

13. There are three excellent studies on the risks associated with epidural: B. Leighton and S. Halpern, "The Effects of Epidural Anesthesia on Labor, Maternal and Neonatal Outcomes," *American Journal of Obstetrics and Gynecology* 186 (2002): 569–77; E. Lieberman and C. O'Donoghue, "Unintended Effects of Epidural Anesthesia during Labor," *American Journal of Obstetrics and Gynecology* 186 (2002): 531–68; and L. Mayberry and D. Clemmens, "Epidural Analgesia Side Effects, Co-interventions, and Care of Women during Childbirth," *American Journal of Obstetrics and Gynecology* 186 (2002): 581–93. In addition, for a thorough review of the risks and benefits of epidural anesthesia for normal labor pain, see Goer, *Thinking Woman's Guide,* pp. 126–48.

14. A review found that women with episiotomies were 53 percent more likely to suffer pain during intercourse three months after giving birth, see K. Hartmann et al., "Outcomes of Routine Episiotomy: A Systematic Review," *Journal of the American Medical Association* 293 (2005): 2141–48. For an argument that routine episiotomy is the Western form of female genital mutilation, see M. Wagner, "Episiotomy: A Form of Genital Mutilation," *Lancet* 353 (1999): 1977–78.

15. There have been no studies on the effects of intentionally delaying birth when the cervix is completely dilated, perhaps because maternity care providers generally do not want to admit that it is done. It is clear, however, that when the cervix is completely open, the baby should be allowed to move on out of the mother's birth canal. Uterine contractions are involuntary. When the uterus continues regular contractions after the cervix is completely dilated, attempts to hold the baby inside mean that the baby's head is repeatedly pushed against the bones of the birth canal, unnecessarily risking head and brain damage.

16. The World Health Organization, the American Medical Association, and the American College of Obstetricians and Gynecologists have all published strong statements supporting the right of a woman giving birth to have fully informed consent over any intervention proposed. In addition, the case described occurred in California, and there is a California state law that explicitly requires that all patients give fully informed consent prior to any medical intervention. Other states have similar laws. Informed consent is further discussed in chapter 7.

17. Only two states have laws mandating public disclosure of maternity practices, achieved only after a long struggle by women's groups and against strong resistance from medical groups. It is the law in Massachusetts that all cases of maternal mortality must be disclosed to the public, and it is the law in New York that hospitals must disclose obstetric intervention rates to the public. Similar regulations have been proposed in other states, but have not yet become law.

18. The high rate of lawsuits against obstetricians is discussed in Daniels and Andrews, "Shadow of the Law." Also see chapter 7.

19. The following data are from "Mothering Perinatal Healthcare Index," *Mothering* 68 (Fall 1993): 44–45, which takes statistics from various official agencies: "Percentage by which U.S. health care expenditures exceed those of Canada, 40%, Germany, 90%, Japan, 100%." The Centers for Disease Control and Prevention also state that the United States spends more than twice per birth on maternity services than these or any other countries do. See www.cdc.gov/nchs/birth. That maternity services are far more expensive when obstetricians attend normal births than when midwives attend normal births is documented by a number of studies reviewed in M. Wagner, "Midwifery in the Industrialized World," *Journal of the Society of Obstetricians and Gynecologists of Canada* 20, no. 13 (1998): 1225–34. For example, studies cited in this review document that the average total cost for care of an obstetrician's patient is $548 higher than the average total cost for care of a midwife's client, and that a large U.S. HMO achieved a 13 percent reduction in payroll costs in its obstetrics and gynecology department by using more midwives.

20. Data on maternal mortality by country is published on the World Health Organization's Web site at www.who.int/reproductive-health. Countries with lower maternal mortality rates than the United States include Australia, Austria, Belgium, Canada, Croatia, the Czech Republic, Denmark, Finland, Germany, Greece, Hungary, Iceland, Ireland, Italy, Japan, Kuwait, Lithuania, New Zealand, Norway, Poland, Portugal, Qatar, Serbia and Montenegro, Slovakia, Spain, Sweden, Switzerland, and the United Kingdom. (France, Israel, and Slovenia have rates equal to those of the United States.)

21. The rates of maternal mortality in the United States, the causes, the fact that many cases go unreported, and the fact that there has been no decrease in maternal mortality in the United States since 1982 can be found in *Safe Motherhood: Preventing Pregnancy-Related Illness and Death* (Atlanta: Centers for Disease Control and Prevention, 2001).

22. The comparison of infant mortality rates and the fact that our infant mortality rate is rising are reported in two op-ed pieces by Nicholas Kristof published in the *New York Times* on January 14 and 17, 2005. The articles cite data from the Centers for Disease Control and Prevention and the latest

C.I.A. World Factbook. Also see www.cdc.gov/nchs/birth. The countries with lower infant mortality rates than the United States include Japan, Sweden, Finland, Switzerland, Canada, Singapore, Hong Kong, Netherlands, France, Ireland, Germany, Denmark, Norway, Scotland, Australia, Northern Ireland, Spain, England and Wales, Belgium, Austria, and Italy. (There is a slight variation from year to year in the rates published in the *Factbook*. On the global list of national infant mortality rates, the United States generally ranks between twentieth and forty-first. In the past ten years the United States has never ranked better than twentieth.)

23. Of the countries with lower maternal and infant mortality rates than those of the United States, those in which the majority of births are attended by midwives include all of the Western and Central European countries, Australia, New Zealand, and Japan.

24. In the Netherlands, which has a lower maternal mortality rate and a lower infant mortality rate than the United States, more than one-third of all births are planned home births attended by a midwife. Other countries with lower maternal and infant mortality rates than the United States and a significant number of planned out-of-hospital births include the United Kingdom and Denmark.

25. For a study of four million births in the United States showing that for low-risk hospital births, midwives are safer than doctors, see M. MacDorman and G. Singh, "Midwifery Care, Social and Medical Risk Factors, and Birth Outcomes in the USA," *Journal of Epidemiology and Community Health* 52 (1998): 310–17. For a review of the scientific literature on midwifery, including research showing the safety of midwives, research showing that midwives use fewer unnecessary interventions during labor and birth than doctors, and research showing that midwives provide higher levels of satisfaction to women, see Wagner, "Midwifery in the Industrialized World."

26. For a discussion of the ways in which midwives have been subjected to witch hunts in modern times, see M. Wagner, "A Global Witch Hunt," *Lancet* 346 (1995): 1020–22.

27. See *National Survey of Obstetric Practices.* Also, data on the number of U.S. births attended by midwives and doctors can be found at www.cdc.gov/nchs.

28. The *Journal of Medical Economics* surveys U.S. physician incomes every few years. In the March 19, 2001, issue, page 141, the survey reported that an obstetrician's *net* income averages close to $200,000; a midwife's income averages less than $100,000. Also see note 19.

29. For further information on the investigation of New York City hospitals and their noncompliance with the state Maternity Information Act, see the Public Advocate for New York City's Web site, http://pubadvocate.nyc.gov/, specifically the report titled "A Mother's Right to Know: New York City Hospitals Fail to Provide Legally Mandated Maternity Information" (July 2005).

30. For further information on the Coalition for Improving Maternity Services and its mission, see www.motherfriendly.org.
31. See www.motherfriendly.org.

TWO. TRIBAL OBSTETRICS

1. Chapter 4 includes a discussion of what underlies this mistake of using Cytotec for induction after previous C-section—the widespread use of the anti-precautionary principle in obstetric practice: an intervention is safe until proven unsafe. But the opposing precautionary principle—unsafe until proven safe—is widely accepted as the basis of medical practice and drug use.
2. For an excellent review of the childbed fever epidemic and the obstetric thinking behind the ninety-year delay in accepting the solution, see J. Murphy-Lawless, *Reading Birth and Death: A History of Obstetric Thinking* (Cork, Ireland: Cork University Press, 1998).
3. For an excellent discussion of tribal rituals and tribal thinking, see V. Turner, *The Ritual Process: Structure and Anti-Structure; The Lewis Henry Morgan Lectures* (London: Routledge & K. Paul, 1969).
4. The results of this experiment were published in J. Moseley et al., "A Controlled Trial of Arthroscopic Surgery for Osteoarthritis of the Knee," *New England Journal of Medicine* 347, no. 2 (2002): 81–88.
5. This survey is discussed in M. Wagner, "Critique of British Royal College of Obstetricians and Gynaecologists National Sentinel Caesarean Section Audit Report of Oct 2001," *MIDIRS Journal* 12, no. 3 (2002): 366–70.
6. For detailed data on childbirth in the United States collected by the federal government, including cesarean section rates, go to www.cdc.gov/nchs/birth.
7. *Dateline NBC*, November 4, 2001.
8. Quotation is from M. McCarthy, "US Maternal Death Rates Are on the Rise," *Lancet* 348 (1996): 394. Data on the rates of maternal mortality in the United States, their causes, and by how much they are underreported can be found in: Centers for Disease Control and Prevention (CDC), "Safe Motherhood: Preventing Pregnancy-Related Illness and Death," *Obstetrics and Gynecology* 88 (2001): 61–67; McCarthy, "US Maternal Death Rates Are on the Rise"; and G. L. Rubin et al., "Maternal Death after Cesarean Section in Georgia," *American Journal of Obstetrics and Gynecology* 139 (1981): 681–85. For further discussion of maternal mortality in the United States, see I. M. Gaskin, *Ina May's Guide to Natural Childbirth* (New York: Bantam Books, 2003), pp. 282–84.
9. A. Panting-Kemp et al., "Maternal Deaths in an Urban Perinatal Network: 1992–1998," *American Journal of Obstetrics and Gynecology* 183 (2000): 1207–12.

10. Data on childbirth are reported annually by the Scottish National Board of Health and are reviewed by the National Perinatal Epidemiology Unit of Great Britain, located at Oxford.

11. The definitive study showing the safety of home birth attended by direct-entry, nonnurse midwives is K. Johnson and B. Daviss, "Outcomes of Planned Home Births with Certified Professional Midwives: Large Prospective Study in North America," *British Medical Journal* 330 (June 2005): 1416. A study showing the safety of home birth attended by nurse-midwives is P. Murphy et al., "Outcomes of Intended Home Births in Nurse-Midwifery Practice: A Prospective Descriptive Study," *Obstetrics and Gynecology* 92, no. 3 (1998): 461–70. For a thorough review of the scientific evidence on alternative birth centers (ABCs), see P. Stephenson et al., *Alternative Birth Centers in Illinois: A Resource Guide for Policy Makers* (Chicago: University of Illinois at Chicago Center for Research on Women and Gender, and the Health and Medicine Policy and Research Group, 1995). The seminal study on ABCs is J. Rooks et al., "The National Birth Center Study," *New England Journal of Medicine* 321 (1989): 1804–11.

12. M. F. Greene, "Vaginal Birth after Cesarean Revisited," *New England Journal of Medicine* 351, no. 25 (2004): 2647–49.

13. M. Landon et al. (NIH), "Maternal and Perinatal Outcomes Associated with a Trial of Labor with Prior Cesarean Section," *New England Journal of Medicine* 351, no. 25 (2004): 2655–59. Based on this study, NIH recommends VBAC as the first choice: see "Labor and Birth after Previous Cesarean," chapter 38, posted on www.nichd.nih.gov.

14. Rita Rubin, "Battle Lines Drawn over C-Sections," *USA Today,* August 24, 2005.

15. M. McMahon, "Comparison of a Trial of Labor with an Elective Second Cesarean Section," *New England Journal of Medicine* 335, no. 10 (1996): 689–95. The study found that, although community and regional hospitals had more repeat cesarean sections and more failed VBACs, there was no difference in mortality rates for these two procedures by type of institution.

16. S. Chauhan et al., "Cesarean Section for Suspected Fetal Distress: Does the Decision–Incision Time Make a Difference?" *Journal of Reproductive Medicine* 42, no. 6 (1997): 347–52.

17. J. Miller and J. Petrie, "Development of Practice Guidelines," *Lancet* 355, no. 9198 (2000): 82–83.

18. A nationwide petition against the ACOG recommendation on the management of VBAC only in larger hospitals is from the consumer organization ICAN, the International Cesarean Awareness Network (www.ican.com). In addition, in December 2005, the National Organization of Women (NOW) passed a resolution that NOW "oppose institutional and health care policies that deny women access to VBAC." See www.now.org.

19. "Trial of Labor after Cesarean (TOLAC), Formerly Trial of Labor versus Elective Repeat Cesarean Section for the Woman with a Previous Cesarean Section: A Review of the Evidence and Recommendations by the American Academy of Family Physicians," March 2005. See "Clinical Guidelines for Maternity Care," posted on www.aafp.org.
20. The study ACOG discussed in its press release of May 2002 is R. Hall et al., "Oral versus Vaginal Midoprostol (Cytotec) for Labor Induction," *Obstetrics and Gynecology* 99 (2002): 1044–48.
21. FIGO Committee for the Ethical Aspects of Human Reproduction and Women's Health, "Ethical Aspects Regarding Cesarean Delivery for Nonmedical Reasons," *International Journal of Gynecology and Obstetrics* 64 (1999): 317–22.
22. W. Harer, "Patient Choice Cesarean," *American College of Obstetricians and Gynecologists Clinical Review* 5, no. 2 (2000): 16–20.

THREE. CHOOSE AND LOSE

1. V. Iovine, *The Girlfriends' Guide to Pregnancy* (New York: Pocket Books, 1995), pp. 217–18.
2. W. B. Harer, "Patient Choice Cesarean," *American College of Obstetricians and Gynecologists Clinical Review* 5, no. 2 (2000): 12–16.
3. ACOG Committee Opinion number 207, "Liability Implications of Recording Procedures or Treatments," published in September 1998.
4. For detailed data on childbirth in the United States collected by the federal government, including birth by the day of the week, see www.cdc.gov/nchs/birth. Cesarean for convenience is discussed in M. Hurst and P. Summary, "Childbirth and Social Class: The Case of Cesarean Section," *Social Science and Medicine* 18 (1984): 621–31. For a fuller discussion of the issue of C-section and doctors' convenience, see M. Wagner, *Pursuing the Birth Machine: The Search for Appropriate Birth Technology* (London: ACE Graphics, 1994), pp. 186–88. Also see M. Wagner, "Choosing Caesarean Section," *Lancet* 356 (2000): 1677–80.
5. For a more thorough discussion of the consequences of obstetricians having experienced only one type of birth, see M. Wagner, "Fish Can't See Water: The Need to Humanize Birth," *International Journal of Gynecology and Obstetrics* 75, supplement (2001): s25–37.
6. World Health Organization, "Having a Baby in Europe," *Public Health in Europe* 26 (1985): 85.
7. M. Enkin et al., *A Guide to Effective Care in Pregnancy and Childbirth*, 3rd ed. (New York: Oxford University Press, 2000), p. 271, reports the results of twelve randomized, controlled trials comparing electronic fetal monitoring (EFM) with intermittent auscultation of the fetal heart rate, involving more

than fifty-eight thousand women in ten centers. C-section rates were higher in the EFM group but there were no differences in outcome for the babies in the EFM and auscultation groups. For an excellent discussion of the limitations of EFM, see H. Goer, *The Thinking Woman's Guide to a Better Birth* (New York: Penguin Putnam, 1999), pp. 85–98.

8. B. Backie and J. Nackling, "Term Prediction in Routine Ultrasound Practice," *Acta Obstetricia et Gynecologica Scandinavica* 73 (1994): 113–18.

9. For information on the mechanical nipple stimulation device, see U.S. Food and Drug Administration Advisory Panel on Obstetrics and Gynecology, minutes, April 4, 1990.

10. For a discussion of the powerful influence social and economic factors have on C-section rates, including a discussion of these studies, see Wagner, *Pursuing the Birth Machine*, pp. 186–88. Nonmedical factors influencing C-section rates were investigated by the World Health Organization; see P. Stephenson, *International Differences in the Use of Obstetrical Interventions* (Copenhagen: World Health Organization European Regional Office, 1992), pp. 6–10.

11. Susan Brink, "Too Posh to Push? Cesarean Sections Have Spiked Dramatically. Progress or Convenience?" *U.S. News and World Report,* August 5, 2002, pp. 42–43.

12. G. Feldman and J. Freiman, "Prophylactic Cesarean Section at Term?" *New England Journal of Medicine* 312, no. 19 (1985): 1264–67.

13. B. Sachs, M. Castro, and F. Frigoletto, "The Risk of Lowering the Cesarean-Delivery Rate," *New England Journal of Medicine* 140 (1999): 54–57.

14. J. Brody, "Warning on Drop in Cesarean Births: 4 Top Specialists Challenge Government's Goal, Citing Dangers," *New York Times,* January 7, 1999; K. Springer, "The Right to Choose. Cesarean Sections Are on the Rise Again. Public-Health Officials Want to Limit Them, but Many Patients and Doctors Are Resisting," *Newsweek,* December 4, 2000, pp. 73–74.

15. See, for example, M. Greene, "Vaginal Delivery after Cesarean Section—Is the Risk Acceptable?" *New England Journal of Medicine* 345 (2001): 54–55.

16. This survey was reported in M. Wagner, "Critique of British Royal College of Obstetricians and Gynaecologists National Sentinel Caesarean Section Audit Report of Oct 2001," *MIDIRS Journal* 12, no. 3 (2002): 366 – 70.

17. The scientific literature on the risks of urinary and fecal incontinence after vaginal birth are reviewed in Wagner, "Critique of British Royal College of Obstetricians and Gynaecologists National Sentinel Caesarean Section Audit Report." As one example, a report of a study in the April 15, 2001, issue of *Ob.Gyn. News* found that one year after giving birth, 3.7 percent of women with spontaneous vaginal birth had urinary incontinence whereas 9.8 percent of women whose babies were delivered with forceps had urinary incontinence. In addition, the risks to women from C-section versus the risks

from vaginal birth are reviewed in detail in three books: Enkin et al., *Guide to Effective Care in Pregnancy and Childbirth;* Goer, *Thinking Woman's Guide to a Better Birth;* and Wagner, *Pursuing the Birth Machine.*

18. Brink, "Too Posh to Push?"

19. G. Buchsbaum et al., "Urinary Incontinence in Nulliparous Women and Their Parous Sisters," *Obstetrics and Gynecology* 106 (2005): 1259–65.

20. By far the most reliable information on the risks of women dying from emergency C-section and elective C-section is in M. Hall and S. Bewley, "Maternal Mortality and Mode of Delivery," *Lancet* 354 (1999): 776. This paper used data from the British Department of Health's confidential enquiries on maternal mortality conducted during the 1990s. See U.K. Department of Health, *Why Mothers Die: Report on Confidential Enquiries into Maternal Deaths* (London: H.M. Stationery Office, 1999).

21. For a discussion of the many risks of C-section to the woman and to the baby, documented with references to the scientific literature, see Wagner, "Choosing Cesarean Section."

22. Personal communication, Ina May Gaskin, as part of her research into cases of maternal mortality in the United States.

23. For a review of risks to woman and baby as a result of C-section, including in subsequent pregnancies, see Wagner, "Choosing Cesarean Section." That the risk of stillbirth in subsequent pregnancies is double with previous C-section is documented in G. C. S. Smith et al., "Cesarean Section and Risk of Unexplained Stillbirth in Subsequent Pregnancy," *Lancet* 362 (2003): 1779–84. The risk of a detached placenta is discussed in E. Hemminki et al., "Long-Term Effects of Cesarean Sections: Ectopic Pregnancies and Placental Problems," *American Journal of Obstetrics and Gynecology* 174, no. 5 (1996): 1569–75.

24. A. Kolaas et al., "Is Planned Caesarean Section Better than Planned Vaginal Delivery for the Child?" submitted for publication, 2005. The authors are affiliated with the University of Oslo and the Norwegian Ministry of Health.

25. See Enkin et al., *Guide to Effective Care in Pregnancy and Childbirth;* O. Hjalmarson, "Epidemiology of Neonatal Disorders of Respiration," *International Journal of Technology Assessment in Health Care* 7, supplement 1 (1991); and J. Lomas and M. Enkin, "Variations in Operative Delivery Rates," in *Effective Care in Pregnancy and Childbirth,* ed. I. Chalmers, M. Enkin, and M. Keirse (Oxford: Oxford University Press, 1989).

26. Harer, "Patient Choice Cesarean."

27. Wagner, "Fish Can't See Water," p. s31.

28. J. Potter et al., "Unwanted Caesarean Sections among Public and Private Patients in Brazil: A Prospective Study," *British Medical Journal* 323 (2001): 1155–58.

29. FIGO Committee for the Ethical Aspects of Human Reproduction and Women's Health, "Ethical Aspects Regarding Cesarean Delivery for Non-medical Reasons," *International Journal of Obstetrics and Gynecology* 64 (1999): 317–22.
30. For detailed data on childbirth in the United States collected by the federal government, including C-section rates, go to www.cdc.gov/nchs/birth.
31. World Health Organization, "Appropriate Technology for Birth," *Lancet* 2, no. 8452 (1985): 436–37.
32. Wagner, "Choosing Cesarean Section." Also see Wagner, *Pursuing the Birth Machine.*
33. F. Notzon, "International Differences in the Use of Obstetric Interventions," *Journal of the American Medical Association* 263, no. 24 (1990): 3286–91.
34. Lomas and Enkin, "Variations in Operative Delivery Rates."
35. Sachs, Castro, and Frigoletto, "Risk of Lowering the Cesarean-Delivery Rate."
36. For a discussion of the process by which the World Health Organization in 1985 determined the optimal C-section rate, see Wagner, "Fish Can't See Water."
37. A. Betran et al., "Rates of Caesarean Section: Analysis of Global and Regional Estimates and Correlation with Indicators of Reproductive Health System Development," presented at the International Forum on Birth, Rome, June 2005, and accepted for publication in *Paediatric and Perinatal Epidemiology.*
38. L. Leeman and R. Leeman, "A Native American Community with a 7% Cesarean Delivery Rate: Does Case Mix, Ethnicity or Labor Management Explain the Low Rate?" *Annals of Family Medicine* 1 (2003): 36–43.
39. In an editorial in the *ACOG Clinical Review,* the then president of ACOG wrote, "The once significant differences in cost between cesarean and vaginal delivery are close to disappearing." Harer, "Patient Choice Cesarean," p. 18.
40. I. M. Gaskin, *Ina May's Guide to Childbirth* (New York, Bantam Books, 2003), p. 234.
41. An excellent review of normal labor pain and factors that influence it is found in Gaskin, *Ina May's Guide to Childbirth,* pp. 150–66.
42. For reviews of the perception of pain in different countries, see I. Senden et al., "Labor Pain: A Comparison of Parturients in a Dutch and an American Teaching Hospital," *Obstetrics and Gynecology* 71 (1988): 4; B. Jordon, *Birth in Four Cultures: A Cross-Cultural Investigation of Childbirth in Yucatan, Holland, and the United States* (Montreal: Eden Press, 1983); and Gaskin, *Ina May's Guide to Childbirth,* pp. 150–53.

43. Goer, *Thinking Woman's Guide to a Better Birth,* pp. 125–48.

44. There are three excellent studies on the risks associated with epidural: B. Leighton and S. Halpern, "The Effects of Epidural Anesthesia on Labor, Maternal and Neonatal Outcomes," *American Journal of Obstetrics and Gynecology* 186 (2002): 569–77; E. Lieberman and C. O'Donoghue, "Unintended Effects of Epidural Anesthesia during Labor," *American Journal of Obstetrics and Gynecology* 186 (2002): 531–68; and L. Mayberry and D. Clemmens, "Epidural Analgesia Side Effects, Co-interventions, and Care of Women during Childbirth," *American Journal of Obstetrics and Gynecology* 186 (2002): 581–93. In addition, an excellent review and summary of the scientific evidence on the risks of using epidural block for normal labor pain is found in Goer, *Thinking Woman's Guide to a Better Birth,* pp. 125–47, 264–76.

45. Lieberman et al., "Changes in Fetal Position during Labor and Their Association with Epidural Analgesia," *Obstetrics and Gynecology* 105, no. 5, part 1 (2005): 974.

46. D. Chestnut et al., "The Influence of Continuous Epidural Bupivacaine Analgesia on the Second Stage of Labor and Methods of Delivery in Nulliparous Women," *Anesthesiology* 66 (1987): 774–80; C. Stavrou, G. J. Hofmeyr, and A. P. Boezaart, "Prolonged Fetal Bradycardia during Epidural Anesthesia: Incidence, Timing and Significance," *South Africa Medical Journal* 77 (1990): 66–68; R. Steiger and M. P. Nageotte, "Effects of Uterine Contractility and Maternal Hypotension on Prolonged Decelerations after Bupivacaine Epidural Anesthesia," *American Journal of Obstetrics and Gynecology* 163 (1990): 808–12.

47. J. Eddleston et al., "Comparison of the Maternal and Fetal Effects Associated with Intermittent or Continuous Infusion of Extradural Analgesia," *British Journal of Anaesthesia* 69 (1992): 154–58.

48. C. M. Sepkoski et al., "The Effects of Maternal Epidural Anesthesia on Neonatal Behavior during the First Month," *Developmental Medicine and Child Neurology* 34 (1992): 1072–80. Also see Goer, *Thinking Woman's Guide to a Better Birth,* p. 271.

49. S. Boschert, "Anesthesiologists Defend Epidural Safety," *Ob.Gyn. News,* July 15, 1998, p. 20.

50. M. Wagner, "Episiotomy: A Form of Genital Mutilation," *Lancet* 353 (1999): 1977–78.

51. Dr. DeLee's remarks are quoted from M. Chase, "Episiotomy, Once Routine, May Not Ease Delivery and Can Slow Recovery," *Wall Street Journal,* March 30, 2000, p. A1.

52. S. Thacker and D. Banta, "Benefits and Risks of Episiotomy: An Interpretive Review of the English Language Literature, 1860–1980," *Obstetrical and Gynecological Survey* 38 (1983): 322–38.

53. World Health Organization, "Appropriate Technology for Birth."

54. Chase, "Episiotomy," includes data from the Cochrane Library review. The Cochrane Library, produced by Update Software in Oxford, England, is the most scientifically respected and valid source of information on obstetric procedures. The best scientists from around the world evaluate the scientific literature and write reviews of the evidence for various obstetric interventions. It is available in nearly every medical library in the United States and comes out four times a year on computer diskette.

55. Chase, "Episiotomy."

56. L. Tarkan, "In Many Delivery Rooms, a Routine Becomes Less Routine," *New York Times,* February 26, 2002.

57. *Listening to Mothers* (New York: Maternity Center Association, 2002), the first national survey of childbearing women in the United States, was conducted by the Maternity Center Association (now called Childbirth Connection), 281 Park Avenue South, New York, NY 10010.

58. K. Hartmann et al., "Outcomes of Routine Episiotomies: A Systematic Review," *Journal of the American Medical Association* 293 (2005): 2141–48.

59. A Swedish study found that when a mother receives three doses of opiates or barbiturates or nitrous oxide gas during her labor, her child is 4.7 times as likely to become addicted to opiate drugs in adulthood. This conclusion was replicated almost exactly in a U.S. study. The Swedish study is B. Jacobson et al., "Opiate Addiction in Adult Offspring through Possible Imprinting after Obstetric Treatment," *British Medical Journal* 301, no. 6760 (1990): 1067–70. The U.S. study is K. Nyberg, "Long-Term Effects of Labor Analgesia," *Journal of Obstetric, Gynecologic, and Neonatal Nursing* 29, no. 3 (2000): 226.

60. For a review of how little is known about possible effects on the baby of ultrasound scanning during pregnancy, including one study suggesting possible minimal neurological damage, see Wagner, *Pursuing the Birth Machine,* pp. 86–92. The study suggesting possible minimal neurological damage is K. Salvesen et al., "Routine Ultrasonography in Utero and Subsequent Handedness and Neurological Development," *British Medical Journal* 307 (1993): 159–64.

61. A. Saari-Kemppainen et al., "Ultrasound Screening and Perinatal Mortality," *Lancet* 336 (1990): 387–91; J. Newnham et al., "Effects of Frequent Ultrasound during Pregnancy: A Randomized Controlled Trial," *Lancet* 342 (1993): 887–91.

62. B. Ewigman, "Effect of Prenatal Ultrasound on Perinatal Outcome," *New England Journal of Medicine* 329 (1993): 821–27.

63. Newnham et al., "Effects of Frequent Ultrasound during Pregnancy."

64. H. B. Meire, "The Safety of Diagnostic Ultrasound," *British Journal of Obstetrics and Gynecology* 94 (1987): 1121–22.

65. R. Salmond, "The Uses and Value of Radiology in Obstetrics," in *Antenatal and Postnatal Care,* ed. F. Browne, 2nd ed. (London: J. and A. Churchill, 1937).

66. J. C. Moir, "The Uses and Value of Radiology in Obstetrics," in *Antenatal and Postnatal Care,* ed. F. Browne, 9th ed. (London: J. and A. Churchill, 1960).

67. A. Stewart et al., "Malignant Disease in Childhood and Diagnostic Irradiation in Utero," *Lancet* 2 (1956): 447.

68. *Lancet* 366, no. 9482 (July 23, 2005): 283.

69. The eight basic, required elements in informed consent are found in FDA regulation 50:25. The list of the most common problems found by the FDA when reviewing informed consent forms is in the FDA Information Sheets, which can be accessed at www.fda.org.

70. The office in the federal government that deals with the abuse of people who are experimented on is the Division of Human Subject Protection of the Office for Protection from Research Risk (OPRR). OPRR is part of the National Institutes of Health, an agency of the Department of Health and Human Services. The quotation is from OPRR, *Guide to Good Clinical Practice,* vol. 3, no. 6, which can be accessed at www.nih.gov.

71. For a fuller discussion of "checkbook science," see D. Zuckerman, "Hype in Health Reporting," *Extra* (the magazine of FAIR, the media watchdog group) 15, no. 4 (2004): 8–11.

72. Enkin et al., *Guide to Effective Care in Pregnancy and Childbirth,* pp. 487–507.

73. D. Petiti et al., "In-Hospital Maternal Mortality in the US," *Obstetrics and Gynecology* 59 (1982): 6–11; D. Petiti et al., "Maternal Mortality and Morbidity in Cesarean Section," *Clinics in Obstetrics and Gynecology* 28 (2001): 763–68; M. Hall and S. Bewley, "Maternal Mortality and Mode of Delivery," *Lancet* 354 (1999): 776.

74. The data showing that the rate of C-section in the United States is nearly twice what it should be are found in Wagner, "Choosing Cesarean Section."

75. Centers for Disease Control and Prevention, *Safe Motherhood: Preventing Pregnancy-Related Illness and Death* (Atlanta: Centers for Disease Control and Prevention, 2001).

76. Discussed in a *New York Times* editorial as reported in the *International Herald Tribune,* October 22, 2002.

FOUR. FORCED LABOR

1. Food and Drug Administration, Adverse Event Reporting System (AERS) Data Base, reported on February 21, 2005.

2. F. G. Cunningham et al., *Williams Obstetrics,* 21st ed. (New York: McGraw-Hill, 2001), p. 447.

3. "Vigorous uterine contractions combined with a long, firm cervix and a birth canal that resists stretch [found in a woman having a first baby] may lead to uterine rupture or extensive lacerations of the cervix, vagina, vulva or perineum. It is in these latter circumstances that the rare condition of amniotic fluid embolism most likely develops." Cunningham et al., *Williams Obstetrics,* p. 447.

4. What is the evidence that there is an increase in AFE deaths in the United States? AFE was once so rare that textbooks estimated its frequency as 1 in every 50,000 to 1 in every 80,000 births. But the Massachusetts Department of Public Health Maternal Mortality and Morbidity Review Committee in 2000 reported AFE as the second most common cause of maternal mortality (*Maternal Mortality and Morbidity Review in Massachusetts: A Bulletin for Health Care Professionals,* no. 1, May 2000).

5. M. Wagner, "From Caution to Certainty: Hazards in the Formation of Evidence-Based Practice. A Case Study on Evidence for an Association between the Use of Uterine Stimulant Drugs and Amniotic Fluid Embolism," *Paediatric and Perinatal Epidemiology* 19, no. 2 (2005): 173–76.

6. For a thorough discussion of the off-label use of drugs in obstetrics, see M. Wagner, "Off-Label Use of Drugs in Obstetrics—A Cautionary Tale," *British Journal of Obstetrics and Gynaecology* 112 (2005): 266–68.

7. W. Rayburn and K. Farmer, "Off Label Prescribing during Pregnancy" *Obstetrics and Gynecology Clinics of North America* 24, no. 3 (1997): 471–78. In this paper, a survey of 731 pregnant and birthing women showed that 22.6 percent had received drugs for off-label indications and none of these women had ever been told that the use was off-label. Such widespread off-label prescribing is not found in other fields of medical practice.

8. Two examples of studies reported in the mid-1990s with insufficient sample size to adequately measure risks are L. Sanchos-Ramos et al., "Labor Induction with the Prostaglandin 1 Methyl Analogue Misoprostol Versus Oxytocin: A Randomized Trial," *Obstetrics and Gynecology* 91, no. 13 (1993): 401–5; and D. Wing and R. Paul, "A Comparison of Differing Dosing Regimens of Vaginally Administered Misoprostol for Preinduction Cervical Ripening and Labor Induction," *American Journal of Obstetrics and Gynecology* 179, no. 1 (1996): 158–64.

9. G. J. Hofmeyr, "Misoprostol Administered Vaginally for Cervical Ripening and Labour Induction with a Viable Fetus," *Cochrane Library,* 2, 1999 (Oxford: Update Software).

10. For detailed data on childbirth in the United States collected by the federal government, including rates of induction of labor, go to the Web site www.cdc.gov/nchs/birth.

11. *Listening to Mothers* (New York: Maternity Center Association, 2002), the first national survey of childbearing women in the United States, was conducted by the Maternity Center Association (now called Childbirth Connection), 281 Park Avenue South, New York, NY 10010.

12. The protocol states, in part, that the hospital's "induction time slots are as follows: (1) Monday through Friday at 0500 [5:00 A.M.], 0700, 1000, or 1200 and for miso [misoprostol, Cytotec] at 2000. Two patients may be scheduled for each time slot. (2) Saturday and Sunday: May schedule up to three patients; time may vary. (3) No 'on call' inductions unless scheduled induction is delayed due to bed availability. . . . (4) Any patient designated by the physician as a medically indicated emergency admission will be accepted for induction at any time. . . . (5) All Misoprostols need to be booked through the ANM, Charge RN, or Induction Nurse in L&D. (6) Induction may be scheduled up to 14 days in advance." There is a waiting list for slots, so the doctor and the woman must plan ahead for the induction, which can be tricky if the induction supposedly is to be done for medical reasons. However, the protocol list of approved reasons for induction includes (albeit at the bottom of the priority list) "social indication," a euphemism for convenience. How dehumanizing this assembly-line approach is can be seen in the way the protocol refers to the woman ("All Misoprostols need to be booked . . .") as well as in the woman's realization that her baby's birthday will be forever determined, not by the optimal physiological moment, but by an empty slot in the hospital's schedule.

13. D. Wing et al., "Disruption of Prior Uterine Incision Following Misoprostol (Cytotec) for Labor Induction in Women with Previous Cesarean Section," *Obstetrics and Gynecology* 91, no. 2 (1998): 828–30.

14. M. Plaut, M. Schwartz, and S. Lubarsky, "Uterine Rupture Associated with the Use of Misoprostol in the Gravid Patient with a Previous Cesarean Section," *American Journal of Obstetrics and Gynecology* 180, no. 6 (1999): 1535–40; H. Blanchette, S. Nayak, and S. Erasmus, "Comparison of the Safety and Efficacy of Intravaginal Misoprostol with Those of Dinoprostone for Cervical Ripening and Induction of Labor in a Community Hospital," *American Journal of Obstetrics and Gynecology* 180, no. 6 (1999): 1543–50.

15. Goldberg, A. B., M. B. Greenberg, and P. D. Darney, "Drug Therapy: Misoprostol and Pregnancy," *New England Journal of Medicine* 344, no. 1 (2001): 38–47.

16. *Dateline NBC,* November 4, 2001.

17. ACOG Practice Bulletin number 10, "Induction of Labor," November 1999.

18. G. J.. Hofmeyr and A. M. Gulmezoglu, "Vaginal Misoprostol for Cervical Ripening and Induction of Labour (Review)," *Cochrane Database of Systematic Reviews,* 1, 2003, art. no. CD000941.

19. Goldberg, Greenberg, and Darney, "Drug Therapy: Misoprostol and Pregnancy."

20. J. Tickner, C. Raffensperger, and N. Myers, *The Precautionary Principle in Action: A Handbook,* Science and Environmental Health Network, posted at www.biotech-info.net/precautionary.

21. P. Saunders, "Use and Abuse of the Precautionary Principle," submission to U.S. Advisory Committee on International Economic Policy, biotech working group, July 13, 2000, posted on the Web site of the Institute of Science in Society, www.i-sis.org.

22. L. Sanchos-Ramos et al., "Misoprostol for Cervical Ripening and Labor Induction: A Meta-Analysis," *Obstetrics and Gynecology* 89 (1997): 633–42.

23. Sanchos-Ramos et al., "Misoprostol for Cervical Ripening and Labor Induction," p. 640.

24. R. Hale and S. Zinberg, "Use of Misoprostol in Pregnancy," *New England Journal of Medicine* 344, no. 1 (2001): 59–60.

25. The FDA alert in May 2005 on the risk of use of misoprostol in labor and delivery may be found at www.fda.gov/cder/drug/infopage/misoprostol.

26. See M. Wagner, "Adverse Events Following Misoprostol Induction of Labor," *Midwifery Today* 71 (Autumn 2004): 9–12.

27. M. Enkin et al., *A Guide to Effective Care in Pregnancy and Childbirth,* 3rd ed. (New York: Oxford University Press, 2000), p. 375.

28. For an excellent review of the indications for induction and the evolution of labor induction, see G. Hart, "Induction and Circular Logic," *Midwifery Today* 63 (Autumn 2002): 24.

29. L. Sanchez-Ramos et al., "Expectant Management versus Labor Induction for Suspected Fetal Macrosomia: A Systematic Review," *Obstetrics and Gynecology* 100, no. 5, part 1 (2002): 997.

30. Wilkes et al., "Premature Rupture of Membranes" (2004), posted on www.emedicine.com; M. Hannah et al., "Induction of Labor Compared with Expectant Management for Prelabor Rupture of the Membranes at Term," *New England Journal of Medicine* 334, no. 16 (1996): 1005.

31. J. McClure-Brown, "Postmaturity," *American Journal of Obstetrics and Gynecology* 85 (1963): 573–82.

32. R. L. Williams et al., "Fetal Growth and Perinatal Viability in California," *Obstetrics and Gynecology* 59 (1982): 624; P. Bergsjo et al., "Comparison of Induced vs. Non-induced Labor in Post-term Pregnancy," *Acta Obstetrica Gynecologica* 68 (1989): 683–87.

33. D. Weinstein et al., "Expectant Management of Post Term Pregnancy: Observations and Outcome," *Journal of Maternal Fetal Medicine* 5, no. 5 (1996): 293–97.

34. For detailed data on childbirth in the United States collected by the federal

government, including rates of induction of labor, go to the Web site www
.cdc.gov/nchs/birth.

35. Information on Cytotec must always make a careful distinction between
Cytotec for medical abortion early in pregnancy, which is thoroughly studied and recommended, and Cytotec for stopping postpartum hemorrhage,
which is also thoroughly studied and recommended, and Cytotec for induction of labor at the end of pregnancy, which is currently under investigation
and not approved because of serious risks.

36. *Dateline NBC,* November 4, 2001; Canadian Broadcasting Company (CBC),
The National, October 2002; CBS Boston affiliate evening news segment,
2005; I. M. Gaskin, *Ina May's Guide to Natural Childbirth* (New York: Bantam Books, 2003), pp. 280–84; H. Goer, *Thinking Woman's Guide to a Better Birth* (New York: Penguin Putnam, 1999), pp. 60–65; "Cytotec: Dangerous Experiment or Panacea?" posted on www.salon.com, July 11, 2000.

37. For a detailed discussion of the issues in the regulation of the newer reproductive technologies such as in vitro fertilization, see P. Stephenson and M.
Wagner, *Tough Choices: In Vitro Fertilization and the Reproductive Technologies* (Philadelphia: Temple University Press, 1993).

38. For more information on the Internet support group for women who survived uterine rupture, see auterineruptturesupportgroup@yahoogroups.com.

FIVE. HUNTING WITCHES

1. Mortality rates for California hospitals for the years 1968 to 1970 are available from the State Department of Health.

2. J. Rooks, *Midwifery and Childbirth in America* (Philadelphia: Temple University Press 1997), an excellent resource on American midwifery, is one of
many books that review the fascinating history of midwifery.

3. For a detailed description of the case of Hanna Porn and an excellent analysis of the witch-hunt against midwives in that era and its similarity to the
present witch-hunt against midwives, see E. Declercq, "The Trials of Hanna
Porn: The Campaign to Abolish Midwifery in Massachusetts," *American
Journal of Public Health* 84, no. 6 (1994): 1022–28.

4. One example is J. van Olphen-Fehr, *Diary of a Midwife: The Power of Positive Childbearing* (Westport, Conn.: Bergin & Garvey, 1998).

5. The two books by nurse-midwives describing their experiences attending
home births are van Olphen-Fehr, *Diary of a Midwife;* and P. Vincent, *Baby
Catcher: Chronicles of a Modern Midwife* (New York: Scribner, 2002). For
information on Citizens for Midwifery, call (888) CFM-4880 or e-mail
cfmidwifery@yahoo.com. For information on the International Cesarean
Awareness Network, see www.ican-online.org. For information on the
Coalition for Improving Maternity Services, see www.motherfriendly.org.

6. E. J. Lehrman, "Nurse-Midwifery Practice: A Descriptive Study of Prenatal Care," *Journal of Nurse-Midwifery* 26, no. 3 (1981): 27–41.

7. Lehrman, "Nurse-Midwifery Practice"; B. K. Cypress, *Office Visits by Women: The National Ambulatory Medical Care Survey* (Hyattsville, Md.: National Center for Health Statistics, 1980). The latter study found that physicians spend an average of only ten minutes on each prenatal visit, 32 percent of their prenatal visits took five minutes or less, and they did little counseling.

8. M. MacDorman and G. Singh, "Midwifery Care, Social and Medical Risk Factors, and Birth Outcomes in the USA," *Journal of Epidemiology and Community Health* 52, no. 5 (1998): 310–17.

9. M. Wagner, "Midwifery in the Industrialized World," *Journal of the Society of Obstetricians and Gynecologists of Canada* 20, no. 13 (1998): 1225–34, is a review of the scientific literature on midwifery, including the research showing the safety of midwives and the research showing that midwives use fewer unnecessary interventions during labor and birth than doctors do.

10. A review of the scientific literature on the advantages and disadvantages of the various positions of women during childbirth is found in M. Wagner, *Pursuing the Birth Machine: The Search for Appropriate Birth Technology* (London: ACE Graphics, 1994), pp. 150–53.

11. Data on the number of U.S. births attended by midwives and doctors and data on the rates of obstetric interventions in the United States can be found on the Web site www.cdc.gov/nchs. Another source of rates of obstetric interventions is *Listening to Mothers* (New York: Maternity Center Association, 2002), the first national survey of childbearing women in the United States, conducted by the Maternity Center Association (now called Childbirth Connection), 281 Park Avenue South, New York, NY 10010. www.childbirthconnection.org.

12. Wagner, "Midwifery in the Industrialized World."

13. See data posted at www.cdc.gov/nchs.

14. For information on doulas, including scientific evidence of the benefits provided by them, contact Doulas of North America (DONA) at www.dona.org.

15. M. Wagner, "A Global Witch Hunt," *Lancet* 346 (1995): 1020–22. Also see D. Korte, "Midwives on Trial," *Mothering,* Fall 1995, p. 54.

16. In the past ten years, I have been personally contacted by dozens of midwives in the United States who have been arrested by local authorities or state attorneys general, investigated by state boards, or fired by obstetric groups or by hospitals. I have testified at state board hearings of midwives or at trials of midwives in several states, including Connecticut, Illinois, Indiana, Vermont, and Washington. I have given advice and sent letters to authorities concerning midwives under attack in many states, including New York,

New Jersey, South Dakota, Oregon, California, and others. And I have read many newspaper accounts of midwives under attack.

17. See Wagner, "Global Witch Hunt."
18. For further discussion of how state quality assurance systems are abused for inappropriate, nonclinical purposes to benefit certain groups of doctors and to punish deviance from the style of practice preferred by those in power, see Wagner, "Global Witch Hunt."
19. I was contacted by the nurse-midwife, had lengthy discussions with her and other home-birth midwives in New Jersey, reviewed her records, and spoke with administrators on the state medical board.
20. ACOG Statement of Policy, "Lay Midwifery," February 2006.
21. The midwife contacted me and I had long discussions with her and other midwives in this state, reviewed records, and attended her state board hearing.
22. See Wagner, "Global Witch Hunt."
23. I was contacted by the midwife and wrote a letter to a newspaper in Las Vegas and continued the contact with this and other midwives in the area throughout the case.
24. W. H. Pearse, past president of ACOG, wrote in the ACOG publication *Obstetrics and Gynecology News* 1, no. 1 (1977), that home delivery is maternal trauma and child abuse. This statement was repeated in 1992 when another past president of ACOG, Dr. Keith Russell, was quoted as saying, "Home birth is child abuse in its earliest form" (P. Warrick, "Midwives to Leave Home: Denied Malpractice Insurance, Women Who Assist Home Births Face Two Choices: Go Establishment, or Go Underground," *Los Angeles Times*, April 28, 1992).
25. G. Judson, "An American Midwife on Trial: With Less Footing Than a Stork, She Fights to Deliver in the Home," *New York Times*, November 4, 1995.
26. For further information on the federal approval of direct-entry midwifery training, contact Susan Hodges, director of Citizens for Midwifery, e-mail: shodgesmwy@negia.net.
27. I have been in contact with the midwives involved and their lawyers.
28. I have been in contact with the midwives involved and their lawyers.
29. In Vermont, I attended a state legislative hearing on a new midwifery law (which passed) declaring that direct-entry midwifery is not the practice of medicine. In Kansas, a case came before the Kansas supreme court in which the opinion of the court was that midwifery is not the practice of medicine.
30. In 1999, a direct-entry home birth midwife in California, Alison Osborn, was arrested for practicing medicine without a license. California Medical Quality Hearing Panel, Office of Administrative Hearings case number I M

9883794. The quotation is from pp. 14–16 of the judge's decision. The judge dismissed the case against Alison Osborn.

31. Van Olphen-Fehr, *Diary of a Midwife*, pp. 8, 218.
32. I was contacted by the family and by their lawyers, reviewed the case, and followed the progress of the litigation to its end.
33. For more information on the case in Utah, contact National Advocates for Pregnant Women, 39 West 19th Street, New York, NY, 10011; telephone (212) 255–9252; e-mail: info@advocatesforpregnantwomen.org.

SIX. WHERE TO BE BORN

1. The cases discussed in this chapter are based on personal communications from midwives, women, and their families, and sometimes from the midwives' attorneys.
2. For more information on ways in which midwives and women birthing out of hospital are attacked by the authorities, including police, see M. Wagner, "A Global Witch Hunt," *Lancet* 346 (1995): 1020–22. Also see D. Korte, "Midwives on Trial," *Mothering*, Fall 1995, pp. 53–59; and J. Mitford, "Teach Midwifery, Go to Jail," *San Francisco Chronicle*, October 21, 1990.
3. ACOG Statement of Policy as issued by the Executive Board, May 1975.
4. C. Burnett et al., "Home Delivery and Neonatal Mortality in North Carolina," *Journal of the American Medical Association* 244 (1980): 2741–45; S. J. Meyers et al., "Unlicensed Midwifery Practice in Washington State," *American Journal of Public Health* 80 (1990): 726–28.
5. ACOG, *Guidelines for Perinatal Care* (Washington, D.C.: ACOG, 2002), pp. 125–26.
6. See M. Wagner, "Fish Can't See Water: The Need to Humanize Birth," *International Journal of Gynecology and Obstetrics* 75, supplement (2001): s25–37.
7. For a detailed exploration of the idea that men have "womb envy" and are afraid of women's unique childbearing gift, see R. S. McElvaine, *Eve's Seed: Biology, the Sexes, and the Course of History* (New York: McGraw-Hill, 2001).
8. McElvaine, *Eve's Seed*.
9. Personal communication from a number of practicing obstetricians.
10. For a thorough review of the scientific evidence on ABCs, see P. Stephenson et al., *Alternative Birth Centers in Illinois: A Resource Guide for Policy Makers* (Chicago: University of Illinois at Chicago Center for Research on Women and Gender, and the Health and Medicine Policy and Research Group, 1995).
11. J. P. Rooks et al., "Outcomes of Care in Birth Centers: The National Birth Center Study," *New England Journal of Medicine* 321, no. 26 (1989): 1804–11.

12. E. Feldman and M. Hurst, "Outcomes and Procedures in Low Risk Births: A Comparison of Hospital and Birth Centre Settings," *Birth and Family Journal* 14, no. 1 (1987): 7–10; G. Baruffi et al., "Investigation of Institutional Differences in Primary Cesarean Birth Rates," *Journal of Nurse-Midwifery* 35, no. 35 (1990): 274–81; U. Waldenstrom and C. Nilsson, "Women's Satisfaction with Birth Centre Care: A Randomized Controlled Study," *Issues in Perinatal Care* 20, no. 1 (1993): 3–13.

13. Stephenson et al., *Alternative Birth Centers in Illinois.*

14. Personal communication, German Midwifery Association.

15. Personal communication from many Japanese midwives and visits to Japanese birth houses and to the National Institute of Public Health in Tokyo.

16. The director of the birth center showed me this letter.

17. The National Association of Childbearing Centers' Web site is www.birthcenters.org.

18. G. Judson, "An American Midwife on Trial: With Less Footing Than a Stork, She Fights to Deliver in the Home," *New York Times,* November 4, 1995.

19. A. Durand, "The Safety of Home Birth: The Farm Study," *American Journal of Public Health* 82 (1992): 450–53; W. Schramm et al., "Neonatal Mortality in Missouri Home Births," *American Journal of Public Health* 77, no. 8 (1987): 930–35; M. W. Hinds, G. H. Bergeisen, and D. T. Allen, "Neonatal Outcome in Planned vs. Unplanned Out-of-Hospital Births in Kentucky," *Journal of the American Medical Association* 253, no. 11 (1985): 1578–82; P. A. Murphy and J. Fullerton, "Outcomes of Intended Home Births in Nurse-Midwifery Practice: A Prospective Descriptive Study," *Obstetrics and Gynecology* 92, no. 3 (1992): 461–70; O. Olsen, "Meta-Analysis of the Safety of Home Birth," *Birth* 24, no. 1 (1997): 4–16.

20. J. Pang et al., "Outcomes of Planned Home Births in Washington State: 1989–1996," *Obstetrics and Gynecology* 100, no. 2 (2002): 253–59.

21. The fact that in Washington State nurses cannot and physicians do not attend home births is detailed in a letter dated May 9, 2002, from the Midwives Association of Washington State (the state's nongovernmental organization of midwives) to Dr. Rowles and the Perinatal Advisory Committee (which is part of the state government). The letter was a clarification to the state about why it is so important for there to be midwives in Washington willing to attend planned home births so that women can have this legitimate choice.

22. Quotation from Pang et al., "Outcomes of Planned Home Births in Washington," p. 257. See Meyers et al., "Unlicensed Midwifery Practice in Washington State."

23. Quotation from Pang et al., "Outcomes of Planned Home Births in Washington," p. 257. The two studies showing a fifty times higher risk of baby

death if the home birth was unplanned are Meyers et al., "Unlicensed Midwifery Practice in Washington State"; and Burnett et al., "Home Delivery and Neonatal Mortality in North Carolina."

24. L. Cawthon, *Planned Home Births: Outcomes among Medicaid Women in Washington State,* Report 7.93 (Olympia, Wash.: Office of Research and Data Analysis, Washington State Department of Social and Health Services, 1996).

25. Pang et al., "Outcomes of Planned Home Births in Washington State," p. 255.

26. O. Olsen, "Meta-Analysis of the Safety of Home Birth."

27. Pang et al., "Outcomes of Planned Home Births in Washington State," p. 259.

28. Editorial in the *New York Times,* reprinted in the *International Herald Tribune,* October 3, 2002.

29. K. Johnson and B. Daviss, "A Prospective Study of Planned Home Births by Certified Professional Midwives in North America," *British Medical Journal* 330, no. 7505 (2005): 1416.

30. J. P. Bruner, S. B. Drummond, A. L. Meenan, and I. M Gaskin, "All-Fours Maneuver for Reducing Shoulder Dystocia during Labor," *Journal of Reproductive Medicine* 43 (1998): 439–43.

31. S. Chauhan et al., "Cesarean Section for Suspected Fetal Distress: Does the Decision–Incision Time Make a Difference?" *Journal of Reproductive Medicine* 42, no. 6 (1997): 347–52.

32. W. H. Pearse, past president of ACOG, wrote in the ACOG publication *Obstetrics and Gynecology News* 1, no. 1 (1977), that home delivery is maternal trauma and child abuse. This statement was repeated in 1992 when another past president of ACOG, Dr. Keith Russell, was quoted as saying, "Home birth is child abuse in its earliest form" (P. Warrick, "Midwives to Leave Home: Denied Malpractice Insurance, Women Who Assist Home Births Face Two Choices: Go Establishment, or Go Underground," *Los Angeles Times,* April 28, 1992).

33. J. van Olphen-Fehr, *Diary of a Midwife: The Power of Positive Childbearing* (Westport, Conn.: Bergin & Garvey, 1998), p. 116. In addition to excellent descriptions of many home births in the Shenandoah Valley of Virginia, the book includes many insights into maternity politics growing out of the author's involvement in home birth politics in Virginia. In addition to urging you to read this book, I highly recommend a second book by another home-birth midwife: P. Vincent, *Baby Catcher: Chronicles of a Modern Midwife* (New York: Scribner, 2002). This book contains wonderful descriptions of many home births in California.

34. Van Olphen-Fehr, *Diary of a Midwife,* pp. 155–62.

35. ACOG news release, "Home Births Double Risk of Newborn Death," July 31, 2002.
36. Reuters News Service, "Neonates More Likely to Die If Born at Home or If Home Delivery Was Attempted," August 2, 2002; John O'Neil, "Vital Signs: At Risk, Weighing Odds and Babies," *New York Times,* August 6, 2002.
37. See Rapid Responses to Johnson and Daviss, "Prospective Study of Planned Home Births with Certified Professional Midwives," posted at www.bmj .com.
38. See the Web site www.cdc.gov/nchs.

SEVEN. RIGHTS AND WRONGS

1. For more information on cases of litigation following Cytotec (misoprostol) induction involving dead or brain-damaged babies or dead women, see M. Wagner, "Adverse Events Following Misoprostol Induction of Labor," *Midwifery Today* 71 (Autumn 2004): 9–12.
2. ACOG news release, "Nation's Obstetrical Care Endangered by Growing Liability Insurance Crisis," May 6, 2002.
3. ACOG news release, "Nation's Obstetrical Care Endangered by Growing Liability Insurance Crisis."
4. ACOG news release, "Nation's Obstetrical Care Endangered by Growing Liability Insurance Crisis."
5. P. E. Steiner and C. C. Lushbaugh, "Maternal Pulmonary Embolism by Amniotic Fluid as a Cause of Obstetric Shock and Unexpected Deaths in Obstetrics," *Journal of the American Medical Association* 117 (1941): 1245–54, 1341–45.
6. T. Chard and M. Richards, *Benefits and Hazards of the New Obstetrics* (London: Heinemann, 1977).
7. F. Geoghegan and M. O'Driscoll, "Amniotic Fluid Embolism," *Journal of Obstetrics and Gynaecology of the British Empire* 71 (1964): 673; M. Gregory and E. Clayton, "Amniotic Fluid Embolism," *Obstetrics and Gynecology* 42 (1973): 236.
8. M. Morgan, "Amniotic Fluid Embolism," *Anaesthesia* 34 (1979): 20–32.
9. For a detailed analysis of the faulty methodology of Morgan's and Clark's papers, see M. Wagner, "From Caution to Certainty: Hazards in the Formation of Evidence-Based Practice. A Case Study on Evidence for an Association between the Use of Uterine Stimulant Drugs and Amniotic Fluid Embolism," *Paediatric and Perinatal Epidemiology* 19, no. 2 (2005): 173–76.
10. S. Clark, "New Concepts of Amniotic Fluid Embolism: A Review," *Obstetric and Gynecology Survey* 45 (1990): 360–68.
11. ACOG, *Prolog: Obstetrics,* 3rd ed. (Washington, D.C.: ACOG, 1993), p. 94.

12. M. Wagner, "Off-Label Use of Drugs in Obstetrics—A Cautionary Tale," *British Journal of Obstetrics and Gynaecology* 112 (2005): 266–68.

13. S. L. Clark et al., "Amniotic Fluid Embolism: Analysis of the National Registry," *American Journal of Obstetrics and Gynecology* 172 (1995): 1158–67.

14. Clark has testified in legal depositions that he destroyed these records because he had no space to store them.

15. F. Cunningham et al., *Williams Obstetrics,* 20th ed. (Stamford, Conn.: Appleton & Lange, 1997).

16. Cunningham et al., *Williams Obstetrics,* p. 792.

17. ACOG, *Prolog: Obstetrics,* 4th ed. (Washington, D.C.: ACOG, 1998), p. 99.

18. R. W. Martin, "Amniotic Fluid Embolism," *Clinical Obstetrics and Gynecology* 39 (1996): 101–6.

19. ACOG Practice Bulletin number 10, "Induction of Labor," November 1999.

20. D. Wing and R. A. Paul, "A Comparison of Differing Dosing Regimes of Vaginally Administered Misoprostol for Preinduction Cervical Ripening and Labor Induction," *American Journal of Obstetrics and Gynecology* 175 (1996): 158–64; Wagner, "Adverse Events Following Misoprostol Induction of Labor"; Medwatch: The FDA Medical Products Reporting Program (see www.fda.gov/medwatch); Searle Pharmaceutical Co., Searle Drug Experience Reports (see www.pfizer.com; Searle is now part of Pfizer); M. Friedman, "(Searle) Manufacturer's Warning Regarding Unapproved Uses of Misoprostol," *New England Journal of Medicine* 344 (2001): 61.

21. M. Wagner, "From Caution to Certainty: Hazards in the Formation of Evidence-Based Practice. A Case Study on Evidence for an Association between the Use of Uterine Stimulant Drugs and Amniotic Fluid Embolism," *Paediatric and Perinatal Epidemiology* 19, no. 2 (2005): 173–76.

22. M. Kramer et al., "Amniotic Fluid Embolism and Medical Induction of Labor," accepted for publication in *The Lancet.*

23. S. Daniels and L. Andrews, "The Shadow of the Law: Jury Decisions in Obstetrics and Gynecology Cases," in *Medical Professional Liability and the Delivery of Obstetrical Care,* ed. V. P. Rostow and R. J. Bulger (Washington, D.C.: National Academy Press, 1989), 2:161–93.

24. B. Sachs, M. Castro, and F. Frigoletto, "The Risks of Lowering the Cesarean-Delivery Rate," *New England Journal of Medicine* 340, no. 1 (1999): 54–57.

25. Sachs, Castro, and Frigoletto, "Risks of Lowering the Cesarean-Delivery Rate."

26. ACOG news releases: "ACOG Statement on Senate Failure to Pass Liability Reform," April 7, 2004; "Medical Liability Pressures Hurt Career Satisfaction among Ob-Gyns," April 30, 2004; "Medical Liability Survey Reaffirms More Ob/Gyns Are Quitting Obstetrics," July 16, 2004; "ACOG's Red Alert on Ob/Gyn Care Reaches 23 States," August 26, 2004; "Statement Regarding Medical Liability Reform by ACOG President," March 15, 2005;

"ACOG Endorses Bipartisan Legislation, 'Fair and Reliable Medical Justice Act,'" July 1, 2005; "Wisconsin Supreme Court Ruling Eliminating Caps on Non-economic Damages Will Have Devastating Consequences," July 14, 2005; "Statement of ACOG on the State of the Union Address," February 1, 2006.

27. Wagner, "Adverse Events Following Misoprostol Induction of Labor."

28. P. Baker, "Bush Campaigns to Curb Lawsuits: President Says 'Junk' Litigation Is Driving Small-Town Doctors Out of Business," *Washington Post,* January 6, 2005.

29. J. Queenam, "Professional Liability: Our Role and Responsibility," *Obstetrics and Gynecology* 100, no. 2 (2002): 217–18; quotations are from p. 217.

30. ACOG news release, "Nation's Obstetrical Care Endangered by Growing Liability Insurance Crisis."

31. ACOG news release, "Medical Liability Survey Reaffirms More Ob/Gyns Are Quitting Obstetrics."

32. ACOG news release, "Statement of ACOG on the State of the Union Address."

33. Sachs, Castro, and Frigoletto, "Risk of Lowering the Cesarean-Delivery Rate."

34. The data on the rates of maternal mortality in the United States, their causes, and how much they are underreported can be found in Centers for Disease Control and Prevention (CDC), "Safe Motherhood: Preventing Pregnancy-Related Illness and Death," *Obstetrics and Gynecology* 88 (2001): 61–67; M. McCarthy, "US Maternal Death Rates Are on the Rise," *Lancet* 348 (1996): 394; and G. L. Rubin et al., "Maternal Death after Cesarean Section in Georgia," *American Journal of Obstetrics and Gynecology* 139 (1981): 681–85. That the real rate of maternal mortality is twice that reported is from the McCarthy paper.

35. M. Hall and S. Bewley, "Maternal Mortality and Mode of Delivery," *Lancet* 354 (1999): 776; U.K. Department of Health, *Why Mothers Die: Report on Confidential Enquiries into Maternal Deaths* (London: H.M. Stationery Office, 1999).

36. ACOG editorial, "Use of Misoprostol in Pregnancy," *New England Journal of Medicine* 344, no. 1 (2001): 59–60.

37. I wish to thank Dr. K. Prown for her excellent work on pregnant women's legal rights and for her generosity in permitting me to use some of her material in the following pages.

38. See K. Prown, "Childbirth and the Law," posted at www.birthpolicy.org.

39. See www.dgcenter.org/acp/pdf/psda.pdf.

40. See www.health.state.ny.us/nysdoh/consumer/patient/patient.htm.

41. See www.forensic-sych.com/articles/artmedmal.html.

42. For further information, see K. Prown, "Childbirth and the Law," posted at www.birthpolicy.org; or contact National Advocates for Pregnant Women, 39 West 19th Street, New York, NY, 10011, telephone (212) 255–9252, e-mail: info@advocatesforpregnantwomen.org.

43. For further information, see K. Prown, "Childbirth and the Law," posted at www.birthpolicy.org; or contact National Advocates for Pregnant Women, 39 West 19th Street, New York, NY, 10011, telephone (212) 255–9252, e-mail: info@advocatesforpregnantwomen.org.

44. For further information, see K. Prown, "Childbirth and the Law," posted at www.birthpolicy.org; or contact National Advocates for Pregnant Women, 39 West 19th Street, New York, NY, 10011, telephone (212) 255–9252, e-mail: info@advocatesforpregnantwomen.org.

45. ACOG, "Ethical Principles" section of "Surgery and Patient Choice," in *Ethics in Obstetrics and Gynecology,* 2nd ed. (Washington, D.C.: ACOG, 2004), posted at www.acog.org/from_home/publications/ethics/.

46. ACOG Committee Opinion number 306, "Informed Refusal," *Obstetrics and Gynecology* 104 (2004): 1465–66, available for download (for a fee) at www.greenjournal.org/cgi/reprint/104/6/1465.

47. "Jehovah's Witnesses, Pregnancy, and Blood Transfusions: A Paradigm for the Autonomy Rights of All Pregnant Women," posted at www.aslme.org/aslmesecure/shop/show_product.php?prod_id = 500.

48. ACOG news release, "Nation's Obstetrical Care Endangered by Growing Liability Insurance Crisis."

EIGHT. VISION OF A BETTER WAY TO BE BORN

1. For further information on the Coalition for Improving Maternity Services and its mission, see www.motherfriendly.org.

2. M. Wagner, "Fish Can't See Water: The Need to Humanize Birth," *International Journal of Gynecology and Obstetrics* 75, supplement (2001): s25–37.

3. E. K. Adams et al., "Transitions in Insurance Coverage from before Pregnancy through Delivery in Nine States," *Health Affairs Journal* 22, no. 1 (2003): 219–29.

4. See data on www.cdc.gov/nchs.

5. A. Enthoven, "Employment-Based Health Insurance Is Failing: Now What?" *Health Affairs Journal,* Web exclusive, May 28, 2003.

6. Data on the rates of maternal mortality in the United States, their causes, and by how much they are underreported can be found in Centers for Disease Control and Prevention (CDC), "Safe Motherhood: Preventing Pregnancy-Related Illness and Death," *Obstetrics and Gynecology* 88 (2001): 61–67; M. McCarthy, "US Maternal Death Rates Are on the Rise," *Lancet* 348

(1996): 394; and G. L. Rubin et al., "Maternal Death after Cesarean Section in Georgia," *American Journal of Obstetrics and Gynecology* 139 (1981): 681–85.

7. See www.fda.gov.

8. U. Reinhardt et al., "U.S. Health Care Spending in an International Context," *Health Affairs Journal* 23, no. 3 (2004): 10–25.

9. G. Anderson et al., "It's the Price, Stupid: Why the United States Is So Different from Other Countries," *Health Affairs Journal* 22, no. 3 (2003): 89–105. Emphasis added.

10. See www.cdc.gov; www.nih.gov; www.who.int/reproductive-health.

11. Anderson et al., "It's the Price, Stupid."

12. R. Lu and W. Hsiao, "Does Universal Health Insurance Make Health Care Unaffordable? Lesson from Taiwan," *Health Affairs Journal* 22, no. 3 (2003): 77–88.

13. P. Krugman, "First, Do More Harm" (op-ed), *New York Times*, January 16, 2006.

14. The case is *Meador v. Stahler and Gheridian.*

15. See data on www.cdc.gov. Click on HAI.

16. M. Wagner, "Choosing Caesarean Section," *Lancet* 356 (2000): 1677–80.

17. Wagner, "Choosing Caesarian Section."

18. See www.cdc.gov. Click on MRSA.

19. I was contacted by the midwife, by other midwives in the area, and by local and regional media.

20. A. d'Oliveria et al., "Violence against Women in Health-Care Institutions: An Emerging Problem," *Lancet* 359 (2002): 1681–85.

21. D'Oliveria et al., "Violence against Women in Health-Care Institutions," p. 1683.

22. Personal communication, Rudy Fedrizzi, M.D., and Heidi Rinehart, M.D., obdocs@bellsouth.net.

23. A. M. Durand, "The Safety of Home Birth: The Farm Study," *American Journal of Public Health* 82 (1992): 450–53.

24. B. Starfield et al., "The Effects of Specialist Supply on Population's Health: Assessing the Evidence," *Health Affairs Journal*, Web exclusive, March 15, 2005.

25. Many obstetricians have told me that their insurance premiums have risen if they provide backup to midwives, and they often use this as an excuse to refuse to provide backup.

26. J. Queenan, "Professional Liability: Our Role and Responsibility," *Obstetrics and Gynecology* 100, no. 2 (2002): 217–18; quotation is on page 218.

27. I attended the inquest and then, when the recommendation was made to the government to look into the reestablishment of midwifery, the government consulted me—a full-time WHO staff member at the time—about mid-

wifery. At my suggestion, the government sent a group to several European countries to study midwifery, and I assisted this study-tour. I then continued to stay in touch with midwives, lawyers, and government officials as midwifery evolved in Canada.

28. M. Wagner, "Midwifery in the Industrialized World," *Journal of the Society of Obstetricians and Gynecologists of Canada* 20, no. 13 (1998): 1225–34.

29. See "History Information" on the Web site of the Frontier Nursing Service, at www. frontiernursing.org/history/history.shtm.

30. Personal communication from a contact in the professional education division of the Department of Health and Human Services. In 2005, I had a series of telephone discussions with various individuals responsible for programs to provide funding of hospital postgraduate training for obstetric residents.

31. Personal communication from ACOG staff involved in ACOG's efforts to appraise obstetric manpower needs and make recommendations to the federal government.

32. J. P. Bruner, S. B. Drummond, A. L. Meenan, and I. M Gaskin, "All-Fours Maneuver for Reducing Shoulder Dystocia during Labor," *Journal of Reproductive Medicine* 43 (1998): 439–43.

33. Personal communication from a professor of obstetrics in the Philippines.

NINE. HOW TO GET WHERE WE NEED TO BE

1. See data at www.who.int/reproductive-health.

2. P. Krugman, "Pride, Prejudice, Insurance," originally an op-ed piece in the *New York Times,* reproduced in the *International Herald Tribune,* November 8, 2005; www.cdc.gov/nchs.

3. Personal communication from the president of the German midwives organization. In 1990, I visited the only out-of-hospital birth center in Germany, located in West Berlin. In 2004, I talked with the then president of the German Midwifery Association, who told me about the exodus of German midwives from hospitals and that there were now more than seventy out-of-hospital birth centers staffed with some of these midwives.

4. When making a visit to New Zealand in the early 1990s, I talked with many midwives and doctors and journalists who confirmed the story of the randomized experimental trial and its effect on women and politicians.

5. See www.who.int; also see A. Betran et al., "Rates of Caesarean Section: Analysis of Global and Regional Estimates and Correlation with Indicators of Reproductive Health System Development," paper presented at the International Forum on Birth, Rome, June 2005, and accepted for publication in *Paediatric and Perinatal Epidemiology.*

6. D. Rattner, "Sobre a hipotese de estabilizacao das taxas de cesarea do Estado

de Sao Paulo, Brasil," *Rev. Saude Publica* 30, no. 1 (1996): 19–33; Secretariat of Health, Sao Paulo State, Brazil, 1999.

7. World Health Organization, "Appropriate Technology for Birth," *Lancet* 2, no. 8452 (1985): 436–37.

8. For a summary of the conference and the resolution, see M. Wagner, "Fish Can't See Water: The Need to Humanize Birth," *International Journal of Gynecology and Obstetrics* 75, supplement (2001): s25–37.

9. Wagner, "Fish Can't See Water."

10. J. Potter et al., "Unwanted Caesarean Sections among Public and Private Patients in Brazil: A Prospective Study," *British Medical Journal* 323 (2001): 1155–58.

11. B. Shields, *Down Came the Rain: My Journey through Postpartum Depression* (New York: Hyperion, 2005); Tom Cruise interview on *Today* (NBC), June 25, 2005; B. Shields, "War of Words" (op-ed piece), *New York Times,* July 1, 2005.

12. The reporter in San Francisco eventually found me and after interviewing me told me the reactions of the other doctors she had interviewed.

13. *Dateline NBC,* November 4, 2001.

14. Susan Brink, "Too Posh to Push? Cesarean Sections Have Spiked Dramatically. Progress or Convenience?" *U.S. News and World Report,* August 5, 2002, pp. 42–43.

15. The FDA alert in May 2005 on the risk of use of misoprostol in labor and delivery may be found at www.fda.gov/cder/drug/infopage/misoprostol; the article covering it is B. Tansey, "Ending the Silence: FDA Moves to Warn Patients of Drug's Possible Side Effects," *San Francisco Chronicle,* June 9, 2005.

16. D. Goodman, "Forced Labor," *Mother Jones,* January/February 2001, pp. 17–19.

17. I. M. Gaskin, "Induced and Seduced: The Dangers of Cytotec," *Mothering,* July/August 2001, pp. 51–55.

18. For documentation linking litigation and obstetricians attending low-risk birth, see S. Daniels and L. Andrews, "The Shadow of the Law: Jury Decisions in Obstetrics and Gynecology Cases," in *Medical Professional Liability and the Delivery of Obstetrical Care,* ed. V. P. Rostow and R. J. Bulger (Washington, D.C.: National Academy Press, 1989), 2:161–91. For documentation linking obstetricians attending low-risk birth with unnecessary interventions, see M. Wagner, "Midwifery in the Industrialized World," *Journal of the Society of Obstetricians and Gynecologists of Canada* 20, no. 13 (1998): 1225–34. For documentation linking obstetricians attending low-risk births with increasing infant and maternal mortality or other adverse outcomes in low-risk births, see M. MacDorman and G. Singh, "Midwifery

Care, Social and Medical Risk Factors, and Birth Outcomes in the USA," *Journal of Epidemiology and Community Health* 52, no. 5 (1998): 310–17.

19. M. Wagner, "The Public Health versus Clinical Approaches to Maternity Services: The Emperor Has No Clothes," *Journal of Public Health Policy* 19 (1998): 1, 25–35.
20. For further information on this book, see www.citizen.org/hrg.
21. See www.medicalconsumers.org.
22. For more information on the case in Utah where a woman was charged with murder after refusing a cesarean section, contact National Advocates for Pregnant Women, 39 West 19th Street, New York, NY, 10011, telephone (212) 255–9252, e-mail: info@advocatesforpregnantwomen.org.
23. See auterinerupturesupportgroup@yahoogroups.com.
24. See www.ican-online.org.
25. T. Parker-Pope, "Growing Number of Physicians Warn of Serious Risks from Vaginal Deliveries," *Wall Street Journal,* June 4, 2002.
26. "Birth Trauma Is Result of Interfering with Nature," letter to the editor, *Wall Street Journal,* June 25, 2002.
27. See www.cfmidwifery.org.
28. The largest is the International Childbirth Education Association. See www.icea.org.
29. See www.motherfriendly.org.
30. In January 2006, the Maternity Care Association changed its name to Childbirth Connection, and its Web site is now www.childbirthconnection.org.
31. See www.childbirthconnection.org.
32. "The Nature and Management of Labor Pain," supplement to *American Journal of Obstetrics and Gynecology* 186, no. 5, part 2 (2002).
33. Maternity Center Association, *What Every Pregnant Woman Needs to Know about Cesarean Section* (New York: Maternity Center Association, 2004). See www.childbirthconnection.org.
34. Potter et al., "Unwanted Caesarean Sections among Public and Private Patients in Brazil."
35. See www.childbirthconnection.org.
36. See www.whiteribbonalliance.org.
37. See www.motherfriendly.org.
38. See www.babyfriendlyusa.org.
39. Wagner, "Public Health versus Clinical Approaches to Maternity Services."
40. Data are from "Mothering Perinatal Healthcare Statistics," *Mothering* 68 (Fall 1993): 44–45.
41. The data table from which I am drawing was published in 1993 and so of course the data are dated. But I know of no more recent such table and all indications are that things have gotten steadily worse the last decade-plus:

costs are certainly way up given the rapid rise in C-sections, the use of epidurals for normal labor pain, and so on.

42. The reason the ranking of the United States on the global list of national infant mortality rates has varied in this book between ranking number 20 and ranking number 41 is because there is a slight variation from year to year in the rates. In any case, in the past ten years the international ranking of the United States in infant mortality has never been better than twentieth.

43. This statistic has been updated from the table published in 1993 from which I drew the other statistics.

44. Personal communication, D. Rattner, National Ministry of Health of Brazil, Brasilia.

45. Betran et al., "Rates of Caesarean Section."

46. MacDorman and Singh, "Midwifery Care, Social and Medical Risk Factors, and Birth Outcomes in the USA."

47. K. Johnson and B. Daviss, "A Prospective Study of Planned Home Births with Certified Professional Midwives in North America," *British Medical Journal* 330, no. 7505 (2005): 1416.

48. J. Pang et al., "Outcomes of Planned Home Births in Washington State: 1989–1996," *Gynecology and Obstetrics* 100, no. 2 (2002): 253–59.

49. See www.midirs.org.

50. M. Wagner, "Whose Data Is It Anyway?" *Paediatric and Perinatal Epidemiology* 2 (1988): 7.

51. See M. Wagner "Creating Your Birth Plan," Penguin, New York, 2006.

INDEX

American Public Health Association (APHA), 231, 242
amniotic fluid embolism (AFE), 72, 73–74, 155–59
amniotic sac rupture, 53, 93–94
anesthesia, 68. *See also* epidural block
antibiotic-resistant infections, 189
anti-precautionary principle, 52, 59–60, 74, 82, 87–89, 98
APHA (American Public Health Association), 231, 242
artificial reproductive services, 97
attention deficit disorders, 68, 247
authoritative knowledge, 168
autism, 68–69, 247
autonomy of birthing women, 12, 104–6, 122–24, 130, 147–48; ACOG guidelines, 176–77; global cycles in, 212–19; high-risk births, 204. *See also* control issues; informed consent; patients' rights
autonomy of childbirth educators, 236
autonomy of midwives, 103, 112, 197, 214, 215, 218–19, 227–28

Baby Friendly Hospital Initiative, 239
battery, 174–75, 180
Beth Israel Hospital (Boston), 92
birth certificate data, 138, 139
birthing beds/chairs, 40–41, 108
birth position: of baby, 55, 109, 209; of mother, 40–41, 108
blood pressure drops, epidural block and, 55
board qualification, 17, 168
book recommendations, 222–23
brain damage. *See* fetal brain damage
Brazil, 46, 194, 216–18, 245
breast-feeding, 41, 135, 239
Breckenridge, Mary, 102
breech position, 109, 209
Britain. *See* United Kingdom
British Medical Journal, 142, 150, 151
Bush, George W., 165, 166

California: midwife investigations/prosecutions, 120, 126–29; midwifery legislative hearings, 35

California Medical Association, 35
California State Board of Medical Quality Assurance, 127, 128
Canadian health care spending, 186, 243
Canadian maternity care, 4, 100, 101, 104, 192, 199–200
Carder, Angela, 176, 178
CDC (Centers for Disease Control and Prevention), 47, 170
Center for Medical Consumers, 232
Center for Medicare and Medicaid Service conditions of participation (CoP), 179, 180
Centers for Disease Control and Prevention, 47, 170
cerebral palsy, 72, 74, 85
certified midwives (CMs), 114. *See also* direct-entry midwives
certified nurse-midwives (CNMs), 125. *See also* nurse-midwives
certified professional midwives (CPMs), 114, 118, 119, 230; Johnson-Daviss home birth study, 142–43, 150–51, 247. *See also* direct-entry midwives
cesarean section, 37–50; claimed benefits, 43–44; costs, 49–50, 244; doctors' promotion of, 38–44; EFM and, 154; epidural block and, 54–55; forced or refused, 122–24, 175–76; labor induction and, 85; maternal/perinatal mortality, 38, 44, 47–48, 68, 244; right to refuse, 175–76, 178, 179; risks of, 44–45, 68. *See also* cesarean section rates; elective cesarean section; VBAC
cesarean section rates: activism to reduce, 216–17, 234–35; hospital vs. ABC births, 135; international statistics, 46, 194, 216, 219, 244; low-rate countries/populations, 49, 216, 244; media coverage/controversy, 42–43, 234–35; New York disclosure law, 11; optimal rates, 42–43, 47–49, 244; perinatal mortality and, 47–48; U.S. statistics, 42–43, 49, 135, 244; U.S. trends, 22, 29, 42–43, 85; women blamed for, 238
checkbook science, 64
Chicago maternal mortality rates, 26

child abuse, home birth equated with, 116, 148

childbed fever, 14–15

childbirth: autonomic nature of, 104–5, 131–32; intimate nature of, 189; medical vs. humanistic views of, 104–5, 106–7, 109, 130–31, 132; men's views of, 131–32. *See also* humanized birth; medicalization of birth

Childbirth Connection, 238. *See also* MCA

childbirth education organizations, 235–38

childbirth educators, 236

China, 214

chiropractors, 229–30

Christilaw, Jan, 42

CIMS (Coalition for Improving Maternity Services), 11–12, 182, 233, 236–37, 239

Citizens for Midwifery, 235

Clark, Steven, 156, 157, 158, 159

clinical judgment, as litigation defense, 167–68

CMs (certified midwives), 114. *See also* direct-entry midwives

CMS conditions of participation (CoP), 179, 180

CNMs (certified nurse-midwives), 125. *See also* nurse-midwives

Coalition for Improving Maternity Services (CIMS), 11–12, 182, 233, 236–37, 239

coalitions, 232–39

Cochrane Library, 57, 65, 77, 87

communications, in doctor-midwife relations, 203–4, 209

community-based maternity services, 191–92, 196

community standard of practice, 32, 34, 131, 166–67, 175

competition for patients, 161–62; from ABCs, 28, 137, 229; from midwives, 112, 122, 126, 196

complaint filing: hospitals, 160–61, 179; state medical boards, 180

conditions of participation (CoP), 179, 180

conferences, 223

congenital defects, in flawed home birth study, 140

Connecticut midwife investigations/ prosecutions, 119–20

consent forms, 178–79, 206–7

consent rights. *See* informed consent

constitutional rights of patients, 173, 225. *See also* informed consent; patients' rights

consumer groups, 232, 234–35

control issues, 104–6, 131–32, 147–48, 153; in doctor-midwife relations, 103, 112, 197; in doctor-patient relations, 105–6, 131–32, 190; litigation and, 153. *See also* autonomy

CoP (conditions of participation), 179, 180

costs of maternity care, 9, 10, 35; cesarean section, 49–50, 244; labor induction, 79; midwife-attended births, 9, 10, 35, 111, 121, 243–44. *See also* health care spending

court-ordered interventions, 174; C-sections, 122–24, 176, 178

CPMs. *See* certified professional midwives; direct-entry midwives

Cruise, Tom, 220

C-section. *See* cesarean section; cesarean section rates; elective cesarean section

Cuba, 212

cultural differences, perception of labor pain, 53

cultural issues, 191

Cytotec: cost of, 79; non-induction uses, 86. *See also* Cytotec induction

Cytotec induction, 2, 14, 70–93, 206; ACOG on, 24–25, 31, 32, 79, 81, 82–83, 92; action to oppose, 96–97; AFE after, 72, 73, 158; case histories, 1–2, 70–73, 84–85; dosage/administration, 78–79, 90; faulty papers on, 86–87, 89; FDA approval status, 2, 24–25, 32, 71, 75, 86–87, 90–91; fetal damage/deaths, 2, 72, 73, 81, 84, 85; history of, 74–78, 156–57; informed consent of patients, 77, 86, 92–93; litigation, 82, 85, 92–93, 97, 163–64, 166–67; maternal deaths, 23, 72, 73–74, 77, 81; media coverage, 23, 24–25, 81–82, 91–92, 93, 96–97, 220–21, 222; reasons for, 78–79, 86–87; statistics, 80 (table); unknown long-term effects, 69,

home birth investigations, 113–17, 119–20, 128. *See also* midwife investigations/prosecutions

home births, 121; ACOG policy, 27, 129–30; backup for, 28, 132, 146, 149, 150; current trends, 151; doctors'/hospitals' antipathy for, 116, 126, 129, 131–32, 145–49; Europe, 143–45, 192–94; hospital transfers, 139, 143, 146, 148; legality, 115; media reporting, 137; outcome research, 130, 137–43, 150–51, 247; planned vs. unplanned, 138–39, 240; safety, 35, 130, 143; shift away from, 41, 56, 129; VBAC, 29. *See also* midwife-attended births; out-of-hospital births

home health care, postpartum, 193

Horney, Karen, 131

hospital-acquired infections (HAIs), 188–89

hospital birth centers, 133

hospital births: vs. ABC births, 133–34; safety/risks of, 134–35, 188–89; transferred out-of-hospital births, 139, 143, 146, 148, 204; videotaping, 24, 168–69. *See also* interventions; medicalization of birth; *specific procedures*

hospital consent forms, 178–79, 206–7

hospital IRBs, 61, 62–63

hospital peer review committees, 23, 26, 162–63

hospitals, 17–18, 187; advertising hype, 161–62, 206; antipathy for out-of-hospital births, 145–47; complaint processes, 113, 160–61, 179; lack of transparency, 9, 23–24, 160, 162–63, 205–6; legal duties to patients, 174, 179; Mother/Baby Friendly Hospital Initiatives, 239; nurse-midwives in, 110–14; patient authority in, 105–6, 188; patient dumping, 179; patient liaisons, 23, 160; state reporting by, 24, 206, 232; tribal loyalties in, 23–24; VBAC prohibitions, 29, 178

humanized birth: activism and advocacy groups, 10–12, 32, 214–18, 226–39; fundamental principles, 130–31, 182–83;

global cycles, 212–19. *See also* improving maternity care

husbands, damage awards for, 175

hyperstimulation. *See* uterine hyperstimulation

hypoxia. *See* fetal oxygen deprivation

iatrogenic adverse outcomes, 2, 13–15, 25–26, 74. *See also* litigation; malpractice

ICAN (International Cesarean Awareness Network), 234–35

Illinois ABC ban, 136

improving maternity care, 182–211; activism examples, 215–18, 229; appropriate role of obstetricians, 4–5, 195–96, 202, 203; better accountability/transparency, 205–9, 230–32; coalitions and advocacy groups, 11, 232–39; educating care providers, 207–9, 223–24; encouraging out-of-hospital births, 187–95; fundamental principles, 182–83; high-risk care, 203–4; individual actions, 248–49; involving public health departments, 240–42; midwives for low-risk births, 195–202; national health care, 183–87, 206, 207, 232; political action, 226–30; potential cost savings, 242–45; preserving litigation rights, 224–26; public education, 200, 209–11, 218, 220–23; research improvements, 246–48

Ina May's Guide to Childbirth (Gaskin), 195

incontinence, 43, 58

induction. *See* labor induction/augmentation; Cytotec induction

infant formula, 41

infant mortality rates, 9, 145, 212, 243. *See also* perinatal mortality

infection, 14–15, 68, 93–94, 188–89

information disclosure: improving, 205–7; inadequate, 9, 23–24, 160–61, 162–63, 173, 205, 230–31; maternal mortality, 25, 163–64, 169–71, 184, 206; national health care and, 184, 206; patients' right to, 173–74; state laws, 9, 11, 170–71, 184, 206, 231. *See also* informed consent

informed consent, 46–47, 105–6, 161, 204; case law, 175–76; drug approval status,

24–25, 93; drug-induced labor, 8, 77, 86, 92–93, 95–96; elective cesarean section, 46–47, 178; epidural block, 55–56; hospital consent forms, 178–79, 206–7; legal bases of, 173–75; research subjects, 59–60, 63–64, 76

insurance fraud, elective cesarean section, 38, 50

insurance industry, 159, 186–87. *See also* malpractice insurance

international birthing practices, 243–44; changes in, 212–19; worthy models, 144–45, 192–95, 198–200. *See also specific countries and regions*

International Cesarean Awareness Network (ICAN), 234–35

International Conference on Humanization of Birth, 183, 217

International Federation of Gynecology and Obstetrics (FIGO), 33–34, 47

international mortality rates, 9, 212, 243

Internet support groups, 98, 234

interventions: ABC vs. hospital births, 135; common unsupported interventions, 66–67 (table); court-ordered, 122–24, 174, 176, 178; EFM and, 154; factors driving use of, 39–41, 153–54; HAI risk and, 188–89; lack of scientific basis, 50–52, 65, 69; low-tech interventions, 145–46, 203–4, 209; midwife-attended births, 109, 143, 145–46, 203–4; new, approaches to introducing, 52, 59–60, 74, 87–89; prenatal screenings, 106; prevalence statistics, 51 (table), 108–9; research needs, 247; right to refuse, 173, 174, 176–77, 178, 179; unknown long-term effects, 58, 68–69, 74, 247. *See also specific interventions*

intrauterine brain damage, 147

intrauterine growth retardation, 93

Inuit people, midwifery among, 104, 192

IRBs (institutional review boards), 61, 62–63

Italy, 218, 219

Japanese birth houses, 135–36, 192, 198–99

Japanese health care spending, 243

Johnson, Kenneth, home birth study, 142–43, 150–51, 247

Journal of the Society of Obstetricians and Gynecologists of Canada, 200

Kaiser Permanente, 121

Kitzinger, Sheila, 223

Krugman, Paul, 186–87

labor: autonomic nature of, 104, 132; mother's position during, 40–41, 108; myths about, 145

labor and delivery nurses, 6–7, 102, 109, 232–33

labor care, 5–6, 7, 145–46; ABCs vs. hospitals, 133–34; case histories, 1–4, 7–8; continuous care, 7, 198, 202; doulas, 109–10; midwives, 107; obstetricians, 5, 30, 107, 134

labor induction/augmentation, 39, 78; ABC vs. hospital births, 133–34, 135; AFE and, 73, 155–59; alternative stimulation methods, 41, 134; case histories, 1–4, 70–73, 84–85; C-section and, 85, 95; informed consent, 95–96; labor pain and, 39, 53; litigated cases, 95; medical indications, 3, 78, 93–94; for post-term pregnancies, 3, 94–96; risks of, 7, 39, 83 (table), 93–94; U.S. rates/trends, 78, 85, 94, 96. *See also* Cytotec induction

labor pain, 39, 53–54, 133. *See also* epidural block

The Lancet, 31, 63

Latin America, 214. *See also* Brazil

lawsuits. *See* litigation

lawyers, 34, 153

lay midwives, 114, 117. *See also* direct-entry midwives

L&D nurses, 6–7, 102, 109, 232–33

leaking urine, 43

learning disabilities, 68, 247

life expectancy, 185

litigation, 152–72; against midwives, 110, 114–15, 117, 119–20, 171–72; Cytotec induction cases, 82, 85, 92–93, 97, 163–64, 166–67; doctors as witnesses, 23, 159,

Sanchos-Ramos, Luis, 69, 89
Saunders, Peter, 88
Scandinavia, 198, 209, 218, 219. *See also*
 Denmark
scientific method, in research, 60
Scruggs, Mary Ann, 192
Searle Pharmaceutical, 75, 90; Cytotec
 induction warning letter, 90–91, 158. *See
 also* Cytotec
Semmelweiss, Ignaz, 15
service role of medical providers, 197–98
settlement caps, 159, 165–66
settlements, 163–64
sex, 189; painful intercourse, 44, 56, 58
Shields, Brooke, 220
shoulder dystocia, 145–46, 209
single-payer health care. *See* national
 health care
South Carolina maternal death audit
 system, 170–71
South Dakota, 201
standards of practice, 32, 34, 131, 166–68
Staphylococcus aureus, 189
state law: ABCs, 136; disclosure and reporting, 9, 11, 170–71, 184, 206, 231; legislative hearings, 228, 229, 240–41; midwifery, 35, 101, 102, 114–15, 118–19, 124,
 125, 227–30; patients' rights, 161, 174
state legislators, 226–27
state medical boards: filing complaints
 with, 180; midwifery regulation/
 investigations, 111–12, 113, 115–16,
 128, 201, 228; physician malpractice
 investigations, 184–85
state midwifery boards, 201, 228
state nursing boards, 115–16, 201, 228
Steiner, P. E., 155
stillbirths, C-section and, 44
surgeons, obstetricians as, 21
surgery, 22, 44, 154. *See also* cesarean
 section; cesarean section rates; elective
 cesarean section

Taiwan, 186
Tatia French Foundation, 227, 229
technology: obstetricians' faith in, 40–41.
 See also interventions; medicalization of
 birth

teenage pregnancy, 210
thalidomide, 74, 130
time of birth: delays/scheduling for convenience, 8, 27, 38–39; neonatal mortality rates and, 5
tort reform efforts, 159, 165, 166, 225–26
transparency. *See* information disclosure

UCLA Hospital, 89
ultrasound scanning, 40, 58–59, 68–69
UNICEF Baby Friendly Hospital Initia-
 tive, 239
United Kingdom, 207, 209; health care
 spending, 186; maternal mortality inves-
 tigation process, 163; midwifery in, 200,
 208
U.S. Department of Education midwife
 training accreditation, 102, 118, 224
U.S. Department of Health and Human
 Services: C-section rate recommenda-
 tions, 244; VBAC policy, 28
U.S. Food and Drug Administration. *See*
 FDA
U.S. health care quality, 184–87
U.S. health care spending, 186–87, 242–45
U.S. military, 241–42
U.S. National Birth Center Study, 134
University of Maryland Hospital, 90
urinary incontinence, 43
urinary retention, 54
uterine hyperstimulation, 71, 72, 73, 158;
 Cytotec-related, 72, 75, 77, 83–85
uterine rupture, 1–2, 7; C-section and, 44;
 Cytotec-related, 1–2, 14, 28, 77, 79, 81,
 82, 83 (table); support groups, 98, 234;
 VBAC and, 2, 28–29
uterine stimulants: AFE and, 155–59;
 hyperstimulation and, 158. *See also*
 Cytotec induction; labor induction/
 augmentation
uterine tachysystole. *See* uterine
 hyperstimulation

vacuum extraction, 4, 8, 39, 43, 54, 143
vaginal birth: claimed risks, 43–44, 234;
 maternal mortality, 68, 244. *See also*
 VBAC
van Olphen-Fehr, Juliana, 121, 149–50

TEXT:
Adobe Garamond
DISPLAY:
DINEngschrift, Adobe Garamond
COMPOSITOR:
Bookmatters, Berkeley
INDEXER:
Thérèse Shere
PRINTER AND BINDER: